Handbook of Food Allergies

Handbook of Food Allergies

Edited by Jimmy Gordon

hayle medical

New York

Hayle Medical,
750 Third Avenue, 9th Floor,
New York, NY 10017, USA

Visit us on the World Wide Web at:
www.haylemedical.com

ISBN: 978-1-63241-812-8

The publisher's policy is to use permanent paper from mills that operate a sustainable forestry policy. Furthermore, the publisher ensures that the text paper and cover boards used have met acceptable environmental accreditation standards.

Printed in China.

Cataloging-in-Publication Data

Handbook of food allergies / edited by Jimmy Gordon.
p. cm.
Includes bibliographical references and index.
ISBN 978-1-63241-812-8
1. Food allergy. 2. Allergy. 3. Food intolerance. 4. Food--Toxicology. I. Gordon, Jimmy.
RC596 .H36 2019
616.975--dc23

Table of Contents

Preface

This book has been an outcome of determined endeavour from a group of educationists in the field. The primary objective was to involve a broad spectrum of professionals from diverse cultural background involved in the field for developing new researches. The book not only targets students but also scholars pursuing higher research for further enhancement of the theoretical and practical applications of the subject.

The abnormal immune system reaction occurring after eating some specific foods is known as food allergy. The symptoms of the reactions can be both mild and severe, and usually occur within minutes to few hours of exposure. Some of the common symptoms include vomiting, itching, diarrhea, low blood pressure, swelling of the tongue and trouble in breathing. Wheat, peanuts, cow's milk, rice, soy, fish, fruits and eggs are examples of common foods causing allergic reactions. Diagnostic methods include examination of medical history, oral food challenge, skin prick test and elimination test. Epinephrine, steroids and antihistamines are effective in treating food allergies. This book provides significant information about food allergies to help develop a good understanding of their treatment methods. It presents researches and studies performed by experts across the globe. The book is appropriate for students seeking detailed information in this area as well as for experts.

It was an honour to edit such a profound book and also a challenging task to compile and examine all the relevant data for accuracy and originality. I wish to acknowledge the efforts of the contributors for submitting such brilliant and diverse chapters in the field and for endlessly working for the completion of the book. Last, but not the least; I thank my family for being a constant source of support in all my research endeavours.

Editor

The development and implementation of a training package for dietitians on cow's milk protein allergy in infants and children based on UK RCPCH competencies for food allergies

Liane Reeves[1,2*], Rosan Meyer[3], Judith Holloway[2] and Carina Venter[2,4,5]

Abstract

Background: Many food allergy guidelines have been published worldwide over recent years. The United Kingdom National Institute of Health and Clinical Excellence guidelines and The Royal College of Paediatrics and Child Health food allergy care pathways require dietitians to assist with the diagnosis and management of food allergies, which highlighted the need for further education of dietitians to meet these competencies. The aim of this study was to design a competence based one day education course for dietitians on the diagnosis and management of cow's milk protein allergy in infants and children.

Methods: A one day training course was developed. Dietitians' knowledge was assessed via multiple choice questions before and on the day of the course and retention of knowledge was assessed one month after the course. Pre course reading was given once the first assessment was completed.

Results: Thirty seven dietitians attended the course and 32 completed all three assessments. A significant improvement in assessment scores was seen between the pre course and on the day assessments of 7.2% ($p < 0.001$) and between pre course and post course assessments of 8.9% ($p < 0.001$). In delegates who rated their perceived level of knowledge as *high*, a significant increase was seen between pre course and on the day and between pre course and post course (both $p < 0.001$). Actual increase in knowledge was seen alongside a significant increase in *high* rating of perceived level of confidence between pre course and on the day and between pre course and post course (both $p < 0.001$).

Conclusions: Educating dietitians using the format of one day teaching with pre and post course assessment has improved both knowledge and competencies in the diagnosis and management of cow's milk protein allergy. Further courses in other areas of food allergy could be developed using this approach within the UK and worldwide.

Keywords: Competencies, Cow's milk protein allergy, Dietitian, Training

Background

A number of food allergy guidelines have been published internationally in the past few years aimed at improving both the diagnosis and management of food allergies. These include the World Allergy Organisation (WAO) Diagnosis and Rationale for Action against Cow's Milk Allergy (DRACMA) [1], the United States' National Institute of Allergy and Infectious Diseases (NIAID) guidelines [2], the United Kingdom (UK) National Institute of Health and Clinical Excellence (NICE) guidelines [3] and the European Society for Paediatric Gastroenterology, Hepatology and Nutrition (ESPGHAN) guidelines on the diagnostic approach and management of cow's milk allergy in 2012 [4]. More recently the European Academy of Allergy and Clinical Immunology (EAACI) also produced guidelines on the diagnosis and management of food allergy [5]. The Royal College of Paediatrics and

* Correspondence: liane.reeves@nhs.net
[1]Community Nutrition & Dietetic Department, East Oxford Health Centre, Cowley Road, Oxford OX4 1XD, UK
[2]MSc Allergy, University of Southampton, Southampton General Hospital, Tremona Road, Southampton SO16 6YD, UK
Full list of author information is available at the end of the article

Child Health (RCPCH) in the UK followed up the NICE guideline with allergy care pathways for children not only on the diagnostic process, but also on management with defined competencies [6]. Both these UK guideline documents recommend that health professionals, including dietitians, meet competencies in order to identify food allergies and provide optimal management strategies.

Although the majority of guidelines suggest that dietitians are ideally placed to give nutritional advice, the NICE food allergy guideline [3] is the only document recommending that dietitians with the relevant competencies should provide nutritional advice. In particular, competent dietitians, as defined by the RCPCH, may help with the choice of appropriate hypoallergenic formulas/milk alternatives in cow's milk protein allergy (CMPA). The UK Milk Allergy in Primary Care (MAP) Guideline [7] also highlights how dietitians can provide guidance on milk avoidance and suitable alternative foods to achieve adequate nutritional status, as well as performing challenges for the initial diagnosis of CMPA and to determine development of tolerance. Adequate allergy training for dietitians is therefore vital for the effective management of the CMPA patient.

The level of general dietetic training varies between countries and the UK is the only country to offer MSc level training in allergy to dietitians (www.southampton.ac.uk/medicine/allergy and www1.imperial.ac.uk/departmentofmedicine/postgraduate/allergyprogramme/). Dietitians' allergy knowledge therefore varies within and between countries. Surveys of dietitians in South Africa [8], the United States [9], the UK and Australia [10,11] found that further training was needed for dietitians in the management of food allergies. Specifically, perceived knowledge of diagnosing food allergy and developing food challenge protocols tended to be rated as moderate or low in the Australian and United States surveys whilst the majority of respondents rated their knowledge of the definitions, clinical features and dietetic management as either moderate or high [12]. A survey of UK dietitians' learning needs in relation to food allergies and intolerances found that 39% felt they needed further training on CMPA. Sixty one percent preferred face to face combined with web based learning and 68% preferred training to be undertaken in less than 2 days [10]. We have used information from this UK survey to design our one-day educational course. Financial burdens in healthcare along with time pressures have lead to the need to develop affordable and easily accessible training courses for dietitians.

In light of international guidelines and dietitians' perception of needing to improve level of knowledge, we set out to design a pilot course for dietitians based on national competencies [6]. The course focused on the diagnosis and management of CMPA in infants and children and intended to provide a 'step-up' from the traditional one day courses to enable dietitians to show competency in the management of this allergy. The course was supported by the Food Allergy and Intolerance Specialist Group (FAISG) of the British Dietetic Association (BDA) (www.bda.uk.com/regionsgroups/groups/foodallergy/home).

Methods

Ethical approval was not required.

Course development and execution

Assessment questions

The definition of 'competence' for this study denotes being able to diagnose and manage patients with allergies safely and effectively as per NICE guidelines [3]. This definition was kept in mind when developing the assessment tool. Twenty-eight multiple choice questions were designed to relate to each objective and competence. Questions were a combination of fact based e.g. 'what is the best definition of.....' and case scenarios in design. All questions required the participant to choose one best answer and were marked out of a possible score of 31 as one question contained 4 parts.

The assessment questions were developed by comparing the knowledge of two groups of volunteer dietitians recruited via emailing FAISG members; 10 with little or no experience in allergy and 10 who were experienced allergy dietitians. The assessment was delivered online via www.surveymonkey.co.uk and the dietitians were given the opportunity to answer and comment on each question via this electronic form. Once completed, responses were reviewed and the wording of some questions adjusted to clarify or adjust the difficulty of the question.

Pre course reading

Delegates were asked to read the NICE food allergy quick reference guide [13].

Course format and assessment

Presentations were designed to meet the course objectives outlined in Table 1 and speakers were selected according to their experience in the diagnosis and management of CMPA.

Delegates were recruited via advertisement in the BDA magazine and website and contacted the BDA to book a place. Places were charged at the standard BDA rate of £95. Delegates were asked to complete online assessment questions prior to the course (pre course assessment) using their unique number given at registration in order to remain anonymous for analysis. Assessment questions were completed again at the end of the day on paper, and online a month after the course (post course assessment) in order to measure whether knowledge had been retained. Based on clinical competencies,

Table 1 Objectives for each session

Timing & Topic	Competences/objectives	
	Once completed, dietitians should:	
	Know	**Be able to:**
9.30-10.00 Background to allergy	• the major categories of adverse reactions to foods	• recognise that food allergy may present in a variety of ways ranging from immediate allergic reactions to more chronic presentations such as eczema or gastro-intestinal symptoms
	• that food allergy may present in a variety of ways	
	• that many common childhood conditions e.g. eczema, gastro-oesophageal reflux may have an allergic aetiology	
	• that food allergy is more common in children with early onset eczema, particularly mild to moderate eczema	• recognise the risk factors for allergic aetiology of presenting features such as family or personal history of atopy
	• the common foods which are responsible for most food allergies in children	• differentiate different types of adverse reactions to food based on findings from history and examination
10.00-11.15 Diagnosis & interpreting tests	• that the level of sIgE varies and should not be used in place of oral food challenges to determine allergy e.g. cow's milk	• take and interpret an allergy focused clinical history
	• that skin prick tests and sIgE have a poor predictive value for non-IgE mediated allergies	• differentiate different types of adverse reactions to food based on findings from the history
	• that atopy patch tests are available but that their role in the diagnosis of food allergy remains unclear	• gather information on relevant exposures to other potential food allergens and take a dietary history including the interpretation of a food and symptom diary
	• that complementary and alternative medicine allergy tests, including kinesiology, serum sIgG and vega tests have no place in the diagnosis and/or management of food allergy	• interpret SPT results in the context of the clinical history • interpret serum sIgE results in the context of the clinical history
11.30-12.45 Diagnostic diets & food challenges	• which diagnostic diet is appropriate to use according to symptoms	• advise about the safe reintroduction of cow's milk following a negative food challenge
	• which formulas are available for managing CMP allergy and lactose intolerance	• recommend an appropriate formula according to symptoms and clinical history
	• which oral challenges may be done as open challenges, which need medical supervision and which are suitable for home	
	• when it is appropriate to challenge and how to decide on challenge outcome	
13.30-14.30 Dietary management	• what foods (including catering, manufactured ingredients and manufactured foods) are likely to contain trigger foods	• advise on appropriate dietary exclusion and alternatives including practical individualised advice (e.g. appropriate to age, culture etc.)
	• clinically relevant cross-reactivities	• educate patients, parents and carers about effective food allergen avoidance including high risk situations e.g. eating out
	• common situations when allergen exposure is most likely to occur (e.g. eating out)	• advise patients, parents and carers of issues relating to risk in specific situations e.g. school
	• the risks inherent to specific situations (e.g. home, school, eating out and hospital settings)	• provide support to patients and families to help minimise the impact of food allergy on quality of life through education, ongoing access and patient queries
14.30-15.30 Nutritional issues & weaning	• how to recognise that faltering growth is a result of food allergy	• give practical advice on weaning the cow's milk allergic infant
	• when it is appropriate to refer to other health care professionals	• provide details of resources including patient charities, websites and local support groups
		• ensure the nutritional requirements of infants and children on a CMP free diet are met
		• manage nutritional deficiencies and faltering growth
15.45-17.00	**Case studies discussion and final assessment**	

CMP; cow's milk protein, sIgE; specific IgE, sIgG; specific IgG, SPT; skin prick tests.

achieving ≥90% in the post course assessment questions was considered sufficient to pass the course and receive a competence certificate. Delegates were informed of the criteria prior to the course and the reason for completing assessments at each stage. They were also asked to complete a general evaluation at the end of the day to assess speakers, venue and overall satisfaction with the course.

At each assessment, delegates were asked to state their perceived level of knowledge of allergies on a Likert scale of none, a little, a fair amount or a lot. They were also asked to rate their level of confidence in managing children with CMPA on a Likert scale of 1 (not at all confident) to 5 (very confident). Following completion of the post course assessment, all delegates were asked to answer one online question to indicate whether they had completed any of the recommended reading prior to answering the post course questions.

A summary of the process of designing and implementing the course can be found in Figure 1.

Statistical analysis

Power calculation

Results from the 20 volunteer dietitians who trialled the questions were assessed. Seven dietitians identified themselves as being proficient in the management of food allergy and these were compared to 7 dietitians with no experience in managing food allergies. The remaining six dietitians stated that they had a little allergy management knowledge and were not included in the calculation. Mean scores were 26.28 (out of 31) in the experienced group and 19.85 in the non-experienced group (effect size 6.43 and SD 4.2). Based on these results a power calculation determined that with 13 delegates in each group, or 26 in total, we would be able to detect a significant difference between pre and post assessment scores at a significance level of 0.01 and 90% power. It was agreed that we would aim for 30 delegates to allow for any drop-outs.

Statistical analyses were performed using SPSS version 19 for Windows (IBM, New York, USA). The Wilcoxon signed rank test was used to determine whether there were significant differences between assessment scores and perceived level of confidence between assessments. The McNemar test was used to determine whether there was a significant change in perceived level of knowledge between assessments and the Fishers exact test was used to determine the relationship between previous training and whether delegates passed or failed.

The Chi-square test was used to investigate the relationship between the NHS grade delegates were employed at (and therefore their level of experience) and passing or failing the post course assessment. A p value of ≤ 0.05 was considered to be statistically significant.

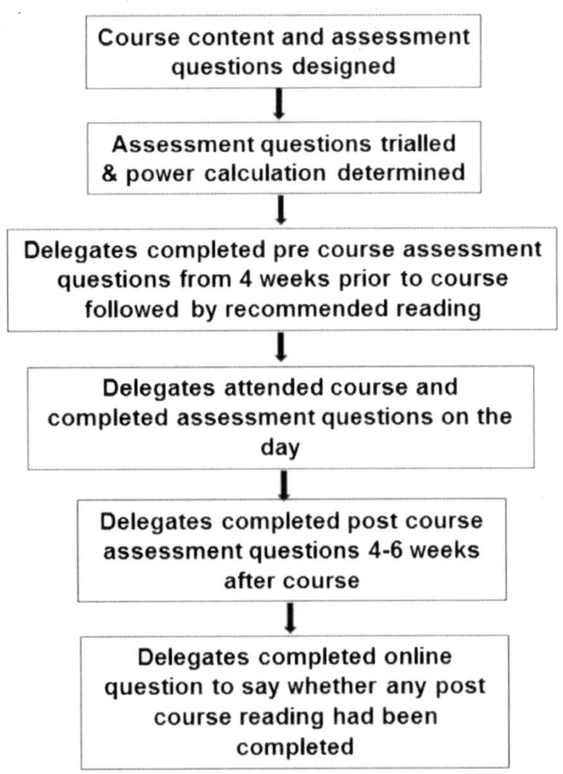

Figure 1 Process of designing and implementing course.

Results

Subjects

Thirty seven dietitians attended the course. Thirty two delegates completed all 3 assessments and results from these candidates were compared. Table 2 illustrates the delegates' characteristics.

Assessment results

The assessments were marked out of a possible 27 points after 4 questions were removed due to the subject matter not being covered adequately. Twenty four (75%) delegates achieved a pass rate of ≥90% on the post course assessments. Eight (25%) delegates therefore did not pass the post course assessment. Mean results for the pre-course, on the day and post course assessments were 84%, 91% and 93% respectively.

A significant improvement in scores was seen between the pre course assessments and on the day assessments of 7.2% ($p < 0.001$) and between the pre course assessments and post course assessments of 8.9% ($p < 0.001$). However there was no significant change in the scores between the on the day assessment and post course assessment, indicating that the information had been retained by the delegates ($p = 0.175$).

Twenty (62.5%) delegates completed some recommended reading after the course. Of the 24 delegates who passed,

Table 2 Characteristics of delegates who completed pre course, on the day and post course assessments

Practice Setting (N = 32) (delegates could choose more than one)	N	%
Hospital outpatients	12	37.5
Hospital inpatients	17	53
Community	14	44
Private Practice	4	12.5
Other (does not practice/industry)	1	3
Current Post NHS Band		
5 (Basic Grade)	8	25
6 (Specialist)	15	47
7 (Advanced)	5	16
Not given	4	12
Type of patients usually seen		
Paediatric	13	41
Adult	4	12
Both paediatric and adult	14	44
Not given	1	3
Previous training in allergy (delegates could choose more than one)		
No previous allergy training	17	53
Specialised one day food allergy conferences	9	28
BDA Paediatric Course	4	12
Post graduate cert/dip/MSc	1	3
Other:		
Shadowing experienced dietitians	3	9
Not given	2	6

BDA; British Dietetic Association, N; number of delegates.

12 (50%) had read some of the recommended reading and 2 (8%) had read all.

Perceived level of knowledge in managing allergies

A significant difference in delegates rating their perceived level of knowledge as high was seen between pre course and on the day ($p < 0.001$) and pre course and post course ($p < 0.001$). The increase between the day of the course and post course perceived knowledge was not significant ($p = 0.5$). Figure 2 shows the change in perceived level of knowledge of allergies at each assessment.

Perceived level of confidence in managing CMPA

A significant increase in delegates rating their perceived level of confidence as high in managing children with CMPA was seen between pre course and on the day ($p < 0.001$), on the day to post course ($p = 0.008$) and between pre course and post course ($p < 0.001$). Figure 3 shows the change in perceived level of confidence in managing CMPA at each assessment.

Previous training

Thirty (94%) delegates gave information on previous food allergy related training they had attended. Of those that failed the post course assessment, 6 (75%) had no previous training in food allergy, 1 (12.5%) had a post graduate qualification in allergy and 1 (12.5%) had shadowed other dietitians.

Of those that passed the post course assessment, 11 (50%) had no previous training in food allergy, 5 (23%) had attended specialised one day food allergy conferences, 4 (18%) had attended both specialised one day food allergy conferences and the BDA paediatric course, and 2 (9%) had shadowed colleagues.

There was no significant relationship between the amount of previous training and whether delegates passed or failed ($p = 0.221$). There was a trend for the

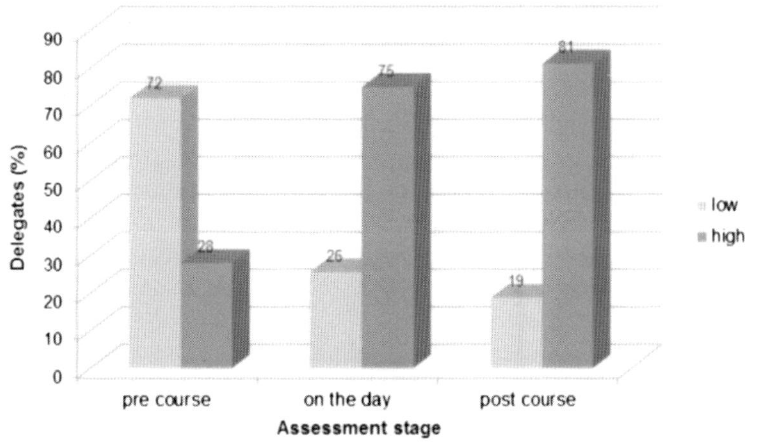

Figure 2 Perceived level of knowledge at pre course, on the day and post course assessments.

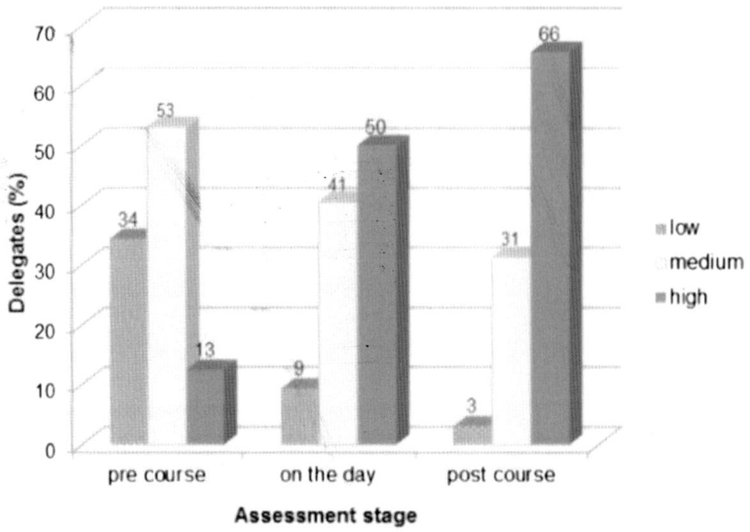

Figure 3 Perceived level of confidence in managing CMPA at pre course, on the day and post course assessments.

more skilled dietitians employed at higher NHS bands to have a higher pass rate (p = 0.038).

Assessment questions

Table 3 shows the number of correct answers given for each question at each assessment. The biggest improvements between pre course and post course assessments were seen in questions relating to: eczema and food allergy (35%), symptoms (25%), milk ingredients (28.5%) and sIgE (22%).

Two questions showed a decrease in correct answers between pre and post course assessments; on sIgE (12.5%) and on appropriate resources (6%).

Three questions were answered correctly by all delegates in all three assessments on: food challenges, managing CMPA in schools and hidden sources of milk.

Evaluation of the course

All delegates gave a score of 8 or more out of 10 on the evaluation forms for enjoyment of the event, met expectations and resources available to take away.

Discussion

The NICE food allergy guidelines and The RCPCH food allergy care pathway [3,6] were designed to improve knowledge and competencies of health professionals managing children with food allergies in order to improve patient care. We designed a one day course for dietitians consisting of 5 lectures and case study discussion that based session objectives on these national competencies. We have shown that dietitians' knowledge of CMPA can be improved and retained by the delivery of a course in this format. Actual level of knowledge, perceived level of confidence and perceived knowledge all improved and knowledge was retained after one month. Satisfaction with the course was high and 75% achieved the required ≥90% to pass the post course assessment.

To our knowledge this is the first study looking at food allergy education for dietitians based on competencies, focusing on CMPA. The format was based on a survey of dietitians' learning needs in the area of food allergies and intolerances [10]. Other studies have looked at food allergy education for physicians; Springston et al. [14] designed an online 'Food Allergy Comprehension Tool' (FACT) which consisted of multiple choice questions (MCQs) and case studies. Their brief education tool significantly improved knowledge in some of the areas addressed, however this did not involve any face to face education and was not based on competencies as in our study. The WAO have produced online learning modules [15] on different allergy topics which can be accessed by any health care professionals, but are not particularly tailored towards the needs of dietitians. They also use case scenarios to educate the participant but there is no a formal method of assessment to show that participants have met designated competencies.

Yu et al. [16] designed a one hour food allergy education programme for primary care physicians caring for teenagers and adults in the US. They based their program on lectures and a practical demonstration in a similar way to ours although much shorter in length. That study showed that knowledge could be improved using this approach. An intensive 'boot camp' format for residents and fellows in training is described by Elizalde et al. [17], where knowledge was assessed before and after the education sessions for six participants. Although they had a small sample size, a significant improvement in knowledge was shown from educating this

Table 3 Number (percentage) of correct answers given for each question on each assessment

Question topic	Pre course correct N (%)	On the day correct N (%)	Post course correct N (%)
Allergy definition	26(81)	31(97)	31(97)
Anaphylaxis	32(100)	31(97)	32(100)
Eczema & food allergy	32(100)	30(94)	32(100)
Eczema & food allergy	18(56)	17(53)	29(91)
Symptoms	23(72)	31(97)	31(97)
Allergy vs intolerance	28(87.5)	32(100)	30(94)
Milk formulae	29(91)	31(97)	32(100)
Milk formulae	26(81)	28(87.5)	31(97)
Milk formulae	25(78)	28(87.5)	31(97)
Milk formulae	29(91)	32(100)	32(100)
Which formula to recommend (case scenario)	30(94)	30(94)	31(97)
Which formula to recommend (case scenario)	18(56)	25(78)	21(66)
Which formula to recommend (case scenario)	26(81)	28(87.5)	29(91)
Diagnosis	28(87.5)	32(100)	32(100)
Skin prick testing	25(78)	28(87.5)	27(84)
Specific IgE	15(47)	21(66)	22(69)
Specific IgE	28(87.5)	23(72)	24(75)
Food challenges	32(100)	32(100)	32(100)
Cross reactions	28(87.5)	31(97)	32(100)
Cross contamination	25(78)	32(100)	32(100)
Milk ingredients	20(62.5)	29(91)	29(91)
Managing CMPA in schools	(32(100)	32(100)	32(100)
Appropriate resources	32(100)	31(97)	30(94)
Food challenging	28(87.5)	32(100)	32(100)
Food challenging	31(97)	30(94)	31(97)
Hidden sources of milk	32(100)	32(100)	32(100)
When to refer on	26(81)	27(84)	27(84)

group in this way. Similarly Swan et al. [18] also showed that knowledge could be improved by the delivery of a one day study day to health professionals by the assessment of knowledge before and at the end of the day.

However the strength of our study remains the proven retention of knowledge, which all the above quoted studies did not perform [14,16,17].

Our study included multiple choice questions marked out of a possible 27 points designed to assess the competencies linked to CMPA, which were completed before, at the end of the study day and repeated again 1 month after. Swan et al. [18] based their assessment on only 7 questions and used audience response pads rather than paper or online assessments. This method provides an immediate way of assessing knowledge and provides instant feedback to delegates. However, this may not suit all delegates as some may prefer to take more time to consider their responses. Assessment of knowledge at the end of the day reflects what has been learned but not what has been retained. An assessment after a time interval can determine whether the improvement in knowledge has been maintained. In our study, assessment results from a month after the course increased from assessment results on the day. Although this increase was not significant it shows that knowledge had been retained. Learning can also be reinforced by suggesting that delegates follow up with recommended reading after the course, although in our study only 58% of those who passed the post course assessment had read any of the recommended reading.

When planning and designing training, it is important to consider what will be the most suitable format to enable the group being taught to learn effectively. We designed our course to be delivered in one day in response to results of the UK dietitians survey [10]. Similar to other studies [14,16,17] we found that knowledge could be improved by designing and implementing training appropriate to the needs of our group following a needs assessment survey.

We have shown that delegates' overall perceived level of knowledge and confidence improved occurring alongside actual increase in knowledge; an essential combination which ensures that correct advice can be given with confidence. Overall satisfaction with the day was high. However, discussions during the case studies at the end of the day and evaluations afterwards highlighted that there was still some confusion over the introduction of soya which may have impacted on confidence scores post asessment. It was also noted that the number of correct responses to one of the formulae questions improved between pre course and on the day answers (56% to 78%) but dropped again on the post course assessment (to 66%) suggesting that this area could have been covered more clearly. The course content has been amended to clarify these areas in more detail for future courses by altering slides and including more opportunity for discussion.

Dietitians valued the fact that the course provided more than a basic study day and that they would be awarded a certificate to show they had met the competencies if they achieved the required level in the assessments. This will provide a valuable addition to their CPD portfolios as well as improve quality of care to patients with CMPA. It may also help to raise the profile of dietitians with other health professionals.

Limitations

In common with Springston et al. [14] and Yu et al. [16], our assessment questions included case scenarios in an attempt to ask delegates to use what they had learned in a fictional but practical example. This is a standard method of introducing the 'student' to examples of problems they may face in a real clinical setting. This method can also be used via online learning modules such as the WAO online food allergy module [15]. However, they are not an equal subsititute for advising a patient in person so the ability to put knowledge into practice in a clinical setting has not been evaluated. This could be considered as being the only way that competence can truly be measured but it is not practical for every dietitian or health professional to be monitored and tested in a real clinical setting at this level of training. Assessment by using questions relating to practical scenarios may be the closest alternative.

Although presentation content was determined by set objectives, the delivery of the presentations may vary between different speakers. In order to ensure that all key points are made, future course material will contain additional notes for speakers.

Although level of knowledge was shown to have been retained after one month, we have not assessed level of knowledge again at a later date. Future courses could reassess a year afterwards to measure ongoing retention of knowledge and find out how this has impacted on practice.

Future use

The course package has been updated, further dates have been arranged for running more courses and is now available for rolling out. This package format could be used in other countries with only small adjustments made to allow for differences in available products in order to deliver training in CMPA. Courses in other areas of food allergy could be designed using the same format, thus improving competencies in a wider range of food allergies both in the UK and worldwide. As competencies are developed in other medical disciplines both in the UK and worldwide, this course format could also be used to deliver courses in other subjects.

Conclusion

Following international guidelines on the diagnosis and management of food allergies and the international need for further training we have developed and implemented a training course for dietitians based on national competencies. The course provides a 'step-up' from standard one day courses. This format could be used to educate dietitians in other areas of food allergy as highlighted in the UK, US and Australian dietitians surveys [9,10,12] and will help to improve the standard of care to patients with food allergies in the UK and worldwide.

Competing interests

The authors declare that they have no competing of interests.

Authors' contributions

The article was written by LR. RM, CV and JH critically revised drafts of the article and approved the final version for publication. LR, RM and CV designed the content of the course, presentations and assessment questions, and interpretation of the data.

Acknowledgements

The authors would like to thank Laura King, British Dietetic Association for her help and support in organising the course; Dr Trevor Brown (Ulster Hospital, Northern Ireland) and Sally-Ann Denton (Portsmouth Hospitals NHS Trust) for help in delivering the course, Scott Harris, Medical Statistician (University of Southampton), for his help with the statistics and finally, all the dietitians who trialled the questions and attended the course.

Funding

This study was supported by the Food Allergy and Intolerance Specialist Group of the BDA. The BDA received financial support from an academic grant from Nutricia and Mead Johnson.

Author details

[1]Community Nutrition & Dietetic Department, East Oxford Health Centre, Cowley Road, Oxford OX4 1XD, UK. [2]MSc Allergy, University of Southampton, Southampton General Hospital, Tremona Road, Southampton SO16 6YD, UK. [3]Department of Gastroenterology, Great Ormond Street Hospital for Sick Children, London WC1N 3JH, UK. [4]University of Portsmouth, James Watson West, 2 King Richard 1st Road, Portsmouth PO1 2FR, UK. [5]The David Hide Asthma and Allergy Research Centre, St Mary's Hospital, Newport, Isle of Wight PO30 5TG, UK.

References

1. Fiocchi A, Brozek J, Schünemann H, Bahna SL, Von Berg A, Beyer K, et al. World allergy organization (WAO) diagnosis and rationale for action against cow's milk allergy (DRACMA) guidelines. Pediatr Allergy Immunol. 2010;21:1–125.
2. Boyce JA, Assa'ad A, Burks AW, Jones SM, Sampson HA, Wood RA, et al. Guidelines for the diagnosis and management of food allergy in the United States: report of the NIAID-sponsored expert panel. J Allergy Clin Immunol. 2010;126:1105–18.
3. National Institute for Health and Clinical Excellence. NICE Clinical Guidelines CG116. London: National Institute for Health and Clinical Excellence; 2011.
4. Koletzko S, Niggemann B, Arato A, Dias JA, Heuschkel R, Husby S, et al. Diagnostic approach and management of cow's-milk protein allergy in infants and children: ESPGHAN GI Committee practical guidelines. J Pediatr Gastroenterol Nutr. 2012;55:221–9.
5. Muraro A, Werfel T, Hoffmann-Sommergruber K, Roberts G, Beyer K, Bindslev-Jensen C, et al. EAACI Food Allergy and Anaphylaxis Guidelines: diagnosis and management of food allergy. Allergy. 2014;69:1008–25.
6. Royal College of Paediatrics and Child Health. Allergy care pathways for children - Food Allergy. [http://www.rcpch.ac.uk/allergy/foodallergy] 2011.
7. Venter C, Brown T, Shah N, Walsh J, Fox AT. Diagnosis and management of non-IgE-mediated cow's milk allergy in infancy - a UK primary care practical guide. Clin Transl Allergy. 2013;3:23.
8. Stear G, Potter P, Labadarios D, Motala C. Management of food allergies in children in South Africa - determining aspects of knowledge and practices of dietitians and medical practitioners. Curr Allergy Clin Immunol. 2011;24:145–55.
9. Groetch ME, Christie L, Vargas PA, Jones SM, Sicherer SH. Food allergy educational needs of pediatric dietitians: A survey by the consortium of food allergy research. J Nutr Educ Behav. 2010;42:259–64.
10. Reeves L, Meyer R, Hollway J, Venter C. Learning needs of registered dietitians working with individuals with food hypersensitivities in the UK. Clin Exp Allergy. 2012;42:1833.

11. Venter C, Meyer R, Reeves L, Swain A, Stuart-Smith W, Christie L, et al. Food allergy knowledge and educational needs of dietitians around the globe. Sidney, Australia: ASCIA Conference; 2012.
12. Maslin K, Meyer R, Reeves L, Mackenzie H, Swain A, Stuart-Smith W, et al. Food allergy competencies of dietitians in the United Kingdom, Australia and United States of America. Clin Transl Allergy. 2014;4:37.
13. National Institute for Health and Clinical Excellence. Food allergy in children and young people:quick reference guide. [http://pathways.nice.org.uk/pathways/food-allergy-in-children-and-young-people] 2011.
14. Springston EE, Lau CH, Patel P, Warrier MR, Sohn MW, Pongracic J, et al. A brief intervention to improve food allergy knowledge among US pediatricians: Lessons learned. Pediatr Allergy Immunol. 2012;23:642–7.
15. World Allergy Organisation. WAO Online Learning and CME modules. [http://worldallergy.org/modules/]
16. Yu JE, Kumar A, Bruhn C, Teuber SS, Sicherer SH. Development of a food allergy education resource for primary care physicians. BMC Med Educ. 2008;8:45.
17. Elizalde A, Perez EE, Sriaroon P, Nguyen D, Lockey RF, Dorsey MJ. Intensive educational course in allergy and immunology. Allergy. 2012;67:1085–6.
18. Swan K, Perkin MR, Du Toit GFA. Do allergy study days improve delegate knowledge? Clin Exp Allergy. 2012;42:1832–3.

2

Dietary intake and risk of asthma in children and adults

Vanessa Garcia-Larsen[1*], Stefano R. Del Giacco[2], André Moreira[3], Matteo Bonini[4,5], Tari Haahtela[6], Sergio Bonini[7,8], Kai-Håkon Carlsen[9], Ioana Agache[10], João Fonseca[13], Nikolaos G. Papadopoulos[11,12] and Luís Delgado[13]

Abstract

Background: Diet has been proposed to modulate the risk of asthma in children and adults. An increasing body of epidemiological studies have been published in the last year investigating the association between dietary intake and asthma. As part of the Evidence-Based Clinical Practice Guideline Task Force on 'Lifestyle Interventions in Allergy and Asthma' funded by the European Academy of Allergy and Clinical Immunology, we will use a systematic approach to review the evidence from published scientific literature on dietary intake and asthma in children and adults.

Methods: This systematic review will be carried out following the PRISMA guidelines. The protocol has been published in PROSPERO (CRD42016036078). We will review the evidence from epidemiological studies in children (from the age of 2 years) and adults and dietary intake of foods and nutrients.

Discussion: The findings from this review will be used as a reference to inform guideline recommendations.

Keywords: Asthma, Wheeze, Diet, Nutrients, Antioxidants, Children, Adults, Systematic review

Background

Since the late 60 s, a sharp increase in the incidence of asthma was observed, which seems to have reached a plateau in the last 10 years in some countries [1], but it continues to rise in others [2]. Asthma prevalence and poor asthma control [3] represent a major problem of public health and a socio-economic burden, particularly in developed countries as well as in nations with fast growing economies where the highest rates of disease have been reported [3]. This trend has been accompanied by noticeable changes in lifestyle. Improved access to technology and development have led to a more sedentary life. Easier access to food and a shift in the eating patterns from naturally sourced to processed food have been accompanied by a reduced intake of fresh fruits and vegetables, less fibre, and an increased intake foods rich in refined sugar.

It is known that oxidative stress and airway inflammation are central features in the manifestation of asthma [4], which might be exacerbated by the poorer quality of the diet [5]. The possible effect of diet on asthma, particularly in relation to the role of dietary antioxidants and polyunsaturated fatty acids has been investigated in numerous observational studies [6]. Current evidence suggests that antioxidant vitamins C and E and a higher intake of fresh vegetables and fruits might have a protective effect on asthma, but most of the findings are still considered weak due to the cross-sectional design of the studies and the heterogeneity in diet assessment between them [7]. Intervention trials have added little so far to understand the role of nutrients on asthma, which opens the question of whether the sources of nutrients matter (e.g. diet vs supplements). We recently completed an overview of high quality systematic reviews on diet and asthma [8] and found some evidence to suggest that

*Correspondence: v.garcialarsen@imperial.ac.uk
[1] Respiratory Epidemiology, Occupational Medicine, and Public Health Group, National Heart and Lung Institute, Imperial College London, Emmanuel Kaye Building, Manresa Road, London SW3 6LR, UK
Full list of author information is available at the end of the article

intake of fruits and vegetables as well as adherence to a Mediterranean diet during childhood might reduce the risk of asthma in children. The evidence from studies in adults was less clear.

In this systematic review we aim to comprehensively assess the existing scientific literature on the relationship between to dietary intake and the risk of asthma in children and adults, published in the last 5 years. There have been few high quality systematic reviews (AMSTAR score $\geq$ 32) published since 2011 and none included both children and adults as target populations. We will not include maternal or infant dietary intake (solids or breastfeeding) as three large systematic reviews have just been completed covering these age groups (International Prospective Register of Systematic Reviews [PROSPERO http://www.crd.york.ac.uk/PROSPERO/search.asp] references CRD42013003802—REVIEW A; CRD42013004239—REVIEW B; CRD42013004252—REVIEW C).

The scope of our Task Force is to provide evidence on dietary intake and dietary habits in relation to risk of asthma, wheeze (recurrent or persistent), and bronchial hyper-responsiveness (BHR). Our findings will serve as a reference to inform guidelines on dietary habits in susceptible and general population to reduce the risk and/or severity of asthma in children and adults. This systematic review protocol has been prepared following the new PRISMA-P guidelines [9].

Objectives

The aim of this systematic review is to evaluate the association between dietary intake and risk of asthma in children and adults. To this end, we will seek to answer the following questions:

1. Does exposure to diet (as a whole, as grouped or individual foods) during childhood influence the risk of asthma ?
2. Does exposure to diet (as a whole, as grouped or individual foods) in adults influence their risk of asthma ?

Methods

Eligibility criteria

Studies will be selected according to the criteria outlined below.

Study designs

We will include randomised controlled trials (RCT), quasi RCT, as well as cohort (prospective or retrospective) studies, nested case–control studies, other case–control studies and cross-sectional studies (including those with retrospective data).

Participants

We will investigate the role of diet on asthma in children from the age of 2 years old to adulthood. Participants of any age group within this range, unrestricted by disease severity, previous or current treatment, will be included.

Interventions

The objective of this systematic review is to collate the evidence on intake of foods and nutrients on asthma as a baseline for guidelines, a decision was made a priori to examine the evidence from studies that included actual food or nutrients (i.e. not supplements). Observational studies that used a dietary questionnaire to capture dietary intake will be included. Intervention studies with actual food rather than supplementation will also be included. Foods and nutrients will be classified, whenever possible, according to their nutritional properties and/or similarities.

Comparator(s)/control

All comparators will be included in the description of eligible studies. We will include report of different doses of forms of an exposure (e.g. frequency/total daily grams intake). For the studies that only report frequency of intake of foods we will report differences as binary comparisons e.g. weekly versus never, daily versus never.

Outcomes

The primary outcomes are asthma or wheeze. Acceptable definitions of asthma will include 'doctor diagnosed asthma', 'self-reported asthma', 'ever had asthma', 'persistent asthma', 'allergic asthma', 'atopic asthma', 'wheeze in the last 12 months', 'current wheeze', 'recurrent wheeze' or any other definition of asthma clearly documented in the selected study. Outcomes will be collected as reported. Due to possible variations in disease definitions, we will extract definitions of outcomes as reported in individual studies. We will extract outcomes in all data forms (e.g. dichotomous, continuous,) as reported in the included studies.

Timing

Eligible studies will be selected for inclusion regardless of the time length between exposure and outcome. Prospective and retrospective exposure will be considered, as well as cross-sectional.

Setting

There will be no restrictions by type of setting.

Language

We will include articles reported in the English language.

Exclusion criteria

This systematic review is centred on the role that diet might have on asthma outcomes, therefore the exclusion criteria applies to those factors listed below:

1. Non-comparative studies
2. Reviews
3. Non-human study
4. In vitro/In vivo studies
5. Chronic obstructive pulmonary disease (COPD)
6. Chronic bronchitis
7. Allergy/Food allergy
8. Eczema/atopic dermatitis
9. Atopy
10. Exposure in pregnancy (in utero)
11. Breastfeeding
12. Use of nutritional supplements not naturally extracted from the diet (e.g. capsules of vitamin a, C, E, fish oils, fish capsules, mineral, pro- and prebiotic, or herbal supplementation)
13. Food challenge (e.g. white or red wine given as a food challenge rather than studied as usual intake)
14. Food avoidance for allergy prevention (i.e. antigen protein cow milk)
15. Nutrients measured in blood (serum or plasma)
16. Work related exposure to foods (e.g. bakery, bakers)
17. Occupational asthma
18. Obesity/weight loss [low calorie diets]/exercise
19. Indoor pollution (e.g. cooking gas)
20. Medication alone as treatment for asthma (e.g. corticosteroids, montelukast, etc.) but medication combined or in parallel to food intake will be accepted
21. Asthma grouped with other diseases such as COPD or bronchitis
22. Sodium chloride/sodium 0.9 % (as saline solution e.g. intravenous) but dietary or supplemented sodium will be included
23. Ethanol as intravenous or oral supplementation—consumption of alcohol will be accepted
24. Exposure to rural-related environmental risk factors that do not include any specific dietary exposures
25. Inhalation of milk proteins or aerosol-related food particles in the air
26. Studies in which participants where defined by a disease state (other than the relevant outcomes studied here) e.g. children or adults with specific nutritional deficiencies.

Information sources

Literature search strategies have been developed using medical subject headings (MeSH) and text words related to asthma or wheeze. We will search MEDLINE (OVID interface), EMBASE (OVID interface), Web of Science, and the Cochrane Central Register of Controlled Trials (CENTRAL; Wiley interface). The electronic database search will be supplemented by searching for trial protocols of food intervention by searching through metaRegister (http://www.controlled-trials.com/mrct/).

Search strategies

We will search for eligible studies published in the last 5 years (1st January 2011–2nd March 2016). The specific search strategies have been designed by VGL in collaboration with a Librarian at Imperial College with expertise in systematic review searching. The strategies were developed with input from the co-authors to ensure that relevant outcomes and exposure terms were included. The search strategies were also reviewed by a second Librarian, not involved in the project. The search strategies for MEDLINE, Web of Science and Cochrane Library are included in Additional file 1: Appendix. Per reviewed abstracts presented in scientific conferences will also be screened. We will check if these were followed by the corresponding peer reviewed publication. The International Clinical Trials Registry Platform Search Portal and ClinicalTrials.gov will be searched for ongoing or recently completed trials. We will also search for studies in progress or completed but unpublished using http://apps.who.int/trialsearch/. The bibliography of all selected eligible papers will be examined for potential relevant additional publications.

We will also separately search for existing systematic reviews published in the same period as in our review (2011–2016) which cover relevant exposures and outcomes. These findings will be used in the Discussion section as part of the interpretation of our findings.

Data management

Relevant study characteristics and results will be recorded in a spreadsheet file (Excel). We will pilot the file to ensure that the descriptors are clear. A template has been prepared by the research team and a calibration exercise will be undertaken to pilot and refine the screening questions.

Selection process

Two members of the research team (VGL and SDG) will independently review titles and abstracts of all identified studies. The search strategies will be piloted and checked for completeness to ensure that as far as possible, all potentially eligible titles are captured. The full text of the paper will also be independently assessed by VGL and SDG, and will be assessed for eligibility against the inclusion and exclusion criteria. Any discrepancies will be resolved through discussions with the research team. Electronic records will be kept regarding included and excluded studies for audit purposes, specifying reasons for any exclusion. Full text articles will be reviewed in duplicate (by two research team members—VGL and SDG), and studies for inclusion will be selected—any discrepancies will be resolved through discussions with the research team. The reasons for the exclusion of any relevant studies will be recorded. Neither of the review authors will be blind to the journal titles or to the study authors or institutions.

Data collection process

A pilot of the data extraction form will be undertaken using a minimum of 5 papers, after which the extraction form will be amended/updated as necessary. The data extraction form will be used to extract the relevant data fields from each included study independently (by two research team members—VGL and SDG). Data abstracted will include demographic information, methodology, intervention details, and all reported relevant outcomes. Reviewers will resolve disagreements by discussion, and one of two arbitrators (AM or LD) will adjudicate unresolved disagreements. We will contact study authors to resolve any uncertainties. Where appropriate data will be entered into STATA statistical software for meta-analysis.

Data on exposures

We will extract all effect estimates available for any dietary exposure studied, as well as all the relevant study characteristics. If effect sizes cannot be calculated, we will report the results as a narrative. We anticipate to find wide variations in the way dietary data is recorded, both with regards to frequency of consumption and to levels of intake compared. Once the data is entered, we will group exposures according to similarities in time and comparison levels (e.g. weekly vs never; highest quintile of intake vs lowest). Data will be extracted either using raw values, crude estimates of effect (including odds ratios, risk ratios, incidence rate ratios, hazard ratios, mean differences) or as adjusted estimates of effect. Adjusted estimates of effect will be used in preference, where available.

Outcomes and prioritisation

The primary outcome will be asthma or wheeze. In the case of pre-school children 'wheezing illness' will also be accepted as proxy definition for asthma. As a secondary outcome, we will include bronchial hyper-responsiveness (BHR). Lung function measurements will be included as outcomes only if used as a direct measure of asthma status, asthma control, or severity in patients with asthma. In children and adults, any established definition of asthma or wheeze will be accepted.

Risk of bias (quality) assessment

Study level bias

We will only include RCTs if these are food interventions (e.g. Mediterranean diet, high fruit intake intervention). If we identify any such trials, the risk of bias will be assessed using the Cochrane Collaboration risk of bias tool, which includes sequence generation, allocation concealment, blinding, incomplete outcome data, and selective outcome reporting, and other bias [10]. RCTs will be considered at low risk of bias where the risk of bias is judged to be low for all key domains of the Cochrane Handbook for Systematic Reviews of Interventions [11].

The risk of bias in observational studies will be assessed using the National Institute for Clinical Excellence Methodological Checklist for cohort, and case–control and cross-sectional studies, which includes considerations of subject selection, assessment of exposure and outcome, and measures to assess confounding [12]. Studies will be considered at low risk of bias where most of the criteria in the checklist are addressed, and those that are not addressed or not reported are judged unlikely to change the study findings. For both RCTs and cohort studies, a level of <20 % loss to follow up will generally be accepted as representing low risk of bias from incomplete outcome data, if there are no other features to suggest increased risk of bias. For all studies, a summary Table of Study Characteristics according to the PICO guidelines from NICE [13] will be presented, which will include the population characteristics, methods used for assessing exposure and for outcome assessment.

Strategy for data synthesis

Separate analyses will be undertaken for each group of similar outcome assessment methods and for each intervention/exposure. Results for randomised or quasi-randomised controlled trials, prospective cohort or longitudinal studies, or where appropriate retrospective cohort studies, nested case–control studies, case–control and cross-sectional studies will be reported separately for each comparison. If the studies are sufficiently homogeneous in terms of design and comparator, we will conduct meta-analyses using a random-effects model.

Measures of treatment/exposure effect

Data from individual studies will be pooled using the generic inverse variance method. Pooled results for binary outcomes will be presented as relative risks s with 95 % confidence intervals and 2-sided *p* values, and also expressed as risk differences where possible. Relevant results will be presented in Summary of Findings tables. For dichotomous outcomes, we will use odds ratio (OR) with 95 % confidence interval (CI). Continuous outcomes (e.g. BHR slope) will be analysed using weighted mean differences (with 95 % CI) or standardised mean differences (95 % CI) if different measurement scales are used. All analyses will be performed using STATA. Non-quantitative data will be presented descriptively.

Assessment of heterogeneity

We will examine the heterogeneity between studies by considering variability in participant factors (e.g. age, setting, type of diet or dietary exposure studied). Statistical heterogeneity will be quantified using I-squared (I^2; 0–40 % might not be important; 30–60 % may represent heterogeneity; >60 % may represent moderate heterogeneity; >75 % considerable heterogeneity).

Analysis of subgroups or subsets

Increased disease risk—studies of populations at increased risk for asthma will be separately analysed—for example children with a family history of atopic disease.

Narrative synthesis

A systematic narrative synthesis will be provided with information presented in the text and tables to summarise and explain the characteristics and findings of the included studies. The narrative synthesis will explore the relationship and findings both within and between the included studies.

Meta-bias assessment

Publication bias will be assessed using funnel plots and Egger's test. Where asymmetry is evident on the funnel plot, a trim and fill analysis will be used. Possible causes for asymmetry other than publication bias (e.g. between study heterogeneity) will also be considered.

Authors' contributions

VGL is the study guarantor. VGL drafted the protocol following agreement with all co-authors on the scope and objectives set out for the systematic review. VGL developed the search strategies. All authors contributed to the development of the selection criteria, the risk of bias assessment strategy and data extraction criteria. All authors read and approved the final manuscript.

Author details

[1] Respiratory Epidemiology, Occupational Medicine, and Public Health Group, National Heart and Lung Institute, Imperial College London, Emmanuel Kaye Building, Manresa Road, London SW3 6LR, UK. [2] Department of Medical Sciences "M Aresu", University of Cagliari, Cagliari, Italy. [3] Faculty of Medicine, University of Porto and Hospital São João, Porto, Portugal. [4] Department of Public Health and Infectious Diseases, Lung Function Unit, Sapienza University of Rome, Rome, Italy. [5] National Heart and Lung Institute, Imperial College London, London, UK. [6] Skin and Allergy Hospital, Helsinki University Central Hospital, Helsinki, Finland. [7] European Medicines Agency, London, UK. [8] Second University of Naples and IFT-CNR, Rome, Italy. [9] Department of Medicine and Allergology, University of Oslo, Oslo, Norway. [10] Faculty of Medicine, Transylvania University, Brasov, Romania. [11] Institute of Human Development, University of Manchester, Manchester, UK. [12] Allergy Department, 2nd Paediatric Clinic, University of Athens, Athens, Greece. [13] Laboratory of Immunology, Faculty of Medicine, and CINTESIS (Centre for Health Technology and Services Research), University of Porto and Hospital São João, Porto, Portugal.

Competing interests

The authors declare that they have no competing interests.

Registration of protocol This systematic review has been planned following the PRISMA guidelines and the protocol was registered on PROSPERO on 3 March 2016 (Registration Number CRD42016036078).

Support/funding

This work is supported by an unrestricted Grant from the European Academy of Allergy and Clinical Immunology (EAACI) awarded to the EAACI Evidence-Based Clinical Practice Guideline Task Force on 'Lifestyle Interventions in Allergy and Asthma'.

References

1. Simpson CR, Sheikh A. Trends in the epidemiology of asthma in England: a national study of 333,294 patients. J R Soc Med. 2010;103:98–106.
2. Zhang X, Morrison-Carpenter T, Holt JB, Callahan DB. Trends in adult current asthma prevalence and contributing risk factors in the United States by state: 2000–2009. BMC Public Health. 2013;13:1156.
3. Slejko JF, Ghushchyan VH, Sucher B, Globe DR, Lin SL, Globe G, Sullivan PW. Asthma control in the United States, 2008–2010: indicators of poor asthma control. J Allergy Clin Immunol. 2013;49:01641–2.
4. Zuo L, Otenbaker NP, Rose BA, Salisbury KS. Molecular mechanisms of reactive oxygen species-related pulmonary inflammation and asthma. Mol Immunol. 2013;56:57–63.
5. Seaton A, Godden DJ, Brown K. Increase in asthma: a more toxic environment or a more susceptible population? Thorax. 1994;49:171–4.
6. Devereux G, Seaton A. Diet as a risk factor for atopy and asthma. J Allergy Clin Immunol. 2005;115:1109–17.
7. Nurmatov U, Devereux G, Sheikh A. Nutrients and foods for the primary prevention of asthma and allergy: systematic review and meta-analysis. J Allergy Clin Immunol. 2011;127:724–33.
8. Garcia-Larsen V, Del Giacco SR, Moreira A, Bonini M, Charles D, Reeves T, Carlsen KH, Haahtela T, Bonini S, Fonseca J, Agache I, Papadopoulos NG, Delgado L. Asthma and dietary intake: an overview of systematic reviews. Allergy. 2015. doi:10.1111/all.12800.
9. Shamseer L, Moher D, Clarke M, Ghersi D, Liberati A, Petticrew M, Shekelle P, Stewart LA, PRISMA-P Group. Preferred reporting items for systematic review and meta-analysis protocols (PRISMA-P) 2015: elaboration and explanation. BMJ. 2015;349:g7647. doi:10.1136/bmj.g7647.
10. Stroup DF, Berlin JA, Morton SC, Olkin I, Williamson GD, Rennie D, Moher D, Becker BJ, Sipe TA, Thacker SB. Meta-analysis of observational studies

in epidemiology: a proposal for reporting. Meta-analysis of observational studies in epidemiology (MOOSE) group. JAMA. 2000;283:2008–12.
11. National Collaborating Centre for Methods and Tools AMSTAR: assessing methodological quality of systematic reviews. (2011) Hamilton, ON: McMaster University. Retrieved from http://www.nccmt.ca/registry/view/eng/97.html.
12. Higgins JP, Altman DG, Gozsche PC, Juni P, Moher D, Oxman AD, Savovic J, Schulz KF, Weeks L, Sterne JA. Cochrane bias methods group; Cochrane statistical methods group. The Cochrane collaboration's tool for assessing risk of bias in randomised trials. BMJ. 2011;343:d5928.
13. National Insitute for Health and Clinical Excellence (NICE). Methods for development of NICE public health guidance. 2006. http://www.nice.org.uk. Accessed 22 Feb 2016.

3

Further studies on the biological activity of hazelnut allergens

F. Blanc[1], H. Bernard[1], S. Ah-Leung[1], L. Przybylski-Nicaise[1], P. Stahl Skov[2], A. Purohit[3], F. de Blay[3], B. Ballmer-Weber[4], P. Fritsche[4], M. Fernandez Rivas[5], I. Reig[5], A. Sinaniotis[6], E. Vassilopoulou[7], K. Hoffmann-Sommergruber[8], S. Vieths[9], N. Rigby[10], C. Mills[11] and K. Adel-Patient[1*]

Abstract

Background: Sensitization to hazelnut allergens vary depending on the geographic origin and age of the patients. The objective of this study was to further investigate the allergenic activity of hazelnut allergens using sera from patients recruited in various European regions and presenting different sensitization patterns to hazelnut proteins.

Methods: Natural Cor a 11 and Cor a 9 were purified from hazelnut whereas Cor a 1 and Cor a 8 were produced as recombinant proteins (rCor a 1.04 and rCor a 8). Sera from hazelnut allergic patients were collected in France ($n = 5$), Switzerland ($n = 2$), Greece ($n = 11$) and Spain ($n = 3$), within the Europrevall project. Total and allergen-specific IgE were quantified by enzyme allergosorbent test and IgE immunoblot were performed using pooled sera from birch-pollen endemic region or from Greece. Histamine Release (HR) assays were performed with stripped basophils passively sensitized with individual sera and challenged by a hazelnut extract or the different hazelnut allergens.

Results: As previously described, hazelnut allergic patients from Mediterranean countries are mainly sensitized to the nsLTP Cor a 8 whereas patients from France and Switzerland are sensitized to pollen-related allergens. Interestingly, an intermediate profile was evidenced in patients from Madrid. Hazelnut 7S globulin (Cor a 11) and 11S globulin (Cor a 9) were found to be minor allergens, recognized only by patients from Mediterranean countries. The biologic activity of the 4 tested allergens, analysed by HR assay, further confirmed the sensitization patterns, but also demonstrated the very high elicitation potency of Cor a 8.

Conclusions: This work, extending previously published researches, represents a step towards the better understanding of the complexity of hazelnut allergy and provides new data on the biological activity of hazelnut allergens and extracts.

Keywords: Food allergy, Hazelnut, Purified allergens, Sensitization patterns, Biological activity, Cor a 1, Cor a 8

Background

Recently, Europrevall data demonstrated that hazelnut (*Corylus avellana*) is one of the most common trigger of IgE mediated food allergies. In fact, a very high prevalence rate of sensitization to hazelnut was evidenced in adults, reaching a mean value of 9.3 % of the general population aged 20–57 years in eight European centers [1]. Prevalence was however variable between centers, ranging from 1.27 % in Reykjavik to 17.79 % in Zurich. Hazelnut allergy was also the most reported food allergy in Europrevall clinic survey (32 %), with frequencies ranging from 68.4 % in Vilnius to 5.7 % in Madrid [2]. Hazelnut allergy involved different kind of allergens, that is type 1 ("complete") or type 2 ("incomplete") allergens, leading to different symptoms. Allergic reaction induced by type 2 hazelnut allergens occurred in patients primary sensitized to pollen allergens, mainly from birch. The later consumption of hazelnut, containing proteins homologous to the sensitizing aeroallergen, will lead to symptoms localized to the oral cavity (Oral Allergy Syndrome–OAS; [3]). Type 1 allergens are able both to sensitize and to elicit an allergic reaction and induce

* Correspondence: karine.adel-patient@cea.fr
[1]INRA-CEA, Service de Pharmacologie et d'Immunoanalyse, Laboratoire d'Immuno-Allergie Alimentaire, Bât. 136–CEA de Saclay, 91191 Gif-sur-Yvette, France
Full list of author information is available at the end of the article

more severe reactions such as urticaria, angiodaema or anaphylaxis. Those symptoms are evidenced in "true food allergic" patients [4, 5].

IgE sensitization to hazelnut then combined both IgE recognition of allergens cross reacting with pollen allergens of the PR-10 family, i.e., Bet v 1-related (Cor a 1), and profilin (Cor a 2), and true food allergens such as the non-specific Lipid Transfer Protein (LTP) Cor a 8 and the seed storage proteins Cor a 9 (11S globulin), Cor a 11 (7S globulin) and Cor a 14 (2S albumin). In fact, different proteins have been involved as allergens in hazelnut, the prevalence of specific ones being related to geographical origin and age [4, 6, 7]. Predominance of sensitization to the Bet v 1 related protein Cor a 1.04 is mainly observed in birch-endemic region, i.e., Northern and Central Europe, whereas Cor a 8 is more implicated in non-birch endemic Mediterranean regions such as Spain and Greece [2, 4, 5, 8, 9]. Sensitization to Cor a 8 purified from hazelnut was also evidenced in children from birch-endemic area, i.e., the Netherlands, in which it was associated to more severe allergic reaction upon challenge [9]. However, this was not confirmed in a later study using recombinant Cor a 8 (rCor a 8), suggesting a contamination of the natural Cor a 8 by other seed storage proteins [6, 8, 10].

Hazelnut allergy in birch-endemic region was also demonstrated to exhibit age-related sensitization profiles with different clinical outcomes. Young children (<2 years) demonstrated more severe reaction with systemic reaction, without associated birch-pollen allergy. Sixty five percent of these children were sensitized to Cor a 9. Sensitization to Cor a 9 decreased with age, and OAS predominated in adults, 90 % of which were sensitized to Cor a 1.04 [6]. In the same birch-endemic region, out of 34 children of less than 1-year-old demonstrating atopic dermatitis, 20 demonstrated IgE reactivity to hazelnut and 15 to peanut. Of the hazelnut sensitized children, 75 % demonstrated anti-Cor a 9 IgE, whereas no sensitization to Cor a 1 nor Cor a 8 was evidenced [11]. Sensitization to Cor a 9 and Cor a 11 was further evidenced mainly in children with systemic reaction in the same birch-endemic area [7]. Sensitization to Cor a 9 and/or Cor a 14 was later demonstrated to identify almost 90 % of children with generalized reactions [12]. In a Dutch hazelnut-sensitized population, sensitization and levels of specific IgE to Cor a 9 and to the 2S albumin Cor a 14 were also significantly more common in both children and adults patients demonstrating objective symptoms compared to patients with no or subjective symptoms [10]. Sensitization to the basic subunit of an isoform of Cor a 9 was also recently described in an Italian pediatric population demonstrating severe symptoms (urticarial, angioedema and/or anaphylaxis), and may be involved in cross-reactivity between nuts and legumes. In this population, Cor a 8 and Cor a 9 were also recognized by 47 and 80 % of the patients, respectively [13].

The objective of the present study was then to further assess the allergenic activity of the hazelnut allergens using Histamine Release (HR) assays and sera from patients recruited in various European regions, i.e., France, Switzerland, Spain and Greece. Sensitization patterns to hazelnut proteins were first assessed by specific IgE measurement and IgE immunoblots to confirm regional variations.

Methods

Allergic patients

Sera of patients with a self-reported hazelnut allergy have been collected within the Europrevall project in Switzerland (Zurich), East of France (Strasbourg), Greece (Athens) and Spain (Madrid) (Table 1; $n = 21$). A written informed consent was obtained before the serum collection and the performed experiments were approved by the corresponding local ethical committees.

Natural allergen purification and recombinant allergens

Natural Cor a 11 and Cor a 9 were purified from hazelnut as described in [14]. Cor a 1.04 and Cor a 8 were produced as recombinant proteins [15] and kindly provided by the EuroPrevall allergen library. Hazelnut proteins correspond to RefLab Hazelnut extract (Histamine release) or were extracted from hazelnut flour (IgE-immunoblot, The Nutt Ranch, Marlborough, New Zealand; Kindly provided by Dr Justin Marsh, University of Manchester) using 0.3 % Sodium Borate, 10 mM EDTA, 0.9 % n-octyl-β-D-Glucoside pH 9.0 buffer. Protein extraction efficiency was about 80 % considering theoretical protein content of hazelnut flour.

Determination of total and specific IgE concentrations

Total IgE and IgE specific for Cor a 11, Cor a 9, rCor a 1.04 and rCor a 8 were quantified by EAST (enzyme allergo-sorbent test) as previously described [16–18]. Briefly, microtitre plates (96 well microtiter MaxiSorp Nunc, Roskilde, Denmark) were coated by passive adsorption of purified hazelnut proteins (specific IgE) or anti-human IgE antibody (total IgE, clone LE-27) (5 µg/ml in 50 mM phosphate buffer, pH 7.4). After saturation with EIA buffer (0.1 M phosphate buffer, 0.1 % bovine serum albumin, 0.15 M NaCl, 0.01 % sodium azide, pH 7.4), 50 µl per well of serial dilutions of individual serum (1/4 to 1/2500, in EIA buffer) were dispensed. After a 24-h incubation at 4 °C and a wash step, a second anti-human IgE antibody (clone BS17) labelled with acetylcholinesterase (AChE) was used as tracer. After extensive washings, Ellman's reagent was used as enzyme substrate and the absorbance was measured at 414 nm. Limit of detection, corresponding to the mean background

Table 1 Data from Hazelnut allergic patients

Source	Reference	Age	Gender	Hazelnut allergy symptoms	SPT	CAP specific IgE (kU/L)	Other food allergies	Other allergies
Strasbourg, France	1	49	f	Rhinitis, Conjunctivitis, Asthma	++	9.7	kiwi, ananas	no
	2	17	m	Rhinitis, Conjunctivitis	++	>100.0	peanut, apple, celery, soya, walnut, sesame, kiwi, carrot, tomato, cherry, fig	cat
	3	25	f	Rhinitis, Conjunctivitis	++	31.2		no
	4	30	m	Rhinitis, Conjunctivitis, Asthma	+	1		house dust mite
	5	33	f	Rhinitis, Conjunctivitis, Asthma	++	>100.0		cat
Athens, Greece	6	42	f		+	1.7	peanut, cabbage, pepper, honey	Resp Allergy Rhinitis
	7	24	f		–	2.6	almond	Resp Allergy Rhinitis, Asthma
	8	21	m	OAS	+	1.0	eggplant	no
	9	36	m	Asymptomatic sensitization	–	3.0	walnut	Resp Allergy Rhinitis
	10	27	m	OAS	++	5.1	peanut, walnut, almond, cashew, pistachio, peach, apple, appricot, mustard, corn	Resp Allergy Rhinitis, Asthma
	11	21	f	OAS	+	0.5	peach, walnut	Resp Allergy Rhinitis
	12	18	f	Asymptomatic sensitization	–	28.5	cabbage, wheat	no
	13			Hazelnut allergy history				
	14	8	m	OAS	++	n/a	egg	no
	15							
	16			hazelnut allergy history				
Madrid, Spain	17	34	f	urticaria + contact urticaria	++	5.1	lentil, chickpea, bean, pea, soybean, sunflower seed, pine nut	grass and olive pollen allergies - rhinoconjunctivitis and asthma
	18	4	m	OAS	++	2.3	walnut	NO
	19	16	f	tongue angioedema	++	7.3	walnut, vetchling	pollen allergy - rhinoconjunctivitis and asthma - due to grass, cypress and plane tree pollens
Zurich, Switzerland	20							
	21							

Asymptomatic sensitization: SPT results (–,+ or ++ according to the SPT/histamine wheal size ratio) or/and specific IgE (CAP) to hazelnut in the absence of clinical symptoms
No information was available for Zurich patients
OAS Oral Allergy Syndrom

value plus three standard deviation, was 0.1 IU/ml. Total IgE concentration was determined as described in [18] using anti-IgE coated plate and human IgE samples (World Health Organization) at concentrations ranging from 10 to 0.08 IU/ml as standard.

IgE-immunoblot

SDS-PAGE and IgE immunoblot analyses were performed using apparatus and reagents from Invitrogen (Life Technologies, Carlsbad, CA, USA) following provider's recommendation. Samples and molecular-weight markers (See Blue prestained marker) were loaded on a NuPage Novex 4-12 % Bis-Tris Gel (1.0 mm). Electrophoresis was performed using XCell SureLock Mini-Cell in MES Buffer with a constant voltage of 200 V during 40 min. After electrophoresis, gels were stained with SimplyBlue™ Safe Stain or proteins were transferred to PVDF membranes for 60 min at 30 V using a XCell II blot module. The membranes were saturated with TBST (20 mM Tris, pH 8.0, 0.25 M NaCl, 0.5 % Tween) supplemented with 5 % milk powder. Immunoblots were performed with a pool of sera specific for Cor a 1.04 from birch-endemic region, or a pool of sera from Athens specific for Cor a 8, Cor a 9 and Cor a 11. Sera diluted 1/40 in TBST supplemented with 5 % milk powder were incubated overnight at 4 °C. Membranes were then washed using TBST, and a human anti-IgE monoclonal Antibody (Star 96P, Serotec) labelled with peroxidase was incubated for 2 h at room temperature. After several washings using TBS (20 mM Tris, pH 8.0, 0.25 M NaCl), the membrane was incubated with the ECL plus Western blotting detection reagent (Amersham GE Healthcare, Buckinghamshire, UK) for 5 min and images then acquired using VersaDoc Imaging System (BioRad, Hercules, CA).

Basophil histamine release assay

PBMCs were isolated from 20 mL of fresh buffy coats (Blood Bank, National University Hospital of Copenhagen, Denmark) using the lymphoprep isolation method. After isolation PBMCs were washed twice in physiologic saline and IgE were removed by exposing the cell pellet to stripping buffer (RefLab, Copenhagen, Denmark; 4 °C for 5 min). After centrifugation, cells were washed twice with Pipes buffer (RefLab) and finally resuspended to a final volume of 2 mL. Aliquots of 100 μl stripped cells were incubated with 100 μl undiluted patient serum or one sera from non allergic patient as a control for 1 h at 37 °C and then resuspended in 3 mL of a washed erythrocyte obtained from the lymphoprep separation suspension containing IL-3 (2 ng/mL). Twenty-five microliters of the passively sensitized cell suspension was incubated with 25 μl of different concentrations of hazelnut extract or purified hazelnut allergens (Cor a 9, Cor a 11, rCor a 1.04 and rCor a 8) for 1 h at 37 °C on HR-Test Plate (RefLab, Copenhagen, Denmark). Anti-IgE or buffer was used as positive (reference) and negative control, respectively. After washing, released histamine was detected fluorometrically according to the method described by Stahl et al. [19]. A net histamine release > 10 ng/mL was considered as a positive response and histamine release was expressed as percentage of reference release. Results were also given in classes 0–6, taking into account the range of allergen concentration inducing a significant histamine release (the lower this concentration is, the higher the class is).

Results

Sensitization pattern

Total and specific IgE

Whatever the regional origin of the patient, total IgE showed a great variability ranging from less than 15 to 4500 IU/mL (Table 2). Patients' sera were considered positive when specific IgE were detected against at least one of the four allergens, i.e., rCor a 1, rCor a 8, Cor a 9 and Cor a 11. All patient sera from Spain, 9 out of the 11 patient sera from Greece, and 6 out of the 7 patient sera from Switzerland and East of France were positive (Table 2; sensitization pattern depending on geographical area is depicted Fig. 1). Within positive sera, those coming from patients from France and Switzerland demonstrated IgE exclusively directed against rCor a 1.04 whereas none of the positive patient's sera from Greece demonstrated IgE specific to this allergen. Conversely, most of the positive Greek sera (8 out of 9) had specific IgE directed against rCor a 8. Sera from 2 out of the 3 patients recruited in Spain showed intermediate patterns, with both specific IgE to rCor a 8 and rCor a 1.04. The third one demonstrated only Cor a 9-specific IgE (Patient #18).

Only few sera had specific IgE directed against either Cor a 11 or Cor a 9. They all came from patients recruited in Greece (5/11 and 3/11 respectively) and Spain (1/3 in each case). The higher levels of specific IgE against these two allergens were demonstrated in a patient from Greece that demonstrated low levels of anti-rCor a 8 IgE (Patient #14).

IgE immunoblot

Pools of sera from patients sensitized exclusively to Cor a 1.04 (birch-endemic region pool) or from patients sensitized to Cor a 8, Cor a 9 and Cor a 11 (Greek pool) were constituted to further analyse their sensitization pattern by IgE-immunoblot. Far more bands were revealed using sera from Greece when compared to birch-endemic region pool that demonstrated very restricted recognition pattern. As evidenced using sera from the birch endemic region, Cor a 1 was intensively recognized when analysing purified recombinant allergen (Fig. 2b, lane 5). However, Cor a 1 recognition was far less intense within the complex hazelnut extract (Fig. 2b, lane 2). Conversely, another band, at MW below that of Cor a 1, was more intensively revealed by IgE-immunoblot.

Electrophoresis pattern of purified Cor a 11 and Cor a 9 evidenced several bands (Fig. 2a), as previously described [14]. Cor a 11 polypeptides with apparent MW of 47 KDa were evidenced whereas the 31–35 KDa bands were hardly visible, suggesting degradation of the corresponding entities–certainly as several intense bands between 20 and 30 KDa (Fig. 2a, lane 2). All those Cor a 11-related bands were slightly recognized by IgE from Greek pool sera (Fig. 2c, lane 3), and not recognized at all by IgE from birch-endemic region pool (Fig. 2b, lane 3). Basic (21–25 KDa) and acidic chains (31–35 KDa) of 11S globulin Cor a 9 were also clearly evidenced by electrophoresis (Fig. 2a, lane 3), as the same as lower MW polypeptides between 9 and 12 KDa. Basic and acidic

Table 2 Total IgE and Cor a 11-, Cor a 9-, rCor a 1.04- and rCor a 8-specific IgE in sera, depending on the regional origin of the patients

Origin	Reference	Total IgE (IU/mL)	Specific IgE (IU/mL)			
			Cor a 11 (7S globulin)	Cor a 9 (11S globulin)	rCor a 1.04 (Bet v 1 like)	rCor a 8 (nsLTP)
Strasbourg, France	1	19	–	–	2.5	–
	2	183	–	–	84.7	–
	3	52	–	–	10.8	–
	4	<15	–	–	–	–
	5	757	–	–	134.5	–
Athens, Greece	6	176	–	–	–	10.0
	7	891	1.5	–	–	9.3
	8	<15	–	–	–	2.4
	9	189	1.9	–	–	–
	10	898	–	–	–	8.2
	11	118	–	–	–	–
	12	861	0.9	–	–	137.0
	13	500	3.2	4.7	–	9.5
	14	1027	85.4	72.3	–	2.2
	15	1591	–	4.8	–	67.2
	16	29	–	–	–	–
Madrid, Spain	17	779	–	–	2.1	14.0
	18	72	–	0.8	–	–
	19	4537	4.6	–	4.5	10.9
Zurich, Switzerland	20	275	–	–	31.3	–
	21	4350	–	–	109.2	–

(– = < limit of detection (0.1 IU/mL))

bands were recognised by IgE from the Greek pool, as evidenced both using the purified allergen (Fig. 2c, lane 4) and the hazelnut extract (Fig. 2c, lane 2). IgE immunoblot also demonstrated the intense recognition of rCor a 8 only by the Greek pool sera (lane 6: rCor a 8 and lane 2: hazelnut extract). Another band, at MW below that of Cor a 8, was also revealed by IgE-immunoblot with Greek pool.

Histamine release

HR tests were performed for all the sera collected in France/Switzerland ($n = 7$), Spain ($n = 3$) and Greece ($n = 11$). All sera from allergic patients tested induced histamine release after challenge with the hazelnut extract, whereas serum from non allergic patient did not (data not shown). Typical results obtained with 4 sera are shown Fig. 3 and Basophil histamine release classes obtained from all the sera

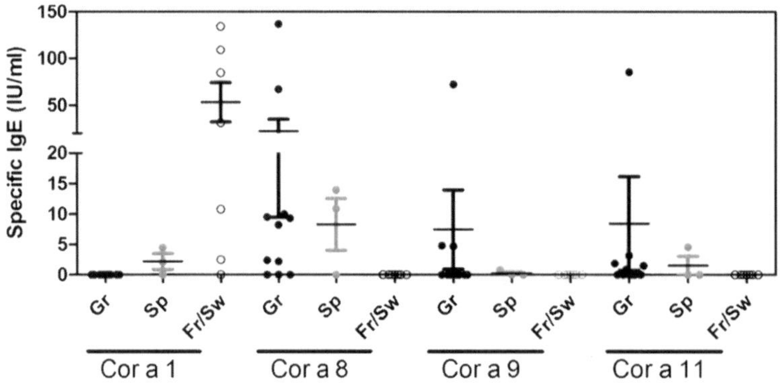

Fig. 1 Sensitization pattern depending on the geographical origin of the patient. Specific IgE against Cor a 11, Cor a 9, rCor a 1.04 and rCor a 8 were assayed by EAST

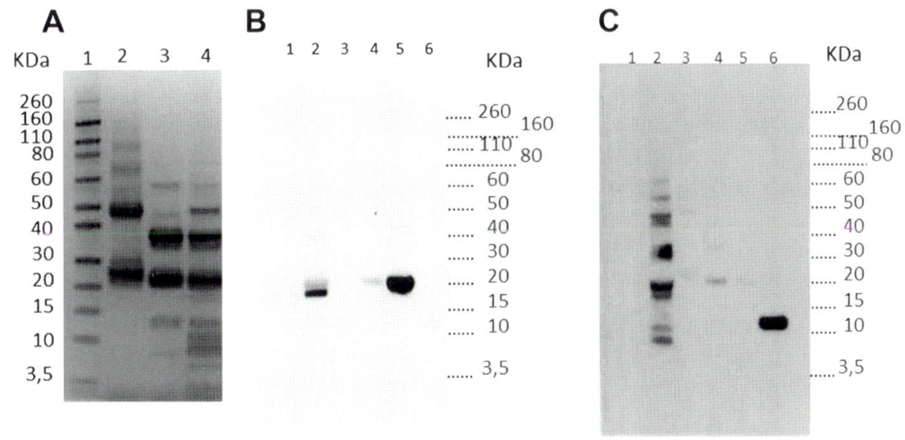

Fig. 2 IgE immunoblot using pooled sera from birch endemic region or from Greece. (**a**) Electrophoresis profile of purified Cor a 11 (*lane 2*), purified Cor a 9 (*lane 3*) and hazelnut extract (*lane 4*). IgE immunoblot using pool of sera from birch-endemic region (**b**) or from Greece (**c**) using hazelnut extract (*lane 2*), purified Cor a 11 (*lane 3*), purified Cor a 9 (*lane 4*), rCor a 1.04 (*lane 5*) or rCor a 8 (*lane 6*). Molecular weights (*lane 1*) are indicated

depending of their geographical origin are gathered Fig. 4. Globally, good correlation was observed between IgE titers (Fig. 1) and HR assay. The 2 sera from Greece (#11 and #16) and sera from Strasbourg (#4) negative for specific IgE demonstrated low HR using the hazelnut extract (BHR class 1), whereas no allergen-specific HR was detected for these sera.

Figure 3a and b shows typical results obtained with 1 serum from Switzerland and France, respectively. Among all sera from patients coming from France and Switzerland, 6 out of 7 demonstrated rCor a 1-specific HR, whereas none of them demonstrated rCor a 8, Cor a 9 nor Cor a 11-specific HR, correlating with specific IgE. Sera in Fig. 3 demonstrated high (patient #21, Fig. 3a) or low (patient #1,

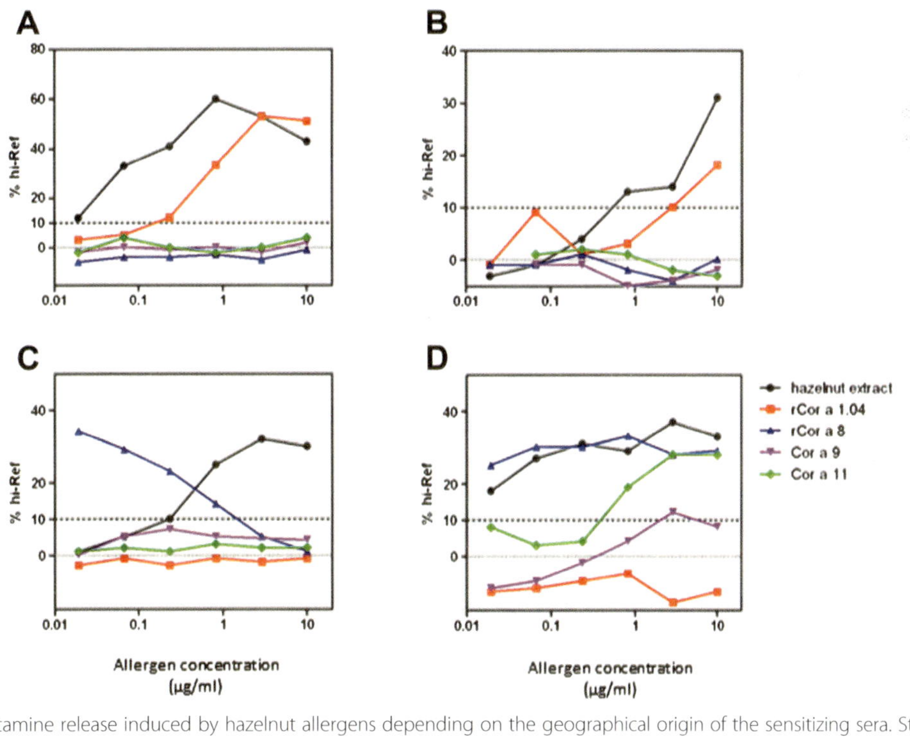

Fig. 3 Basophil histamine release induced by hazelnut allergens depending on the geographical origin of the sensitizing sera. Stripped human basophils were passively sensitized with serum #21 (Zurich–**a**), #1 (Strasbourg–**b**), #8 or #12 (Athens, **c** and **d** respectively) and then incubated with increasing concentration of hazelnut allergens, i.e., hazelnut extract (*black*), rCor a 1 (*red*), rCor a 8 (*blue*), Cor a 9 (*purple*) or Cor a 11 (*green*). Released histamine is represented as percentage of reference release, i.e., induced by anti-IgE

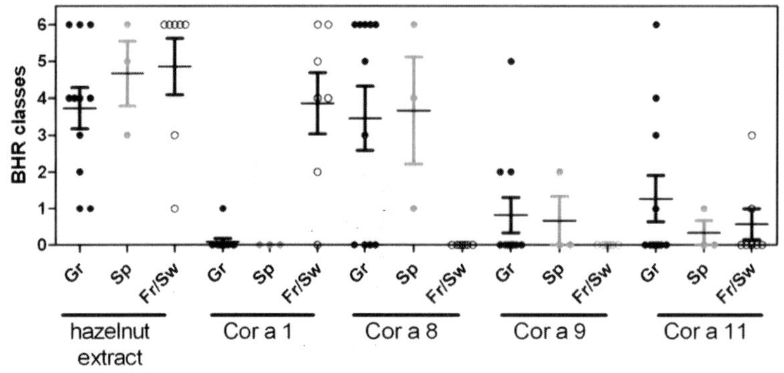

Fig. 4 BHR classes depending on the geographical origin of the sensitizing sera and of the purified allergens. BHR class represent the range of allergen concentration inducing a significant histamine release

Fig. 3b) rCor a 1-specific IgE concentrations (Table 2). Additional results using 3 other sera from France with various specific IgE titers are shown in Additional file 1: Figure S1. No clear correlation between rCor a 1-specific IgE concentrations and HR intensity could be evidenced.

On the opposite, sera from Greek patients induced mainly Cor a 8-specific HR, at very low doses of allergen (Fig. 3c and d showing two sera from Greece), suggesting a high elicitation potency of this allergen. All the sera of patients from Spain induced HR after rCor a 8 challenge (even patient #18 who did not demonstrated specific IgE), but not after rCor a 1 challenge, although rCor a 1 specific IgE were detected in 2 of these 3 sera. One of them demonstrated HR after Cor a 9 and Cor a 11 challenge, but at the highest tested doses. Globally, Cor a 9 and Cor a 11-specific HR were less frequent (Cor a 9: 3 sera from Greek patients, 1 serum from Spain; Cor a 11: 4 sera from Greece, 1 serum from Spain, 2 sera from France; Fig. 4). Considering those allergens, HR occurred at higher doses than those observed for rCor a 8 (Fig. 3d).

Discussion

The results obtained in our adult population confirm that hazelnut allergic patients from Mediterranean countries are mainly sensitized to Cor a 8 whereas patients from Northern Europe are sensitized to pollen-related allergens such as Cor a 1.04 [2, 4, 5, 8]. In fact, in our population, Cor a 1.04 sensitization was clearly evidenced in French and Swiss patients when using EAST or IgE immunoblot with purified recombinant allergen, correlating with the very high frequency of recognition (>80 %) of this allergen within Strasbourg and Zurich cohorts of Europrevall [2]. It is to note however that another IgE-reactive protein is evidenced by IgE immunoblot using Birch-endemic pool, leading to an even more intense signal than Cor a 1 within the hazelnut extract (Fig. 2b). This protein could correspond to another pollen-related allergen such as Cor a 2 (MW 14 KDa vs Cor a 1 MW 17–18 KDa, [4, 20]). In fact, Cor a 2 was also recognized by about 19 % of Zurich and Strasbourg patients within Europrevall cohorts [2], by 26 % of patients form Zurich and Copenhagen [4] and up to 42 % in hazelnut allergic patients from Switzerland or Denmark [8]. Using purified allergens and ImmunoCAP, the IgE concentrations against rCor a 1 were demonstrated to be far higher than that against rCor a 2 [2, 8], but our study suggests that the contents and/or the allergenic activity [21] of the relative allergens within the hazelnut extract have also to be taken into consideration to further assess their relative contribution in hazelnut allergy. This is further confirmed when comparing elicitation potency of rCor a 1.04 vs hazelnut extract (see below).

Conversely, no Cor a 1.04 sensitization was evidenced in the Greek patients whereas Cor a 8 sensitization was observed in 8 out 9 of the sensitized patients from Athens, comforting recent data [2]. Within these 8 patients and considering the allergens we tested, 3 patients were monosensitized to Cor a 8. In a study involving 26 hazelnut patients from Spain, in which 10 patients demonstrated anaphylactic reaction, rCor a 8 was recognized by 62 to 77 % of the patients, most of them being monosensitized, whereas only 1 patient demonstrated IgE against rCor a 1.04 and none against rCor a 2 [5]. Interestingly, the 3 Spanish patients in the present study demonstrated intermediate sensitization profiles, 2 of them demonstrating both rCor a 1.04 and rCor a 8 specific IgE.

We observed sensitization to seed storage proteins Cor a 9 and Cor a 11 in 55 and 33 %, respectively, of the sensitized patients from Athens ($n = 9$), and 1 out 3 patients from Madrid. None of the French nor Swiss patients tested ($n = 7$) demonstrated specific IgE against these proteins. The IgE-immunoblot using the Greek pool confirmed sensitization to Cor a 8, Cor a 9 and Cor a 11. It is to note that purified Cor a 9 used in the present study may also contain isoallergen of Cor a 9, notably its 20.7 KDa IgE reactive subunit recently described in Italian paediatric patients ([13], Fig. 2c).

Others bands suggest also sensitization to the 2S albumin Cor a 14 (MW around 9 KDa, Fig. 2c) in the Greek population, an allergen that allowed identifying almost 90 % of children with generalized reactions to hazelnut [12]. This is in accordance with the fact that all patients sensitized to Cor a 14 were also sensitized to Cor a 9 [2]. Unfortunately, we didn't assay corresponding IgE in individual sera.

Interestingly, the higher sensitization to Cor a 9 and Cor a 11 was observed in one of the 2 children of our population, i.e., patient #14, a 8-year old child from Athens. The other child, a 4-year-old from Madrid was monosensitized to Cor a 9 (patient #18). In our restricted population, none of the adults from the 2 birch-endemic regions were sensitized to these allergens. This is in accordance with the observation that sensitization to Cor a 11 was not or rarely found in hazelnut-allergic adults from birch-endemic region such as the Netherlands and Belgium [7, 22], whereas sensitization to Cor a 11 was evidenced in children of such area, mainly in infants demonstrating severe reaction. In birch-endemic region, Cor a 9 (and Cor a 14) sensitization was evidenced as soon as preschool age in infants with atopic dermatis, preceding sensitization to Cor a 11, and in children demonstrating severe symptoms [7, 11, 12].

The biologic activity of the 4 tested allergens was then analysed by histamine release assay, further confirming the sensitization patterns observed in EAST and IgE immunoblot, and the efficiency of the interaction between these sera and the corresponding specific allergen. We can observe that for some patients and allergens, the presence of specific IgE is not confirmed by HR. For example, rCor a 1.04 specific IgE were detected in 2 patients from Spain (patients #17 and #19), but were not associated with basophil activation. This can reflected IgE cross reactivity with others Bet v 1 pollen allergens, as these two patients were allergic to grass and olive or grass, cypress and plane tree pollens, but not clinical reactivity. The biological activity of nCor a 11 [7] or nCor a 9, rCor a 1 and rCor a 8 [6] was also studied using Basophil activation test and selected sera from birch-endemic region. In this study, the most active allergen, i.e., the allergen activating basophils at the lower dose, was Cor a 1. In the present study we demonstrated that the activity of rCor a 8 is very high in the Athens patients, with elicitation potency and BHR classes higher than that observed for the reference hazelnut extract. In contrast, HR release induced by rCor a 1.04 was far less efficient in patients from France and Switzerland. In these patients, the most efficient release was induced by the hazelnut extract, thus confirming the presence of other IgE reactive protein(s) for these patients in the extract. BHR classes for Cor a 9 and Cor a 11 in respective-sensitized patients were lower. Altogether, this thus suggests that rCor a 8 is a more potent elicitor than the other tested allergens, which can also partially explain the more severe symptoms in the patients sensitized to this allergen [4, 5].

Conclusions

Although based on a limited number of patients, this work extends previously published researches on the sensitizing profiles of hazelnut allergic patients in birch-endemic versus Mediteranean regions and provides new data on the biological activity of hazelnut allergens and extracts. Notably, the present study demonstrates the high biological activity of Cor a 8 and the IgE reactivity and functionality of other pollen-related proteins in hazelnut extract.

Competing interests

The authors declare that they have no competing interests.

Authors' contributions

FB & HB supervised and performed the IgE assays, analysed all the data and participated in the manuscript preparation; SAh-L and LP-N performed the protein extraction from hazelnut flour and the IgE-immunoblot; PSS performed the histamine release tests; AP, FdeB, BB-W, PF, MFR, IR, AS, EV, SV recruited and characterized the patients and provided the sera; KH-S, NR and CM produced/purified the recombinant and natural allergens; KA-P supervised the whole study, analysed the data and wrote the manuscript. All authors read and approved the final manuscript.

Acknowledgements

This work was funded by the EU through the EuroPrevall (FP6, FOOD-CT-2005-514000) and iFAAM (FP7, KBBE.2012.2.4-04) projects.

Author details

[1]INRA-CEA, Service de Pharmacologie et d'Immunoanalyse, Laboratoire d'Immuno-Allergie Alimentaire, Bât. 136–CEA de Saclay, 91191 Gif-sur-Yvette, France. [2]RefLab ApS, Copenhagen, Denmark. [3]Hôpitaux Universitaires de Strasbourg, Strasbourg, France. [4]University Hospital Zurich, Zurich, Switzerland. [5]Hospital Clinico San Carlos, Madrid, Spain. [6]University of Athens & "Sotiria" Regional Chest Diseases Hospital of Athens, Athens, Greece. [7]University of Nicosia, Nicosia, Cyprus. [8]Medical University of Vienna, Vienna, Austria. [9]Paul-Ehrlich-Institut, Langen, Germany. [10]Institute of Food Research, Norwich, UK. [11]University of Manchester, Manchester, UK.

References

1. Burney PGJ, Potts J, Kummeling I, Mills ENC, Clausen M, et al. The prevalence and distribution of food sensitization in European adults. Allergy. 2014;69:365–71.
2. Datema M, Zuidmeer-Jongejan L, Asero R, Barreales L, et al. Hazelnut allergy across Europe dissected molecularly: a Europrevall outpatient clinic survey. J Allergy Clin Immunol. 2015 in press.
3. Hirschwehr R, Valenta R, Ebner C, Ferreira F, Sperr WR, Valent P, et al. Identification of common allergenic structures in hazel pollen and hazelnuts–a possible explanation for sensitivity to hazelnuts in patients allergic to tree pollen. J Allergy Clin Immunol. 1992;90:927–36.

4. Pastorello EA, Vieths S, Pravettoni V, Farioli L, Trambaioli C, Fortunato D, et al. Identification of hazelnut major allergens in sensitive patients with positive double-blind, placebo-controlled food challenge results. J Allergy Clin Immunol. 2002;109:563–70.
5. Schocker F, Luttkopf D, Scheurer S, Petersen A, Cistero-Bahima A, Enrique E, et al. Recombinant lipid transfer protein Cor a 8 from hazelnut: a new tool for in vitro diagnosis of potentially severe hazelnut allergy. J Allergy Clin Immunol. 2004;113:141–7.
6. De Knop KJ, Verweij MM, Grimmelikhuijsen M, Philipse E, Hagendorens MM, Bridts CH, et al. Age-related sensitization profiles for hazelnut (Corylus avellana) in a birch-endemic region. Pediatr Allergy Immunol. 2011;22(1 Pt 2):e139–49.
7. Verweij MM, Hagendorens MM, Trashin S, Cucu T, De Meulenaer B, Devreese B, et al. Age-dependent sensitization to the 7S-vicilin-like protein Cor a 11 from hazelnut (Corylus avellana) in a birch-endemic region. J Investig Allergol Clin Immunol. 2012;22(4):245–51.
8. Hansen KS, Ballmer-Weber BK, Sastre J, Lidholm J, Andersson K, Oberhofer H, et al. Component-resolved in vitro diagnosis of hazelnut allergy in Europe. J Allergy Clin Immunol. 2009;123(5):1134–41.
9. Flinterman AE, Akkerdaas JH, den Hartog Jager CF, Rigby NM, Fernandez-Rivas M, Hoekstra MO, et al. Lipid transfer protein-linked hazelnut allergy in children from a non-Mediterranean birch-endemic area. J Allergy Clin Immunol. 2008;121(2):423–8.
10. Masthoff LJ, Mattsson L, Zuidmeer-Jongejan L, Lidholm J, Andersson K, Akkerdaas JH, et al. Sensitization to Cor a 9 and Cor a 14 is highly specific for a hazelnut allergy with objective symptoms in Dutch children and adults. J Allergy Clin Immunol. 2013;132(2):393–9.
11. Verweij MM, Hagendorens MM, De Knop KJ, Bridts CH, De Clerck LS, Stevens WJ, et al. Young infants with atopic dermatitis can display sensitization to Cor a 9, an 11S legumin-like seed-storage protein from hazelnut (Corylus avellana). Pediatr Allergy Immunol. 2011;22(2):196–201.
12. Faber MA, De Graag M, Van Der Heijden C, Sabato V, Hagendorens MM, Bridts CH, et al. Cor a 14: missing link in the molecular diagnosis of hazelnut allergy? Int Arch Allergy Immunol. 2014;164(3):200–6.
13. Nitride C, Mamone G, Picariello G, Mills C, Nocerino R, Canani RB, et al. Proteomic and immunological characterization of a new food allergen from hazelnut (Corylus avellana). J Proteomics. 2013;86:16–26.
14. Rigby NM, Marsh J, Sancho AI, Wellner K, Akkerdaas J, van Ree R, et al. The purification and characterisation of allergenic hazelnut seed proteins. Mol Nutr Food Res. 2008;52:S251–61.
15. Lauer I, Alessandri S, Pokoj S, Reuter A, Conti A, Vieths S, et al. Expression and characterization of three important panallergens from hazelnut. Mol Nutr Food Res. 2008;52 Suppl 2:S262–71.
16. Bernard H, Paty E, Mondoulet L, Burks AW, Bannon GA, et al. Serological characteristics of peanut allergy in children. Allergy. 2003;58:1285–92.
17. Mondoulet L, Paty E, Drumare MF, Ah-Leung S, Scheinmann P, et al. Influence of thermal processing on the allergenicity of peanut proteins. J Agric Food Chem. 2005;53:4547–53.
18. Grassi J, Didierlaurent A, Stadler BM. Quantitative determination of total and specific human IgE with the use of monoclonal antibodies. J Allergy Clin Immunol. 1986;77:808–22.
19. Skov PS, Mosbech H, Norn S, Weeke B. Sensitive glass microfibre-based histamine analysis for allergy testing in washed blood cells. Results compared with conventional leukocyte histamine release assay. Allergy. 1985;40(3):213–8.
20. Willison LN, Sathe SK, Roux K. Production and analysis of recombinant tree nut allergens. Methods. 2014;66:34–43.
21. Andersson K, Ballmer-Weber BK, Cistero-Bahima A, Ostling J, Lauer I, Vieths S, et al. Enhancement of hazelnut extract for IgE testing by recombinant allergen spiking. Allergy. 2007;62(8):897–904.
22. Hansen KS, Ballmer-Weber BK, Luttkopf D, Skov PS, Wuthrich B, Bindslev-Jensen C, et al. Roasted hazelnuts–allergenic activity evaluated by double-blind, placebo-controlled food challenge. Allergy. 2003;58:132–8.

4

Food allergy in mice is modulated through the thymic stromal lymphopoietin pathway

Christophe P. Frossard[1], Simone C. Zimmerli[2,3], José M. Rincon Garriz[1,4] and Philippe A. Eigenmann[1*]

Abstract

Background: Thymic stromal lymphopoietin (TSLP) is involved in the pathogenesis of allergic reactions in the skin and the lung. Nevertheless, data on the role of TSLP in food allergy are scarce. We explored the role of TSLP in a mouse model with oral sensitization and oral challenge eliciting food allergy.

Methods: TSLP receptor (TSLPR)−/− mice and wild type mice were orally sensitized to β-lactoglobulin in presence of cholera toxin (CT) or CT alone. The elicited immune response was characterized in vitro and the mice were subsequently challenged with the antigen. Lymphocytes from various locations in the gut were activated either by the antigen or by CT and assayed for cytokine secretion.

Results: Here we report that TSLPR−/− are less prone to generate food-induced reactions in conjunction with a decreased antigen-specific IgG1, but not IgE response. In addition, mesenteric lymphnode lymphocytes of TSLPR−/− mice were secreting lower quantities of IL-4, IL-5 and IL-10 after in vivo Ag activation, whereas higher numbers of IL-17 secreting cells were observed. Similarly, activation by the Th2-type adjuvant cholera toxin resulted in an increased frequency of IL-12 and IL-17 secreting lamina propria and mesenteric lymphocytes, together with increased production of IL-12 by activated dendritic cells in TSLPR−/− mice.

Conclusions: TSLP can be considered as an essential, but not exclusive, mediator for elicitation of food allergy in mice, as well as a potential target for future therapeutic interventions.

Background

The pathogenesis of food allergy involves various mechanisms, all closely associated with the gut-related immune system [1]. Initiation of IgE-mediated food allergy follows the path of Th2-type sensitization involving antigen presentation and CD4+ T cells, followed by IL-4 and IL-13 facilitated antigen-specific IgE production. Mice models of food allergy with oral sensitization to common food antigens eliciting anaphylactic reactions upon re-exposure have allowed extensive description of Th2-type, gut-related mechanisms of IgE-mediated food allergy [2, 3]. In addition to IgE-dependent pathways of gut-mediated anaphylaxis, other mechanistic pathways have been described, e.g. by involving IgG1 antibodies, or antigen-activated complement [4, 5]. Thymic stromal lymphopoietin (TSLP) dependant mechanisms of food allergy have also been suspected [6, 7].

TSLP has a close four helix structural analogy to IL-7, and can be found secreted in increased amounts in epithelial cells (EC) of the skin, the lung and the gut. TSLP is expressed in presence of the Th2–type cytokines IL-4 and IL-13 [8–13]. TSLP in relation to allergy has been first studied in atopic dermatitis where increased levels have been found in inflamed skin associated with Th2-type cytokines [14]. Similarly, TSLP receptor (TSLPR)$^{-/-}$ mice lacking responsiveness to TSLP fail to express Th2-type cytokines and lung inflammation [15, 16]. It has also been demonstrated that skin-derived dendritic cells are targets of TSLP in the Th2-type immune response in

*Correspondence: Philippe.Eigenmann@hcuge.ch
[1] Inflammation and Allergy Research Group and Department of Pediatrics, University Hospitals of Geneva and University of Geneva, 6 rue Willy-Donzé, 1211 Geneva 14, Switzerland
Full list of author information is available at the end of the article

the skin [17]. In the gut, intestinal EC produce TSLP, and expression of TSLP and the TSLPR are closely linked to inflammation mediated by IL-12, IL-17, and Th2-type cytokines [18, 19].

We hypothesize that, similarly to the skin and the lung, IgE-mediated immunity in the gut is regulated by TSLP and its receptor. For these studies, we used a well characterized mouse model with oral antigen sensitized with β-lactoglobulin (BLG) in presence of the Th2-type adjuvant cholera-toxin (CT). The main characteristic of this widely used model are symptoms of anaphylaxis upon food gavage [20, 21], the most closely reproducing symptoms seen in food allergy in humans. Clinical parameters and biomarkers were measured in wild-type (wt) and TSLPR−/− mice in the light of two specific aims: (1) to investigate if a functional TSLPR was instrumental in eliciting food allergy, and (2) to assess the role of CT in relation to a functional TSLPR in the sensitization process.

Methods

Mice

BALB/c female mice were purchased from Charles River (L'Arbresle, France) and were housed at the Animal Facilities of the University of Geneva, School of Medicine. TSLPR−/− mice [22] were backcrossed to a BALB/c background for eight generations or more. All animals were used between 4 and 5 weeks of age and were fed with standard mice pellets without milk proteins. All experiments were approved by the Animal Studies Ethics Committee and performed in accordance to their guidelines.

Antibodies, reagents and medium

Anti-CD11c (HL3), anti-IL-4 (11B11), anti-IL-5 (TRFK5), anti-IL-10 (JES5-16E3), anti-IL-12p70 (C15.6) and anti-IL-17 (TC11-18H10) were from BD Pharmingen (Allschwil, Switzerland). Anti-IL-13 was from eBioscience (eBio13A) (Vienna, Austria).

CT was from List Biological Labs (Campbell, CA, USA). BLG was from Sigma (Buchs, Switzerland).

RPMI 1640 and DMEM medium were supplemented with 100 U/ml penicillin, 100 μg/ml streptomycin, 2 mM L-glutamine, 100 μg/ml gentamicin, 15 mM HEPES pH 7.4 and 10 % heat-inactivated FCS. In addition, DMEM was supplemented 2×10^{-5} M 2-mercaptoethanol, 1 % nonessential amino acids and 1 mM sodium pyruvate (all reagents from Sigma).

In vivo sensitization, and BLG specific challenge

Mice were sensitized 5 times 1 week apart by oral administration of 10 μg of CT in association with 10 mg of antigen in a solution containing 0.2 M of $NaHCO_3$, pH 9. An oral antigen challenge was performed 1 week after the last sensitization by gavaging 100 mg BLG. A score based on symptoms of anaphylaxis (*0* no reaction; *1* mild reactions: decreased activity, random scratching, myocloni; *2* moderate reactions: marked decreased activity, continuous scratching, abnormal breathing; *3* severe reactions low or absence of reactivity, abnormal breathing leading occasional to death) was assessed [21]. Mice were thereafter sacrificed at the indicated time and their intestinal lymphoid cells isolated.

Measurement of BLG-specific antibodies in mouse serum

Sera were obtained 7 days after the last sensitization by tail vein bleeding. BLG-specific Ab titers were measured by a method adapted from Adel-Patient et al. [23] as described previously [24].

Isolation of lymphocytes

After sacrifice of the mice with CO_2, mesenteric lymph nodes (MLN) were isolated, the small intestine was excised, and Peyer's patches (PP) lymphocytes, lamina propria lymphocytes (LPL), intraepithelial lymphocytes (IEL) and epithelial cells (EC) were isolated using modified methods as previously described [25, 26]. Briefly, the small intestine was opened longitudinally and cut into 5-mm pieces. The tissue was incubated in calcium- and magnesium-free cHBSS containing 2 mM EDTA and 1 mM dithiothreitol (Sigma) for 30 min at 37 °C with magnetic stirring. It was then vigorously vortexed and filtered through a 70-μm nylon filter in order to obtain a cell suspension. The cell population was washed twice and separated by discontinuous 33/40 % Percoll (Bioscience, Uppsala, Sweden) on a lympholyte M gradient (Cederlane, Hornby, Canada) for 20 min at 600 g at room temperature. IELs were harvested on the Percoll 40 % lympholyte M interface, and ECs on the 30 % interface.

Cytokine measurement by ELISPOT

ELISPOT plates were coated with streptavidin overnight at 37 °C, followed by addition of 1 μg of biotinylated BLG for 3 h. Lymphocytes isolated on a Percoll 60/66 % gradient (Amersham, Zurich, Switzerland) were resuspended as 2 and 1×10^6 in Iscove's modified Dulbeco medium supplemented with penicillin, streptomycin, L-glutamine, 100 μg/mL gentamycin, polymixin B + 5 % FCS for 24 h at 37 °C, followed by overnight incubation at 4 °C with the corresponding antibodies. Amino-ethyl-carbazole 100 μl/well was added for 10 min, and the spots were automatically counted by the KS EliSpot 4.2.1 Software (Zeiss, Halbermoos, Germany) and expressed as cell forming units (CFU) per 10^6 cells.

Real-time PCR

Total RNA from PP lymphocytes, LPL, IEL or EC was extracted with Isol-RNA Lysis reagent. 5 x 10^6 cells were first centrifuged 5 min at 1400×g and the pellet was resuspended in 1.0 ml of Isol-RNA Lysis reagent for 5 min., 0.2 ml chloroform was added and tubes were mixed by inversion for 30 s and left for 3 min at room temperature. Samples were then centrifuged for 15 min at 14,000 rpm (4 °C) resulting in a colorless upper aqueous phase that contains the RNA and a lower red organic phase. 0.5 ml isopropyl alcohol was added to the aqueous phase in order to precipitate RNA. After centrifugation, the RNA pellet was washed once in 1 ml 75 % ethanol. At the end of the procedure, the RNA pellet was briefly air-dried and resuspended in 40 µl RNAse-free water.

RNA content of each sample was assessed using a nanodrop ND-1000 spectophotometer. 1 µg of RNA was used to perform the semi-quantitative RT-PCR with specific primers for the mouse TSLP gene. The PCR was realized [using taq DNA polymerase from Invitrogen (Zug, Switzerland)], with the following primers: 5′-GACAGCATGGTTCTTCTCAG-3′ and 5′-CTGGAGATTGACATGAAGG-3′ (30 cycles of 94 °C for 60 s denaturation, 55 °C for 60 s annealing, and 72 °C for 60 s extension). As a control, the same amount of RNA was used to perform a semi-quantitative RT-PCR with specific primers for GAPDH. The final result was expressed as the ratio of the signal obtained for TSLP divided by the signal obtained for GAPDH.

Statistics analysis

Statistical significance between groups was analyzed by using the Wilcoxon rank-sum test for nonparametric unpaired data. For assessment of clinical reactivity, batches of 4–5 mice were challenged simultaneously, and the experiments were repeated twice. Antibody titers measurements and cell experiments were performed with pooled samples from three mice per experiments, and repeated 3 times.

Results

TSLPR−/− mice have less pronounced food allergy symptoms

In order to generate mice with an allergic phenotype to foods, sets of mice were sensitized 5 times at 1 week interval by intra-gastric gavage with BLG in presence of CT. Allergy was characterized by mean of a subsequent oral BLG challenge. Mice were clinically evaluated by a symptom score published earlier [21]. In order to add an objective measure, the severity of anaphylaxis was correlated to the measure of decreased body temperature. We observed that wt mice were showing symptoms of anaphylaxis in form of decreased activity, swelling of the snout, erythema of the face and feet, as well as itching and erected pilli. Increased breathing and severe reactions leading to death were also observed. In correlation to these observations, marked decreased body temperature was seen, peaking at 30 min after gavage (Fig. 1a). Conversely, assessment of TSLPR−/− mice at the same time points showed predominantly mild or no symptoms of anaphylaxis (Fig. 1b) and a faster recovery correlating to only a slight decrease in body temperature. These results suggest that food-mediated allergic reactions are, to a significant extent, mediated by a TSLP-dependent mechanism.

How do antigen-specific serum antibody levels correlate with TSLP?

We were then interested in characterizing BLG-specific antibody production in wt, and TSLPR−/− mice. Serum was collected 7 days after the last oral antigen-sensitization and BLG-specific IgE (Fig. 2a), IgG1 (Fig. 2b) and IgG2a (Fig. 2c) antibody titers were measured by ELISA. Clearly, wt mice had much higher titers of IgG1 (in wt mice: mean 51.0 ± 9.4 AU/ml, TSLPR−/− mice: mean 16.0 ± 2.7 AU/ml), a Th2-type related antibody isotype, while IgG2a, a Th1-type related isotype was increased in TSLPR−/− mice. IgE titers were similar in both groups.

Is the modulation of Th2-type cytokine secretion after in vivo antigen-specific cell activation TSLPR dependent?

In order to correlate cytokine production and TSLP expression after sensitization to BLG, we isolated MLN cells 8 h after infra-clinical antigen gavage given for in vivo cell activation and measured their ex vivo cytokine production by ELISPOT. The presence of the TSLPR was clearly modulating cytokine production, as shown by a decreased secretion of IL-4, IL-5 and IL-10 in TSLPR−/− mice (79 % decrease of IL-4 secretion, 80 % of IL-5, 51 % of IL-10; significant for IL-4 and IL-5 but only trend for IL-10) (Fig. 3). In contrast, we did measure strongly increased levels of IL-17 (4.4 times) in TSLPR−/− mice. IL-12 (not shown) was secreted in similar amounts by MLN cells isolated from both type of mice.

CT activates TSLP in gut epithelial cells

We next investigated whether TSLP RNA expression was related to the CT administration given by gavage during the sensitization. RNA expression of TSLP by gut EC, Peyer's patches cells, lamina propria lymphocytes and intra-epithelial lymphocytes from wt mice was measured by semi-quantitative RT-PCR at various time points after CT administration. Only EC (other cells not shown) were found to express TSLP RNA after administration of CT

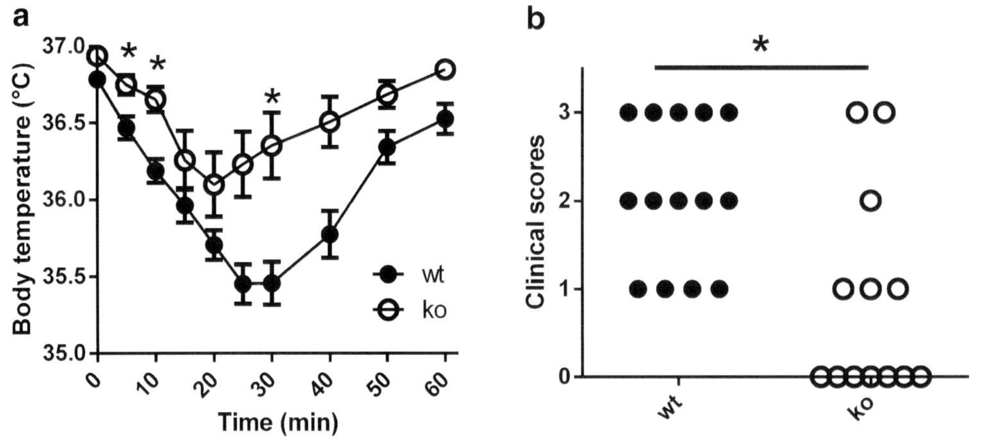

Fig. 1 Reduced severity of anaphylactic reaction in CT-sensitized TSLPR−/− mice. BLG-sensitized mice, either wild type (wt) and TSLPR−/− mice (ko) are challenged by oral gavage with 100 mg of BLG 7 days after the last sensitization, the body temperature is recorded on the ear (**a**). In addition symptoms of anaphylaxis were clinically assessed (*0* no reaction to *3* severe reaction) (**b**). The results are expressed as a pool of data from independent experiments. *p < 0.05

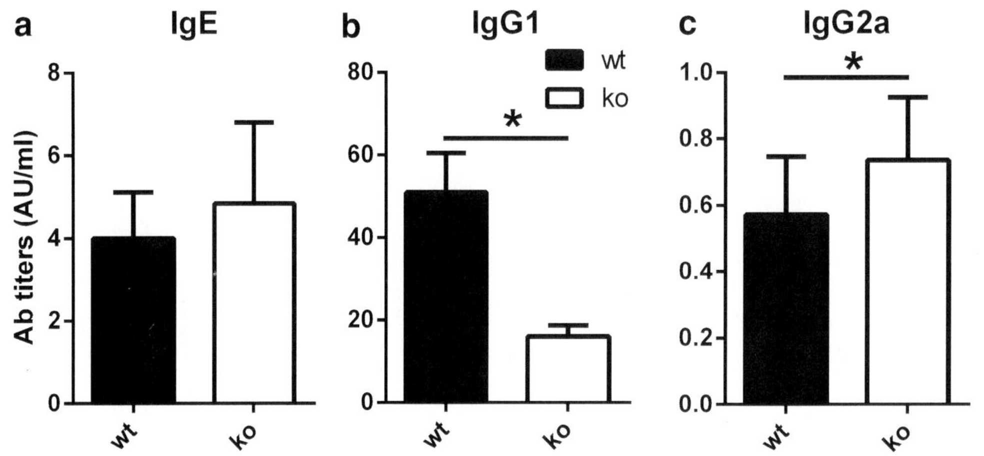

Fig. 2 Th2-related and Th1-related Ab profiles in BLG-sensitized wild type and TSLPR−/− mice. Serum IgE (**a**), IgG1 (**b**) and IgG2a (**c**) Abs specific for BLG in BLG-sensitized wild type (wt) and TSLPR−/− mice (ko) 7 days after the last sensitization. The results are expressed as arbitrary units from three independent experiments. *p < 0.05

(Fig. 4a). Figure 4b shows the progressively increased expression of TSLP RNA with a peak at 48 h post CT administration, clearly showing a CT-related TSLP RNA expression in gut EC of wt mice.

Does the TSLPR regulate CT-induced inflammation in the gut?

Next we explored if and to what extent, the TSLPR was regulating CT-induced inflammation. By ELISPOT, *we* measured ex vivo CT-induced cytokine production of mesenteric lymph node (MLN) cells and lamina propria cells (LPL) from wt and TSLPR−/− mice after oral gavage with CT. Figure 5 shows a clear modulation of IL-12 secretion by TSLP in both MLN and LPL as IL-12 is increased in TSLPR−/− mice (MLN cells in wt mice: mean 38.6 ± 14.9 spots/10^6 cells, TSLPR−/− mice: mean 137.8 ± 4.9 spots/10^6 cells; LPL in wt mice: mean 12.2 ± 8.3 spots/10^6 cells, TSLPR−/− mice: mean 45.7 ± 15.3 spots/10^6 cells). Similarly, IL-17 expression was strongly increased in TSLPR−/− mice (MLN in wt mice: mean 62.8 ± 13.4 spots/10^6 cells, TSLPR−/− mice: mean 156.9 ± 16.5 spots/10^6 cells; LPL in wt mice: mean 20.5 ± 2.9 spots/10^6 cells, TSLPR−/− mice: mean 47.0 ± 18.8 spots/10^6 cells). IL-13 secretion was strongly decreased in TSLPR−/− mice, but only in LPL. IL-10 secretion was not influenced by the absence of expression

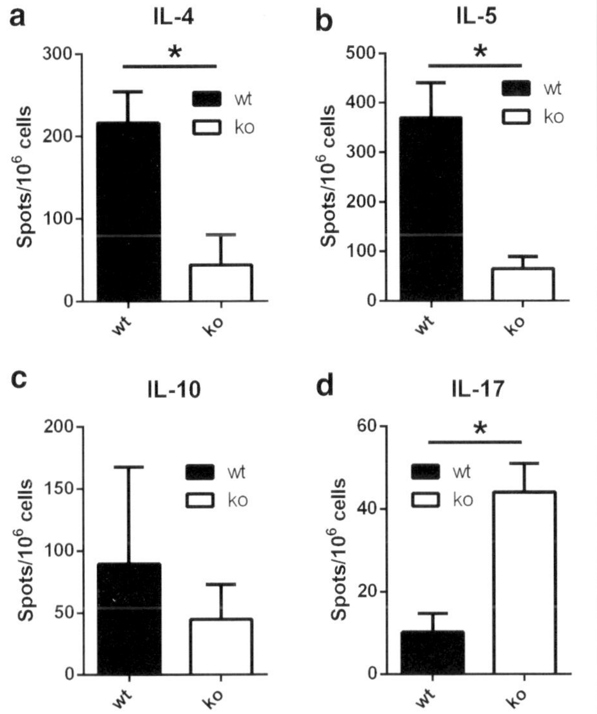

Fig. 3 Reduced Th2 cytokines and increase of IL-17 in BLG-sensitized TSLPR−/− mice by ELISPOT. Ex vivo cytokines secretion by mesenteric lymphnode lymphocytes 8 h after oral boost with 20 mg of BLG in $NaHCO_3$ in wild type (wt) and TSLPR−/− (ko) mice. The results are expressed as number of cytokines forming spots/10^6 cells from three independent experiments. *$p < 0.05$

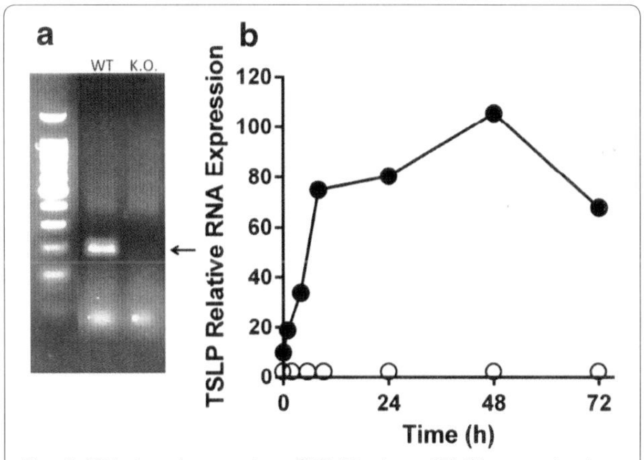

Fig. 4 CT induced expression of TSLP in vivo. **a** TSLPR expression in epithelial cells from wild type (WT), and TSLPR−/− mice (K.O.). The band representing TSLP is marked by an *arrow*. **b** Relative TSLP mRNA expression by intestinal epithelial cells from WT mice (*close circles*) and from K.O. mice (*open circles*) after oral administration of 10 mg of cholera toxin. The results (in %) are normalized to GAPDH expression

of the TSLP receptor. These results are suggesting that IL-12 and IL-17-driven inflammation in the current model is regulated by TSLP in the gut.

Discussion

Experiments presented here clearly show that food allergy in mice induced after oral antigen sensitization in presence of CT followed by an oral antigen challenge is strongly, but not exclusively, dependent on a functional TSLP pathway. Absence of TSLP receptor expression in knock-out mice biases antigen and CT sensitization towards a reduced Th2/increased Th17-type profile, and influences dendritic cells to promote a Th1-type antigen presentation. TSLP can be considered as a protein contributing to modulating food allergy in the mouse model described here.

The pathogenesis of immediate-type food allergy is strongly Th2-type oriented with subsequent IgE production and IgE-mediated immediate-type symptoms. We and others have previously described that intestinal T cells produce Th2-type cytokines, and that the gut-associated lymphoid structures are strongly involved in the pathogenesis of the disease [2, 3]. Nevertheless, IgE-independent mechanisms have also been described, involving IgG antibody isotype or complement-driven inflammation [4, 5]. TSLP in the context of allergy has so far been more extensively studied in atopic dermatitis and asthma. In these diseases, it has been shown that in the skin TSLP is essential for eliciting a Th2-type skin sensitivity, as TSLPR−/− mice were unable to mount a Th2-type cytokine production, with the resulting absence of antigen-specific IgE production, and of skin inflammation upon re-exposure to the antigen [17]. In the experiments we report here, we were able to show similar results in the gut. We observed that not only TSLP is essential for the secretion of the Th2-type cytokines IL-4 and IL-5, but also that the Th1 and Th17 pathways are TSLP dependent, as IL-12 and IL-17 were strongly increased in TSLPR−/− mice. These results are in line with previous publications which have shown increased Th1 and Th17 responses in TSLPR−/− mice [18, 19]. In this regard, we have not seen a modified IgE response in TSLPR−/− mice, while IgG1 was significantly lower in TSLPR−/− mice. This finding is correlated to previous studies reporting that in mice mechanisms independent of IgE might be involved in the pathogenesis of food allergy [27], and suggests that TSLP might be linked to them. It is also well known in humans that sensitization to IgE might appear independently of clinical food allergy [28].

Gut intraepithelial lymphocytes constitutively express IL-17 [26], and it has been clearly shown that this cytokine is involved in inflammation in the gut. In addition, it has been shown that TSLP expression and IL-17A is linked, as disruption of the TSLP-TSLPR pathway

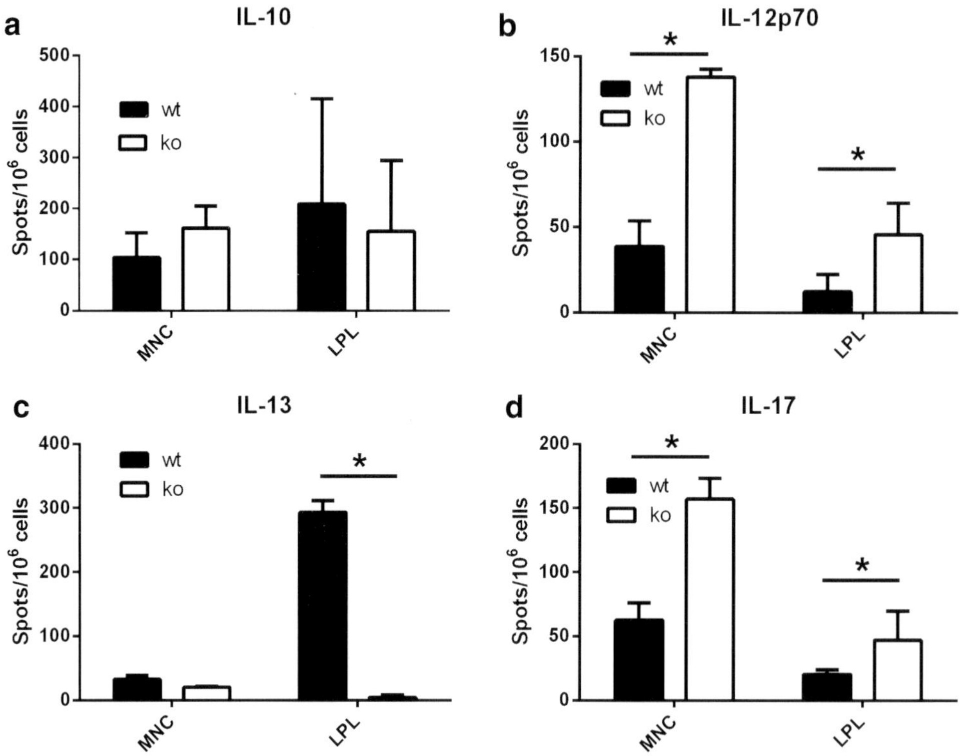

Fig. 5 Increased frequency of IL-12 and IL-17 producing cells in CT-sensitized TSLPR−/− mice by ELISPOT. *Ex vivo* cytokine secretion by mesenteric lymphnode (MLN) or lamina propria (LPL) lymphocytes 24 h following oral gavage with 10 μg of CT in $NaHCO_3$ in wild type (wt) and TSLPR−/− (ko) mice. The results are expressed as number of cytokines forming spots/10^6 cells from three independent experiments. *$p < 0.05$

resulted in increased expression of IL-17A, and the development of severe gut inflammation [19]. In relation to food allergy, the study by DeLong et al. reports activation with the major peanut allergen Ara h 1 of T cell-lines and clones from peanut allergic subjects. While all cells produced IL-4, IL-17 secreting cells were also found. Interestingly, the percentage of cells co-producing IL-4 and IL-17 was minimal, suggesting similarly to our study an antagonistic role for IL-4 and IL-17 [29]. Decreased IL-17 secretion has also been observed in antigen-activated CD4+ cells from food allergic children when compared to tolerant controls [30]. This suggests that in humans, IL-17 may be involved to some extent in the regulation of food allergy. Similarly to food allergy, in eczema and asthma the paradigm of the dysbalance of Th1 and Th2 cells has been completed by increased knowledge of the role of Th17, as well as other T cell sub-types [31].

The role of TSLP has been ascertained in the regulation of various experimental types of allergy, e.g. in models of skin allergy, such as atopic dermatitis [32] or nickel allergy [33], or in allergic airway diseases [15, 16]. Similar observations have been made in human studies [14, 34]. Several investigations addressed the role of TSLP in food allergy. Hong et al. have suspected a role for TSLP, as a specific single nucleotide polymorphism of the TSLP gene was correlated with an increased sensitization to common food allergens in correlation to breastfeeding [35]. Also, eosinophilic esophagitis, an inflammatory disease of the esophagus associated with food allergy characterized by esophageal eosinophilia, has been associated with TSLP gene polymorphisms [36]. Links between the skin and the gut have also been explored. TSLP-associated antigen sensitization through the skin has been shown to induce diarrhea and anaphylaxis after oral reexposure to the same antigen [37]. Also, TSLP has been found to modulate allergy through antigen exposure on the skin and subsequent allergic reactions similar to our model [6]. In the gut, TSLP is also produced by DCs, and protects against inflammatory colitis [38]. Exploring the role of TSLP in two separate murine food allergy models, Blazquez et al. have found that allergen-induced diarrhea was TSLPR dependent, while the Th2-type sensitization model they used was TSLP independent with similar antigen-specific IgE titers, and absence of decreased anaphylaxis upon allergen reexposure [7]. However, in their studies mice were challenged by i.p. injections, while we gavaged them, this can possibly explain the difference in the antigen-induced anaphylaxis score. Also, antigen-specific IgG1 titers were not measured, and an IgE-independent mechanism cannot be excluded. Chu et al. have observed that after a similar oral sensitization protocol than the one we used, but followed by an i.p. antigen challenge, the procedure elicited a similar anaphylactic response in TSLPR−/− mice than in wt mice [39]. In these studies, besides IgE IgG1 titers were measured and both were found similar in wild type and TSLPR−/− mice. The results in these two studies differ from ours.

Our results suggest that absence of a functional TSLP does only partially prevent food-induced sensitization, as TSLPR−/− mice are able to mount an antigen-specific Ab response. In addition, absence of functional TSLP does not prevent a response to the strong stimulus of i.p. food antigen challenge, while it significantly reduces the anaphylactic response after a more physiological gastric antigen challenge. Altogether, these results suggest that TSLP, in addition to other factors, intervenes in the pathogenesis of food allergy in the mouse models studied here.

It has been well recognized that allergy in general and food allergy in particular is mediated by several, complementary, but independent pathways. Options for treatment or prevention have targeted several of these pathways. In various studies, therapeutic options including oral administration of IL-12 [40], oral administration of a synthetic agonist of Toll-like receptor 9 [41], or blockade of platelet-activating factor and histamine [42] have been investigated for treatment of food allergy. Recently, a preliminary trial in patients with allergen-induced asthma and airway inflammation has found a therapeutic value for an anti-TSLP monoclonal immunoglobulin [43]. Here we define TSLP as a new target for modulation of food allergy. Indeed, we identified TSLP as an essential contributor to the pathogenesis of the Th2-type inflammation elicited after oral sensitization followed by an oral challenge. The immunological parameters correlated with a strong decrease of clinical reactivity upon oral antigen challenge reinforcing a strong dependency of food allergy on TSLP. Defining whether this is due to a lack of direct control of TSLP on T cells or on DCs will need further exploration.

Conclusions

In conclusion, in the set of experiments presented here, we show that food allergy in mice is in part dependent on a functional TSLP receptor, as antigen sensitization in TSLPR−/− mice was biased towards an allergy protective, reduced Th2/increased Th17-type immune response with decreased clinical reactivity. New therapeutic strategies might consider including TSLP as a target for modulation of food allergy.

Authors' contributions

CPF, SCZ, JMRG and PAE designed the study, CPF, SCZ and JMRG performed the experiments, CPF and PAE wrote the manuscript. All authors read and approved the final manuscript.

Author details

[1] Inflammation and Allergy Research Group and Department of Pediatrics, University Hospitals of Geneva and University of Geneva, 6 rue Willy-Donzé, 1211 Geneva 14, Switzerland. [2] Allergy Unit, University Hospitals of Geneva and University of Geneva, Geneva, Switzerland. [3] Present Address: EMD Serono, Billerica, MA, USA. [4] Present Address: Fasteris SA, Plan-les-Ouates, Switzerland.

Acknowledgements

The study was funded by Grant 310030-134904 from the Swiss National Science Foundation.

Competing interests

The authors declare that they have no competing interests.

References

1. Vickery BP, Scurlock AM, Jones SM, Burks AW. Mechanisms of immune tolerance relevant to food allergy. J Allergy Clin Immunol. 2011;127:576–84.
2. Li XM, Serebrisky D, Lee SY, Huang CK, Bardina L, Schofield BH, Stanley JS, Burks AW, Bannon GA, Sampson HA. A murine model of peanut anaphylaxis: T- and B-cell responses to a major peanut allergen mimic human responses. J Allergy Clin Immunol. 2000;106(1 Pt 1):150–8.
3. Frossard CP, Tropia L, Hauser C, Eigenmann PA. Lymphocytes in Peyer's patches regulate clinical tolerance in a murine model of food allergy. J Allergy Clin Immunol. 2004;113:958–64.
4. Strait RT, Morris SC, Finkelman FD. IgG-blocking antibodies inhibit IgE-mediated anaphylaxis in vivo through both antigen interception and Fc gamma RIIb cross-linking. J Clin Invest. 2006;116:833–41.
5. Khodoun M, Strait R, Orekov T, Hogan S, Karasuyama H, Herbert DR, Köhl J, Finkelman FD. Peanuts can contribute to anaphylactic shock by activating complement. J Allergy Clin Immunol. 2009;123:342–51.
6. Noti M, Kim BS, Siracusa MC, Rak GD, Kubo M, Moghaddam AE, Sattentau QA, Comeau MR, Spergel JM, Artis D. Exposure to food allergens through inflamed skin promotes intestinal food allergy through the thymic stromal lymphopoietin-basophil axis. J Allergy Clin Immunol. 2014;133:1390–9 **(1399.e1–6)**.
7. Blázquez AB, Mayer L, Berin MC. Thymic stromal lymphopoietin is required for gastrointestinal allergy but not oral tolerance. Gastroenterology. 2010;139:1301–9.
8. Bogiatzi SI, Fernandez I, Bichet J-C, Marloie-Provost M-A, Volpe E, Sastre X, Soumelis V. Cutting edge: proinflammatory and Th2 cytokines synergize to induce thymic stromal lymphopoietin production by human skin keratinocytes. J Immunol. 2007;178:3373–7.
9. Kato A, Favoreto S Jr, Avila PC, Schleimer RP. TLR3- and Th2 cytokine-dependent production of thymic stromal lymphopoietin in human airway epithelial cells. J Immunol. 2007;179:1080–7.
10. Lee H-C, Ziegler SF. Inducible expression of the proallergic cytokine thymic stromal lymphopoietin in airway epithelial cells is controlled by NFkappaB. Proc Natl Acad Sci USA. 2007;104:914–9.
11. Zhang K, Shan L, Rahman MS, Unruh H, Halayko AJ, Gounni AS. Constitutive and inducible thymic stromal lymphopoietin expression in human airway smooth muscle cells: role in chronic obstructive pulmonary disease. Am J Physiol Lung Cell Mol Physiol. 2007;293:L375–82.
12. Miyata M, Nakamura Y, Shimokawa N, Ohnuma Y, Katoh R, Matsuoka S, Okumura K, Ogawa H, Masuyama K, Nakao A. Thymic stromal lymphopoietin is a critical mediator of IL-13-driven allergic inflammation. Eur J Immunol. 2009;39:3078–83.
13. Tanaka J, Saga K, Kido M, Nishiura H, Akamatsu T, Chiba T, Watanabe N. Proinflammatory Th2 cytokines induce production of thymic stromal lymphopoietin in human colonic epithelial cells. Dig Dis Sci. 2010;55:1896–904.

14. Soumelis V, Reche PA, Kanzler H, Yuan W, Edward G, Homey B, Gilliet M, Ho S, Antonenko S, Lauerma A, Smith K, Gorman D, Zurawski S, Abrams J, Menon S, McClanahan T, de Waal-Malefyt Rd R, Bazan F, Kastelein RA, Liu Y-J. Human epithelial cells trigger dendritic cell mediated allergic inflammation by producing TSLP. Nat Immunol. 2002;3:673–80.
15. Al-Shami A, Spolski R, Kelly J, Keane-Myers A, Leonard WJ. A role for TSLP in the development of inflammation in an asthma model. J Exp Med. 2005;202:829–39.
16. Zhou B, Comeau MR, De Smedt T, Liggitt HD, Dahl ME, Lewis DB, Gyarmati D, Aye T, Campbell DJ, Ziegler SF. Thymic stromal lymphopoietin as a key initiator of allergic airway inflammation in mice. Nat Immunol. 2005;6:1047–53.
17. Larson RP, Zimmerli SC, Comeau MR, Itano A, Omori M, Iseki M, Hauser C, Ziegler SF. Dibutyl phthalate-induced thymic stromal lymphopoietin is required for Th2 contact hypersensitivity responses. J Immunol. 2010;184:2974–84.
18. Zaph C, Troy AE, Taylor BC, Berman-Booty LD, Guild KJ, Du Y, Yost EA, Gruber AD, May MJ, Greten FR, Eckmann L, Karin M, Artis D. Epithelial-cell-intrinsic IKK-beta expression regulates intestinal immune homeostasis. Nature. 2007;446:552–6.
19. Taylor BC, Zaph C, Troy AE, Du Y, Guild KJ, Comeau MR, Artis D. TSLP regulates intestinal immunity and inflammation in mouse models of helminth infection and colitis. J Exp Med. 2009;206:655–67.
20. Li XM, Schofield BH, Huang CK, Kleiner GI, Sampson HA. A murine model of IgE-mediated cow's milk hypersensitivity. JAllergy ClinImmunol. 1999;103(2 Pt 1):206–14.
21. Frossard CP, Hauser C, Eigenmann PA. Oral carrageenan induces antigen-dependent oral tolerance: prevention of anaphylaxis and induction of lymphocyte anergy in a murine model of food allergy. Pediatr Res. 2001;49:417–22.
22. Carpino N, Thierfelder WE, Chang M, Saris C, Turner SJ, Ziegler SF, Ihle JN. Absence of an essential role for thymic stromal lymphopoietin receptor in murine B-cell development. Mol Cell Biol. 2004;24:2584–92.
23. Adel-Patient K, Créminon C, Bernard H, Clément G, Négroni L, Frobert Y, Grassi J, Wal JM, Chatel JM. Evaluation of a high IgE-responder mouse model of allergy to bovine beta-lactoglobulin (BLG): development of sandwich immunoassays for total and allergen-specific IgE, IgG1 and IgG2a in BLG-sensitized mice. J Immunol Methods. 2000;235:21–32.
24. Frossard CP, Steidler L, Eigenmann PA. Oral administration of an IL-10-secreting Lactococcus lactis strain prevents food-induced IgE sensitization. J Allergy Clin Immunol. 2007;119:952–9.
25. Lefrancois L. Carbohydrate differentiation antigens of murine T cells: expression on intestinal lymphocytes and intestinal epithelium. J Immunol. 1987;138:3375–84.
26. Asigbetse KE, Eigenmann PA, Frossard CP. Intestinal lamina propria TcR-gammadelta + lymphocytes selectively express IL-10 and IL-17. J Investig Allergol Clin Immunol. 2010;20:391–401.
27. Miyajima I, Dombrowicz D, Martin TR, Ravetch JV, Kinet JP, Galli SJ. Systemic anaphylaxis in the mouse can be mediated largely through IgG1 and Fc gammaRIII. Assessment of the cardiopulmonary changes, mast cell degranulation, and death associated with active or IgE- or IgG1-dependent passive anaphylaxis. J Clin Invest. 1997;99:901–14.
28. Muraro A, Werfel T, Hoffmann-Sommergruber K, Roberts G, Beyer K, Bindslev-Jensen C, Cardona V, Dubois A, duToit G, Eigenmann P, Fernandez Rivas M, Halken S, Hickstein L, Høst A, Knol E, Lack G, Marchisotto MJ, Niggemann B, Nwaru BI, Papadopoulos NG, Poulsen LK, Santos AF, Skypala I, Schoepfer A, Van Ree R, Venter C, Worm M, Vlieg-Boerstra B, Panesar S, de Silva D, et al. EAACI food allergy and anaphylaxis guidelines: diagnosis and management of food allergy. Allergy. 2014;69:1008–25.
29. DeLong JH, Simpson KH, Wambre E, James EA, Robinson D, Kwok WW. Ara h 1–reactive T cells in individuals with peanut allergy. J Allergy Clin Immunol. 2011;127(1211–1218):e3.
30. Dhuban KB, d'Hennezel E, Ben-Shoshan M, McCusker C, Clarke A, Fiset P, Mazer B, Piccirillo CA. Altered T helper 17 responses in children with food allergy. Int Arch Allergy Immunol. 2013;162:318–22.
31. Souwer Y, Szegedi K, Kapsenberg ML, de Jong EC. IL-17 and IL-22 in atopic allergic disease. Curr Opin Immunol. 2010;22:821–6.
32. Yoo J, Omori M, Gyarmati D, Zhou B, Aye T, Brewer A, Comeau MR, Campbell DJ, Ziegler SF. Spontaneous atopic dermatitis in mice expressing an inducible thymic stromal lymphopoietin transgene specifically in the skin. J Exp Med. 2005;202:541–9.
33. Ashrin MN, Arakaki R, Yamada A, Kondo T, Kurosawa M, Kudo Y, Watanabe M, Ichikawa T, Hayashi Y, Ishimaru N. A critical role for thymic stromal lymphopoietin in nickel-induced allergy in mice. J Immunol. 2014;192:4025–31.
34. Ying S, O'Connor B, Ratoff J, Meng Q, Mallett K, Cousins D, Robinson D, Zhang G, Zhao J, Lee TH, Corrigan C. Thymic stromal lymphopoietin expression is increased in asthmatic airways and correlates with expression of Th2-attracting chemokines and disease severity. J Immunol. 2005;174:8183–90.
35. Hong X, Wang G, Liu X, Kumar R, Tsai H-J, Arguelles L, Hao K, Pearson C, Ortiz K, Bonzagni A, Apollon S, Fu L, Caruso D, Pongracic JA, Schleimer R, Holt PG, Bauchner H, Wang X. Gene polymorphisms, breast-feeding, and development of food sensitization in early childhood. J Allergy Clin Immunol. 2011;128(374–381):e2.
36. Noti M, Wojno EDT, Kim BS, Siracusa MC, Giacomin PR, Nair MG, Benitez AJ, Ruymann KR, Muir AB, Hill DA, Chikwava KR, Moghaddam AE, Sattentau QJ, Alex A, Zhou C, Yearley JH, Menard-Katcher P, Kubo M, Obata-Ninomiya K, Karasuyama H, Comeau MR, Brown-Whitehorn T, de Waal Malefyt R, Sleiman PM, Hakonarson H, Cianferoni A, Falk GW, Wang M-L, Spergel JM, Artis D. Thymic stromal lymphopoietin-elicited basophil responses promote eosinophilic esophagitis. Nat Med. 2013;19:1005–13.
37. Han H, Thelen TD, Comeau MR, Ziegler SF. Thymic stromal lymphopoietin-mediated epicutaneous inflammation promotes acute diarrhea and anaphylaxis. J Clin Invest. 2014;124:5442–52.
38. Spadoni I, Iliev ID, Rossi G, Rescigno M. Dendritic cells produce TSLP that limits the differentiation of Th17 cells, fosters Treg development, and protects against colitis. Mucosal Immunol. 2012;5:184.
39. Chu DK, Llop-Guevara A, Walker TD, Flader K, Goncharova S, Boudreau JE, Moore CL, In TS, Waserman S, Coyle AJ, Kolbeck R, Humbles AA, Jordana M. IL-33, but not thymic stromal lymphopoietin or IL-25, is central to mite and peanut allergic sensitization. J Allergy Clin Immunol. 2013;131(187–200):e8.
40. Lee SY, Huang CK, Zhang TF, Schofield BH, Burks AW, Bannon GA, Sampson HA, Li XM. Oral administration of IL-12 suppresses anaphylactic reactions in a murine model of peanut hypersensitivity. Clin Immunol. 2001;101:220–8.
41. Zhu F-G, Kandimalla ER, Yu D, Agrawal S. Oral administration of a synthetic agonist of Toll-like receptor 9 potently modulates peanut-induced allergy in mice. J Allergy Clin Immunol. 2007;120:631–7.
42. Arias K, Baig M, Colangelo M, Chu D, Walker T, Goncharova S, Coyle A, Vadas P, Waserman S, Jordana M. Concurrent blockade of platelet-activating factor and histamine prevents life-threatening peanut-induced anaphylactic reactions. J Allergy Clin Immunol. 2009;124:307–14 **(314.e1–2)**.
43. Gauvreau GM, O'Byrne PM, Boulet L-P, Wang Y, Cockcroft D, Bigler J, FitzGerald JM, Boedigheimer M, Davis BE, Dias C, Gorski KS, Smith L, Bautista E, Comeau MR, Leigh R, Parnes JR. Effects of an anti-TSLP antibody on allergen-induced asthmatic responses. N Engl J Med. 2014;370:2102–10.

5

The expression of CD123 can decrease with basophil activation: implications for the gating strategy of the basophil activation test

Alexandra F. Santos[1,2,3,4], Natalia Bécares[1,2], Alick Stephens[1,2], Victor Turcanu[1,2] and Gideon Lack[1,2*]

Abstract

Background: Basophil activation test (BAT) reproduces IgE-mediated allergic reactions in vitro and has been used as a diagnostic test. Different markers can be used to identify basophils in whole blood and have implications for the outcome of the test. We aimed to assess changes in the expression of CD123 and HLA-DR following basophil activation and to select the best gating strategy for BAT using these markers.

Methods: BAT was performed in whole blood from 116 children. Peanut extract, anti-IgE, anti-FcεRI or formyl-methionyl-leucyl-phenylalanin (fMLP) was used for stimulation. Surface expression of CD123, HLA-DR, CD63 and CD203c was evaluated by flow cytometry.

Results: In some cases, gating on CD123+/HLA-DR− led to the loss-to-analysis of basophils in conditions where basophils were activated. Adding CD203c as an identification marker restored the cell number. Basophils remained HLA-DR-negative with activation. CD123 expression decreased following stimulation with fMLP ($n = 116$, $p < 0.001$), anti-IgE ($n = 104$, $p < 0.001$) and peanut ($n = 42$, $p < 0.001$). The decrease in the mean fluorescence intensity of CD123 correlated with the up-regulation of basophil activation markers, CD63 ($r_s = -0.31$, $p < 0.001$) and CD203c ($r_s = -0.35$, $p < 0.001$). BAT to peanut gating basophils on CD203c+/CD123+/HLA-DR− reduced the false-negatives (1 vs. 5 %) and showed a higher diagnostic accuracy compared to using CD123+/HLA-DR− (97 vs. 91 %). CD203c+ appeared as an alternative gating strategy allowing two-colour BAT.

Conclusions: Basophils of a subset of patients down-regulate CD123 with activation. The use of CD203c before gating on CD123+/HLA-DR− cells or in isolation ensures the identification of the entire basophil population and accurate assessment of basophil activation, with important diagnostic implications.

Keywords: Basophil activation test, Peanut allergy, CD123, CD63, CD203c, IL-3

Background

The basophil activation test (BAT) is a flow cytometry-based assay that reproduces IgE-mediated allergic reactions in vitro. Following cell stimulation and activation, basophils undergo degranulation with the release of histamine, leukotrienes and cytokines, and up-regulate the expression of activation markers on their surface, such as CD63 and CD203c, which can be measured by flow cytometry [1, 2]. CD63 is a lysosomal-associated membrane protein (LAMP-3) and is not expressed on resting basophils but only after degranulation as the granules fuse with the plasma membrane. Its expression is bimodal, as only a subset of basophils express CD63, therefore it is usually represented as a proportion of positive cells (i.e. %CD63+ basophils). CD203c is constitutively and specifically expressed on the surface of resting basophils, which increases after basophil activation; thus, it can be used as an identification as well as an activation marker [3]. CD203c has been related to piecemeal degranulation and CD63 to anaphylactic degranulation [4, 5]. The BAT has been used primarily as a research tool

*Correspondence: gideon.lack@kcl.ac.uk
[1] Division of Asthma, Allergy and Lung Biology, Department of Pediatric Allergy, St Thomas' Hospital, King's College London, 2nd Floor, Stairwell B, South Wing, Westminster Bridge Road, London SE1 7EH, UK
Full list of author information is available at the end of the article

and its application for clinical use in the diagnosis and monitoring of allergic diseases [6–10], namely following immuno-modulatory treatments such as allergen-specific immunotherapy [11–13] and omalizumab [14–16], is still in development. Our first allergen-specific (peanut) study that is clinically validated and based on double-blind-placebo-controlled-food-challenges (DBPCFC) initially established retrospectively diagnostic cut-off values for CD63 expression (n = 104) and verified this prospectively in a second population (n = 65) [6]. In this study [6], BAT showed 97 % accuracy in the diagnosis of peanut allergy. This enhanced diagnostic performance is in large part due to inclusion of CD203c in the gating strategy.

Different cell-surface markers may be preferred for the identification of basophils in whole blood. One of the commonly used is the combination of CD123 and HLA-DR [1, 2]. CD123 is the low affinity subunit of the IL-3 receptor and is highly expressed on plasmocytoid dendritic cells and basophils, and in low levels on monocytes, eosinophils, myeloid dendritic cells and hematologic progenitor cells. While eosinophils can be excluded by side-scatter, additional staining with anti-HLA-DR discriminates between HLA-DR-negative basophils and HLA-DR-positive dendritic cells and monocytes. To exclude hematologic progenitor cells, an additional marker specific for basophils such as CD203c could be used. In previous studies, the expression of CD123 and HLA-DR were shown to be stable with the atopic status of patients and following basophil activation [2, 17]. However, stimulation of the IL-3 receptor by IL-3 can increase the baseline expression of CD203c and possibly CD63 and maximise the up-regulation of CD63 upon basophil activation [4, 18]. Therefore, we hypothesized that CD123 expression could change in response to basophil activation. With increasing attention given to basophils in the coordination of adaptive immune responses and their possible role in antigen presentation [19–21], we considered that there could be an increase in the expression of HLA-DR by basophils following activation by allergen or other stimulants. Given the important implications for the gating strategy to be adopted for BAT in future studies, we sought to determine whether the expression of CD123 and HLA-DR remained unchanged with basophil activation and to select the best gating strategy using these markers.

Methods

Study population

Results of BAT to peanut performed in children attending our Pediatric Allergy clinic, aged from 5 months to 17 years, performed using the same methodology as part of two clinical studies [6, 10] were analyzed. Peanut allergy was diagnosed based on a positive oral peanut challenge or the combination of a recent clear history of one or more systemic reactions to peanut and a weal diameter on skin prick testing (SPT) $\geq$8 mm and/or serum peanut-specific IgE $\geq$15 KU_A/l [22]. Peanut-tolerance was defined by a negative oral peanut challenge or the ability to eat an age-appropriate quantity of peanut regularly (as defined by a validated food-frequency questionnaire [23]) without developing any allergic symptoms. Ethical approval was obtained from the South East London Research Ethics Committee 2 and parents of all children signed written informed consent.

Whole blood basophil activation test

Heparinized whole blood (100 μl) was stimulated for 30 min at 37 °C with peanut extract (0.1; 1; 10; 100; 1000 and 10,000 ng/ml, ALK Abelló, Horsholm, Denmark) diluted in Rosewell Park Memorial Institute (RPMI, GIBCO, Paisley, UK). Polyclonal goat IgG anti-human IgE (1 μg/ml, Sigma-Aldrich, Poole, UK) and monoclonal mouse anti-human FcεRI (2.5 μg/ml, Ebioscience, San Diego, CA, USA) were used as IgE-mediated positive controls. Formyl-methionyl-leucyl-phenylalanine (1 μM, fMLP, Sigma-Aldrich) was used as a non-IgE-mediated positive control (as it acts via a G-protein-coupled receptor (FPR-1) that activates MAPK pathways and phospholipase C bypassing part of the signalling pathway downstream the IgE receptor FcεRI). RPMI alone was used as a negative control. The reaction was stopped by adding cold ethylenediaminetetraacetic acid. Prior to erythrocyte lysis with BD Pharmlyse (BD Biosciences, San Jose, CA, USA), cells were stained with anti-CD123-fluorescein isothiocyanate (FITC) (Ebioscience), anti-CD203c-phyco-erythrin (PE), anti-HLA-DR-peridinin chlorophyll protein (PerCP) and anti-CD63-allophycocyanin (APC) (Biolegend, San Diego, CA, USA) for 30 min. In selected experiments, anti-CD14-PECy7, anti-CD3-pacific blue (PB), anti-CD19-PB, anti-CD41-PB and anti-CD56-PB (Biolegend) were additionally used. The surface expression of these markers was evaluated using FACS CantoII with FACSDiva software (BD Biosciences, San Jose, CA, USA). Data was analysed with FlowJo software version 7.6.1 (TreeStar, Ashland, OR, USA).

Basophil activation was expressed as a proportion of CD63+ basophils, corrected for the negative control, and as a ratio of the MFI of CD203c-PE of stimulated to unstimulated basophils, the stimulation index of CD203c (SI CD203c). The variation of CD123 was defined as the proportion of the difference between the MFI of CD123-FITC of the negative control and of the stimulated cells and the MFI of CD123-FITC of the negative control, and was calculated using the formula (MFI CD123-FITC of negative control − MFI CD123-FITC of stimulated cells)/MFI CD123-FITC of negative control.

When assessing basophil activation induced by anti-IgE ($n = 104$), patients with non-responder basophils, i.e. basophils which did not respond to any IgE-mediated stimulants but only to fMLP, were excluded. When evaluating the response to peanut, peanut allergic patients with responding-basophils were considered ($n = 42$). In the data analysis, when only one concentration of peanut extract was used, 100 ng/ml was selected unless indicated otherwise.

Statistical analysis

Qualitative variables were represented as number of patients and percentage (taking into account the missing values) and groups were compared using the Fisher's exact test or Chi square test, as appropriate. Continuous variables were represented as median and range and were compared using the Mann–Whitney U test or Kruskall–Wallis test, as appropriate. Wilcoxon-signed rank test was used to compare samples before and after stimulation.

For receiver-operating characteristic (ROC) curve analysis, the performance of the average percentage of CD63-positive basophils at 10 and 100 ng/ml of peanut extract determined using different gating strategies was evaluated against the patients' allergic status to peanut, i.e. in relation to allergy versus tolerance.

All statistical analyses were performed with SPSS 20.0 for Windows. Significance was determined using a two-sided α level of 0.05.

Results

Gating on basophils using CD123 and HLA-DR led to the loss of cells

Identifying basophils with CD123 and HLA-DR (Fig. 1a–d) led to the loss to analysis of cells particularly in conditions where basophils were activated. The baseline number of unstimulated basophils was variable (median = 1721, IQR = 1225–2184) but comparable between atopic and non atopic patients ($p = 0.444$) and between peanut allergic and peanut tolerant children ($p = 0.739$). Following basophil stimulation with fMLP ($p = 0.012$) and anti-IgE ($p = 0.005$), the number of basophils was significantly reduced compared to baseline (Table 1).

Of note, if only patients with non-responder basophils were considered ($n = 12$), the change in basophil number was significant after fMLP stimulation ($p = 0.004$) but not after anti-IgE stimulation ($p = 0.099$), suggesting that the reduction in cell number was dependent on basophil activation. Considering anti-IgE stimulation, 14 % of patients showed more than 25 % decrease in the number of basophils compared to the negative control (Fig. 2).

In 27 % of patients, this number decreased to below 1000 basophils (the minimum number of cells usually required for BAT). Selecting peanut allergic patients, a trend was seen toward a reduction in the basophil number after stimulation with 1000 ng/ml of peanut extract compared to the negative control ($n = 42$, $p = 0.081$). As the starting volume of blood, and thus the starting number of cells, was similar in all experimental conditions, we hypothesized that the expression of the identification markers, CD123 and/or HLA-DR, changed with basophil activation.

CD123 is down-regulated with basophil activation

To evaluate the changes in the expression of CD123 and HLA-DR on the surface of basophils, we used CD203c to gate on the basophil population (Fig. 1a–g). The baseline MFI of CD123-FITC was variable between patients (median = 1082, IQR = 98–1549) but comparable between atopic and non-atopic children ($p = 0.153$) and between peanut allergic and peanut tolerant patients ($p = 0.826$). Down-regulation of CD123 by basophils was seen following stimulation with fMLP ($n = 116$, $p < 0.001$), anti-IgE ($n = 104$, $p < 0.001$) and peanut extract ($n = 42$ peanut allergic patients, $p < 0.001$)—Table 1 and Fig. 3a. In 92.3 % of patients, anti-IgE stimulation led to a decrease in the MFI of CD123-FITC compared to the negative control: in 38.5 less than 25 % decrease, in 26.9 % between 25 and 50 % decrease, in 13.5 % between 50 and 75 % decrease and in 13.5 more than 75 % decrease (Fig. 4a). The down-regulation of CD123 expression on the surface of basophils stimulated by fMLP and by anti-IgE was correlated ($r_s = 0.723$, $p < 0.001$), suggesting this phenomenon happened in the same patients with different stimulants. The decrease in CD123 expression with anti-IgE stimulation was similar between atopic and non atopic ($p = 0.828$) and between peanut allergic and peanut tolerant children ($p = 0.431$). The expression of CD123 was stable when basophils were not activated—for example, after stimulation with peanut in peanut tolerant patients ($p = 0.658$) or after stimulation with anti-IgE in non-responders' basophils ($p = 0.083$), while down-regulation was still observed in this subgroup after stimulation with fMLP ($p = 0.006$).

Basophils were HLA-DR-negative and were distinct from the CD123+ HLA-DR+ population of plasmacytoid dendritic cells. Following basophil activation, the HLA-DR expression did not increase and remained distinct from HLA-DR+ cells.

Decrease in CD123 is correlated with the up-regulation of CD63 and CD203c

Taken together the previous observations indicate that the down-regulation of CD123 by basophils is an activation-dependent phenomenon. A weak statistically significant correlation was observed between the

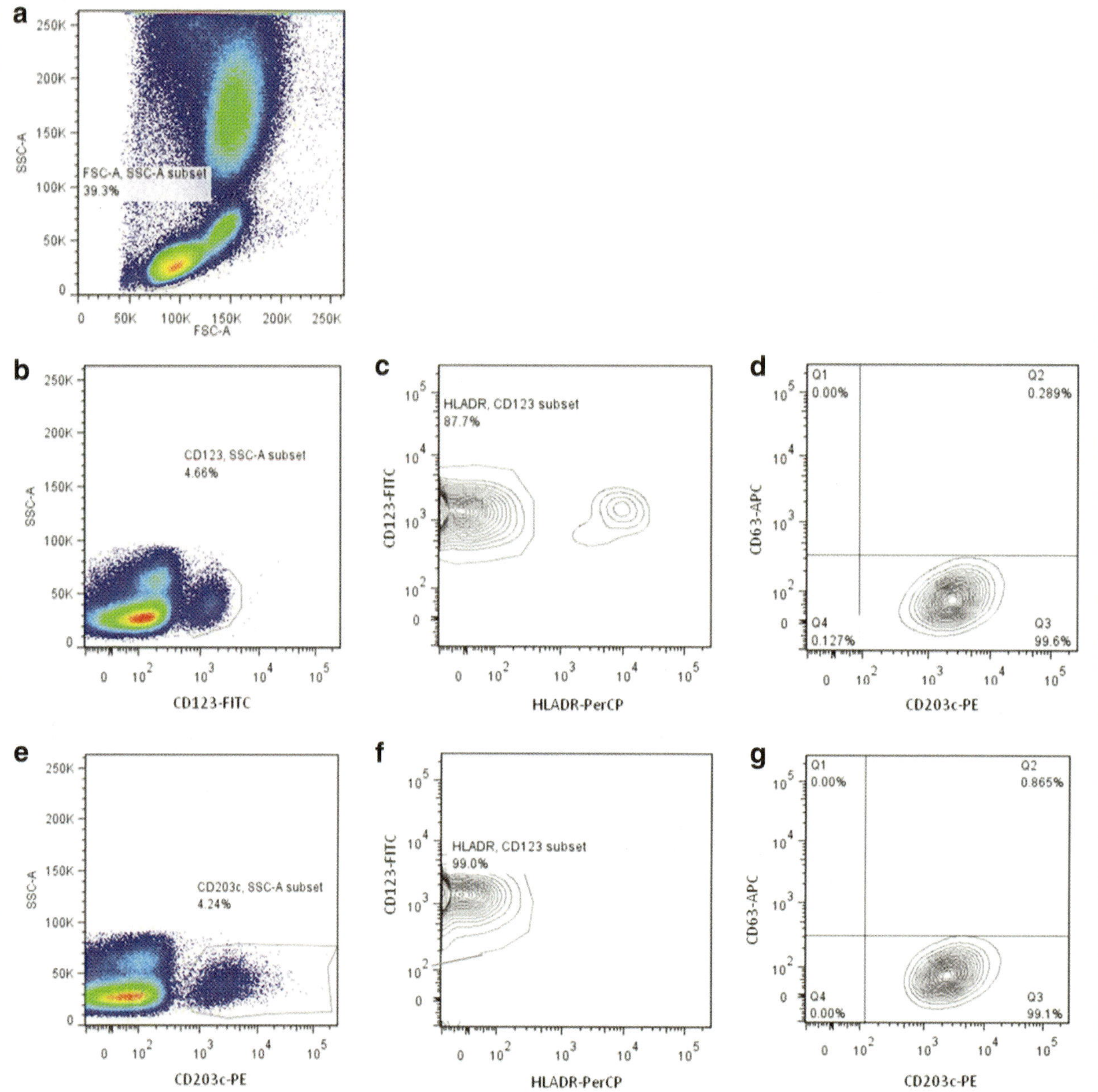

Fig. 1 Basophils were identified in whole blood in the lymphocyte-monocyte area (**a**) as SSC^{low}/CD123+/HLA-DR− (**b, c**) or as SSC^{low}/CD203c+ (**e**) or as SSC^{low}/CD203c+/CD123+/HLA-DR− (**e, f**) cells. CD63 expression was assessed in basophils identified as SSC^{low}/CD123+/HLA-DR− (**d**) or SSC^{low}/CD203c+/CD123+/HLA-DR− (**g**).

decrease in the MFI of CD123 and the up-regulation of basophil activation markers after stimulation with anti-IgE (Fig. 4b) as measured by the stimulation index of CD203c ($r_s = -0.35$, $p < 0.001$) or by the percentage of CD63-positive basophils ($r_s = -0.31$, $p < 0.001$), suggesting that the basophils that down-regulate CD123 the most are also the ones that express more CD63 and CD203c. The correlations between changes in the MFI of CD123-FITC and in the percentage of CD63+ basophils or the SI of CD203c following stimulation with fMLP (−0.191, p = 0.04 and −0.223, p = 0.016, respectively) and following stimulation with peanut extract (−0.229, p = 0.145 and −0.31, p = 0.051, respectively) were less strong.

Table 1 Number of basophils (gated as SSClow/CD123+/HLA-DR− cells) and expression of CD123 on the surface of basophils (gated as SSClow/CD203c+ cells) as measured by MFI of CD123-FITC in different stimulation conditions

Stimulant	n	Pre-stimulation	Post-stimulation	p value
Number of basophils				
fMLP	116	1722 (1226, 2184)	1572 (1037, 2100)	*0.012*
Anti-IgE	104	1722 (1221, 2191)	1414 (972, 1995)	*0.005*
Peanut extract	42	1732 (1212, 2174)	1514 (914, 2041)	0.134
MFI of CD123-FITC				
fMLP	116	1082 (98, 1549)	514 (75, 1020)	*<0.001*
Anti-IgE	104	1081 (95, 1549)	495 (60, 1111)	*<0.001*
Peanut extract	42	1172 (80–2058)	293 (40, 1244)	*<0.001*

Median (inter-quartile range) is represented. p value refers to the comparison of post-stimulation conditions with the negative control

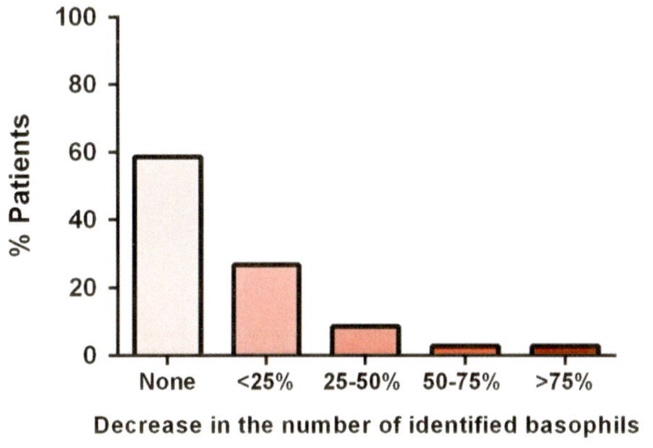

Fig. 2 Variation in the number of identified basophils following anti-IgE stimulation compared to the negative control (n = 104). Variation was calculated as (number of identified basophils pre-stimulation − number of identified basophils post-stimulation)/number of identified basophils pre-stimulation

Additional use of CD203c prevented the loss-to-analysis of activated basophils

The down-regulation of CD123 with basophil activation has important implications in gating strategies that depend on CD123. Identifying basophils using CD123 and HLA-DR led to the loss-to-analysis of basophils, particularly of the ones with higher expression of the activation markers CD63 and CD203c, and thus leading to an underestimation of basophil activation (Table 2; Fig. 5a). Adding CD203c as an identification marker restored the cell number, regardless of the basophil activation status and allowed to include the basophils that were activated the most in the analysis, improving the outcome of the test (Table 2; Fig. 5b). The expression of CD203c remained stable or increased following basophil activation, allowing a good separation from the remaining blood cells (Fig. 3b).

Selecting the optimal gating strategy using CD203c

In order to select the best gating strategy using the available markers, we compared the results of the BAT following the identification of basophils as SSC^{low}/CD203c+ cells, as SSC^{low}/CD123+/HLA-DR− cells or as SSC^{low}/CD203c+/CD123+/HLA-DR−. To combine the three identification markers to gate on basophils, we first selected the SSC^{low}/CD203c+ cells and then gated on the plot CD123/HLA-DR following the contour of the cell population of interest, including $CD123^{low}$ as well as $CD123^{high}$ cells, all HLA-DR− (Fig. 1f).

The gating strategy using CD203c+/CD123+/HLA-DR− proved superior to CD123+/HLA-DR− and similar to what was observed for gating on CD203c+ cells alone (Table 2). The combination of the three markers was superior to CD203c+ in the subgroup of peanut allergic patients improving the detection of basophil activation (Table 2, borderline non-significant p values for %CD63+

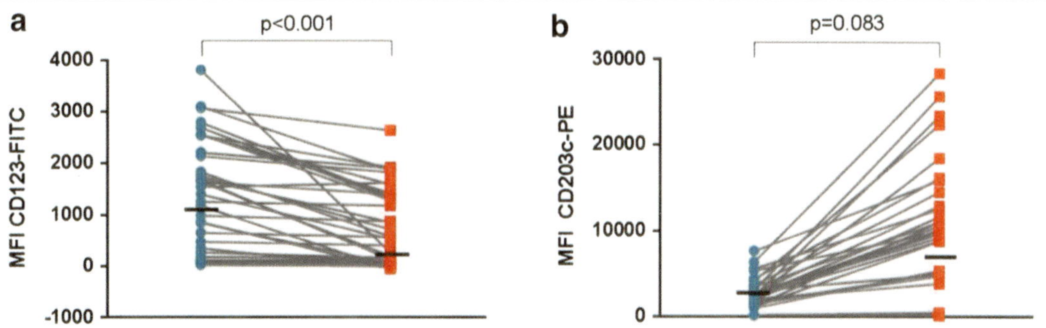

Fig. 3 Changes in the MFI of CD123-FITC (**a**) and in the MFI of CD203c-PE (**b**), following stimulation with 100 ng/ml of peanut extract (n = 42 peanut allergic patients)

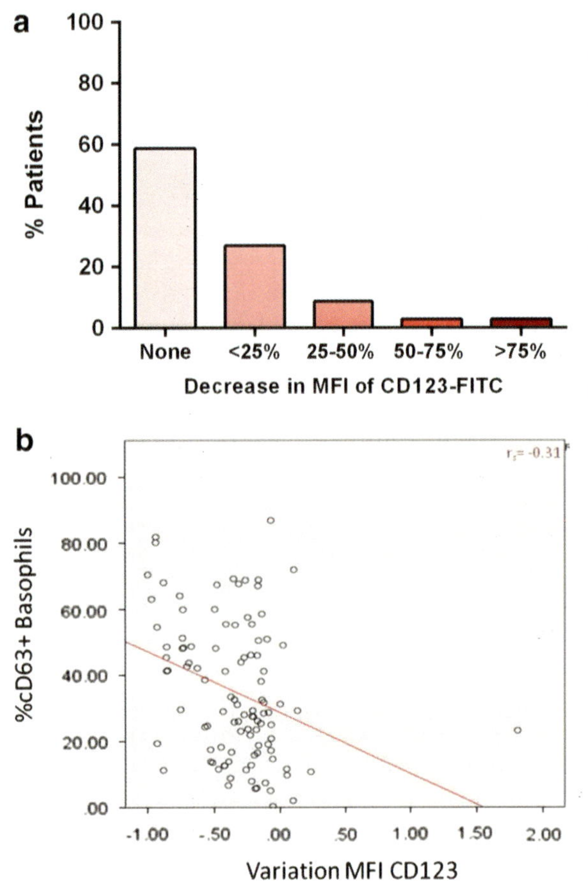

Fig. 4 Down-regulation of CD123 expression with basophil activation. **a** Change in the MFI of CD123-FITC on the surface of basophils following anti-IgE stimulation. **b** Correlation between decrease in CD123 and up-regulation of CD63 on the surface of basophils

basophils, SI CD203c and MFI of CD203c) and in patients with a subset of CD203c+/HLA-DR+ cells thus avoiding contamination with HLA-DR+ cells. However, in the majority of patients, the gating strategies SSC^{low}/CD203c+ and SSC^{low}/CD203c+/CD123+/HLA-DR− were comparable. SSC^{low}/CD203c+ could be used as an alternative gating strategy in a two-colour BAT.

In additional experiments (n = 10) using antibodies anti-CD14, anti-CD3, anti-CD19, anti-CD41 and in six of these experiments also anti-CD56, there was no contamination of the gating strategy using SSC^{low}/CD203c+/CD123+/HLA-DR− with other immune cells nor did they express CD203c. Only in one patient, CD14+ cells were also $CD203^{low}$ and HLA-DR+. In the PB-positive (PB+) population, there was a minor expression of CD63, possibly by CD41+ platelets, but this population was gated out as it did neither express CD123 nor CD203c, and CD63 expression remained stable with activation (data not shown).

Gating strategy of BAT has important diagnostic implications

The diagnostic performance of BAT gating on SSC^{low}/CD203c+/CD123+/HLA-DR− was superior to the one using SSC^{low}/CD123+/HLA-DR− with a larger area under the ROC curve (Fig. 6). The optimal cut-off based on the ROC curve generated using the latter gating strategy resulted in a 91 % diagnostic accuracy with 5 % false-negatives and 3 % false positives (Table 3). Adopting the SSC^{low}/CD203c+/CD123+/HLA-DR− gating strategy resulted in a diagnostic accuracy of 97 %, as we recently reported [6], with 1 % false-negatives and 2 % false-positives. Unusually, this methodological improvement resulted in both enhanced sensitivity and specificity of BAT in the diagnosis of peanut allergy. Figure 5 shows an example of a patient that would be considered false negative if gating was confined to CD123+/HLADR− cells. Furthermore, using this gating strategy, 15 % of patients showed <500 basophils in at least one condition and thus BAT would be uninterpretable.

Discussion

BAT can be used to diagnose allergic disease and to study the underlying immunological mechanisms. The methodology of identification of basophils has important consequences for the outcome of the test. In this study, we showed that CD123 is down-regulated with basophil activation and gating strategies that depend solely on this marker lead to the loss-to-analysis of activated basophils and to the underestimation of basophil activation. Using CD203c in addition to CD123/HLA-DR or in isolation proved superior to gating on CD123/HLA-DR, reducing the number of false-negatives and false-positives and improving the diagnostic accuracy from 91 to 97 %. When BAT is used as an allergy test, the gating strategy adopted has diagnostic implications in the assessment of individual patients. Basophils have been identified with CD123 and HLA-DR in previous studies, using flow cytometry and other techniques [24], and CD123 expression was reported to be stable with the atopic status of the patient and following basophil activation, although no direct comparisons were made [2, 17, 25]. In our study, the MFI of CD123-FITC was comparable between atopic and non atopic patients, but there was a decrease in the MFI of CD123-FITC with basophil activation. This is in contrast to previous studies [2, 17, 25] and is probably related to differences in the study population (e.g. adults vs. children), in the disease models studied (e.g. patients with respiratory vs. food allergies) and in the study design (e.g. basophils stimulated with allergen in vivo vs. in vitro, which can have different kinetics). We do not believe compensation played a role in the observed

Table 2 Comparison of different strategies to gate on basophils

Parameters	Stimulants	CD123+ HLA-DR−	CD203c+	CD203c+ CD123+ HLA-DR−	Overall p value	p value[1]	p value[2]	p value[3]
Number of basophils	Negative control[a]	1722 (1226, 2184)	1782 (1334–2239)	1697 (1268–2134)	0.635	0.390	0.436	0.908
	Anti-IgE[b]	1414 (972–1995)	2156 (1620–3097)	1939 (1452–2877)	*<0.001*	*<0.001*	0.06	*<0.001*
	fMLP[a]	1572 (1037, 2100)	2146 (1684–2940)	1891 (1447–2715)	*<0.001*	*<0.001*	0.084	*<0.001*
	Peanut extract[c]	1514 (914–2041)	2351 (1748–3062)	2104 (1615–2752)	*<0.001*	*<0.001*	0.348	*0.001*
%CD63 + basophils	Anti-IgE[b]	24.8 (10.7, 42.5)	29.4 (17.3–48.9)	32.0 (17.1–53.9)	*0.021*	*0.020*	0.809	*0.013*
	fMLP[a]	28.2 (15.9, 42.3)	41.1 (26.3–53.4)	41.4 (26.9–56.9)	*<0.001*	*<0.001*	0.644	*<0.001*
	Peanut extract[c]	32.3 (10.9, 56.2)	41.0 (18.0–56.9)	42.1 (20.0–68.5)	0.185	0.220	0.561	0.074
MFI CD63	Anti-IgE[b]	104.0 (26.3–195.2)	148 (36, 345)	159.3 (45.4–350.8)	*0.019*	*0.029*	0.611	*0.009*
	fMLP[a]	139 (37, 284)	285 (76, 683)	307 (81, 708)	*<0.001*	*<0.001*	0.678	*<0.001*
	Peanut extract[c]	138.4 (24.8–270.7)	190 (37, 513)	202.9 (42.6–567.4)	0.267	0.271	0.629	0.113
SI CD203c	Anti-IgE[b]	2.4 (1.5–3.8)	2.9 (2.0–4.2)	3.2 (2.0–4.6)	*0.004*	*0.028*	0.191	*0.002*
	fMLP[a]	2.3 (1.7–3.1)	2.6 (2.2–3.7)	2.8 (2.2–4.1)	*<0.001*	*0.001*	0.280	*<0.001*
	Peanut extract[c]	3.3 (1.8–5.3)	3.8 (2.4–4.8)	4.3 (2.4–5.4)	0.193	0.386	0.260	0.088
MFI CD203c	Anti-IgE[b]	2331 (197–5633)	4833 (254, 9020)	5013 (29–9161)	*0.008*	*0.011*	0.677	*0.005*
	fMLP[a]	2763 (216–5139)	4549 (279, 7961)	4908 (334–8270)	*0.001*	*0.002*	0.813	*0.001*
	Peanut extract[c]	3631.6 (179.4–8491.4)	5312 (206, 11,976)	7012 (236–11,857)	0.173	0.14	0.714	0.083

Median and inter-quartile range are represented. Medians were compared between the three groups using Kruskall–Wallis test and between two groups using Mann–Whitney U test

[a] n = 116

[b] n = 104 (non-responders were excluded)

[c] n = 42 (peanut allergic)

[1] CD123+/HLA-DR− versus CD203c+

[2] CD203c+ versus CD203c+/CD123+/HLA-DR−

[3] CD123+/HLA-DR− versus CD203c+/CD123+/HLA-DR−

changes as this phenomenon only happened in a subset of patients and in other patients the expression of CD123 was stable regardless of the increase in the expression of CD63 and CD203c. Furthermore, while the spectrum of CD203c-PE overlapped with CD123-FITC, the spectra of CD123-FITC and of CD63-APC did not overlap and we performed compensation before running the samples, used the same compensation matrix during acquisition of all samples for each patient and did not see any differences in compensation within the same experiment. Although the size and the granularity of basophils change with activation and degranulation [5, 26], these modifications do not lead to cell loss in the FSC/SSC gate and basophil numbers are stable with and without stimulation using identification markers such as CD203c. With respect to HLA-DR, basophils were HLA-DR-negative and kept distinct of HLA-DR-positive cells in all conditions. These findings are consistent with previous reports [17] and with recent studies that did not confirm a role for basophils in antigen-presentation in humans [27, 28].

The expression of CD123 being dependent on basophil activation raises the question as to whether CD123 can be used as a basophil activation marker. However, this phenomenon is significant in only a subset of patients and the dose–response with increasing concentrations of the stimulant is subtle; thus, CD123 does not seem to offer any advantage to the existing activation markers, such as CD63 and CD203c.

The combination of the three identification markers, CD203c/CD123/HLA-DR, proved superior to using CD123/HLA-DR. We compared the diagnostic performance of BAT to peanut identifying basophils as CD123+/HLA-DR− cells and as CD203c+/CD123+/HLA-DR− cells and the latter resulted in a greater area under the ROC curve (0.96 vs. 0.99) and improved diagnostic accuracy (91 vs. 97 %). Furthermore, if we took into consideration a minimum number of basophils as exclusion criteria, 15 % of patients would be inevaluable using CD123+/HLADR−. The consequences of the gating strategy adopted are clinically relevant as the purpose of the BAT is to diagnose peanut allergy in individual patients. An example is illustrated in Fig. 5, where with basophils gated as CD123+/HLA-DR−, BAT would be considered negative at the diagnostic concentration of 100 ng/ml but in fact it was clearly positive when basophils were selected using the three markers' strategy. This would be a false-negative with potential serious consequences, as it could lead to liberalization of peanut consumption with the risk

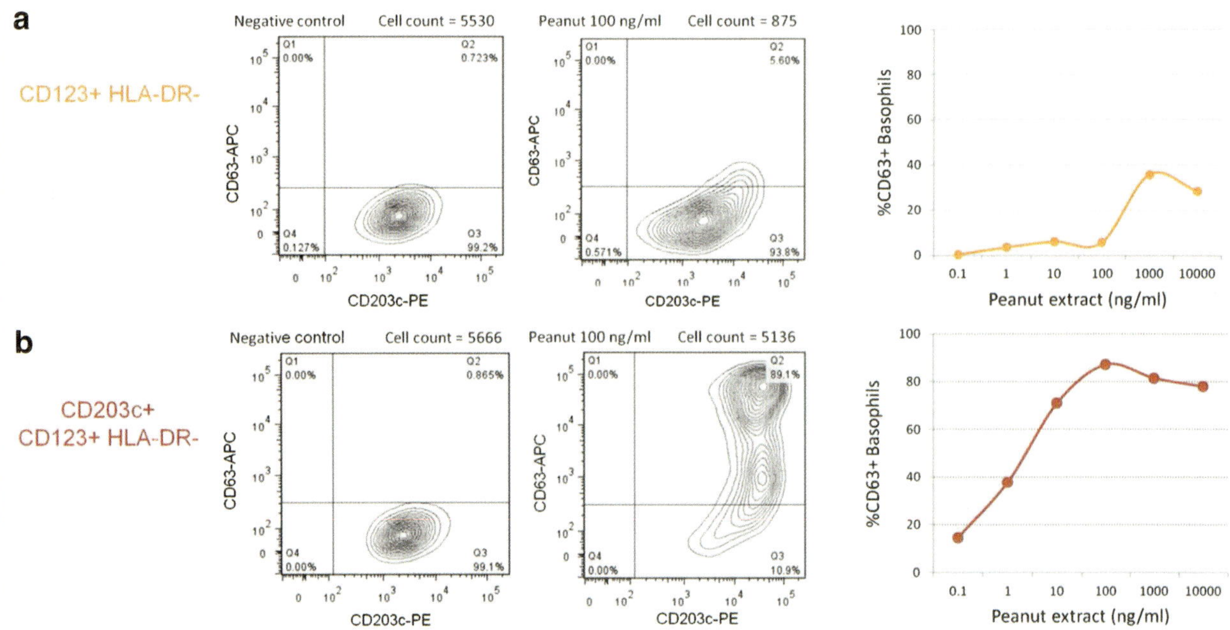

Fig. 5 Gating with CD123/HLA-DR led to the loss-to-analysis of basophils and underestimation of basophil activation. In a representative experiment, basophils were gated as SSClow/CD123^{bright}/HLA-DR− (**a**) or SSC^{low}/CD203c+/CD123+/HLA-DR− (**b**). The percentage of CD63+ basophils is represented in different conditions: negative control, peanut extract 100 ng/ml and peanut-dose–response curve. Note the bi-exponential display [38]

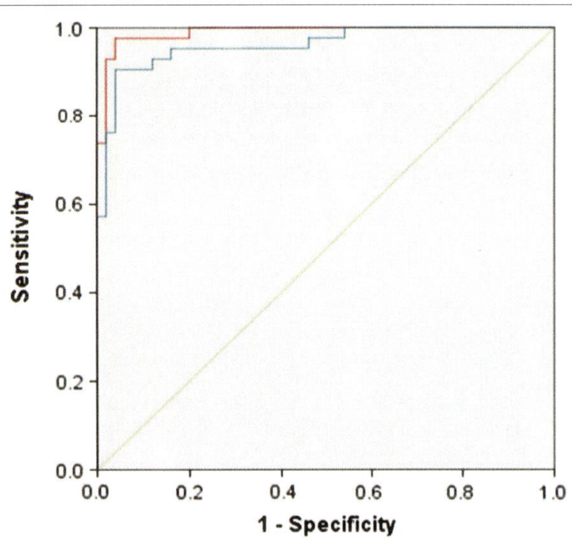

Gating strategy	AUC	95% CI
CD203c+ CD123+ HLADR-	0.99	0.975-1.0
CD123+ HLADR-	0.96	0.922-0.998

Fig. 6 ROC curve of the average %CD63+ basophils at 10 and 100 ng/ml of peanut extract using different basophil gating strategies: SSC^{low}/CD203c+/CD123+/HLA-DR− (*red*), SSC^{low}/CD123+/HLA-DR− (*blue*)

of allergic reactions that are potentially severe. The loss-to-analysis of cells and/or the underestimation of basophil activation have important implications for the final outcome of the test and thus for the diagnosis of individual patients. The same applies to other clinical applications, such as monitoring of treatment, and to mechanistic experiments. The fact that we detected no contamination of the gating with other immune cells suggests that there would be no advantage in using a lineage negative antibody mixture to exclude other immune cells before gating on the CD203c+/CD123+/HLA-DR− cells as basophils.

Identifying basophils with CD203c alone lead to comparable outcome in terms of number of basophils and basophil activation markers to using CD203c+/CD123+/HLA-DR− and was also superior to using CD123+/HLA-DR−, as represented in Table 2. CD203c is a basophil specific marker in whole blood. Its constitutive expression is increased in patients with atopic eczema and food allergy [29–31], as previously described in terms of histamine release [32] suggesting it is a marker of underlying basophil activation, possibly reflecting ongoing piecemeal degranulation. This enhances the separation of CD203c+ basophils from the other blood cells in populations of highly atopic children [6]. The majority of patients in our study had eczema

Table 3 Diagnostic accuracy of the basophil activation test to peanut using different gating strategies

	Gating strategy	
	CD123+ HLADR−	CD203c+ CD123+ HLADR−
Optimal cut-off	6.8	8.1
AUC ROC for the cut-off	0.91	0.97
Accuracy (%)	91	97
Sensitivity (%)	88	98
Specificity (%)	94	96
PPV (%)	93	95
NPV (%)	90	98
%True positives	40	45
%False positives	3	2
%True negatives	51	52
%False negatives	5	1
LR+	14.7	24.4
LR−	0.13	0.02

The optimal cut-off was determined for the %CD63+ basophils following stimulation with 100 ng/ml of peanut extract

PPV positive predictive value, *NPV* negative predictive value, *LR+* positive likelihood ratio, *LR−* negative likelihood ratio

and other food allergies in addition to suspected peanut allergy and this represents a population where CD203c would be constitutively expressed at a higher level than in other children allowing a clear differentiation between CD203c+ basophils and other blood cells. The conjugation to the bright fluorochrome PE may have also contributed to the good identification of cells expressing CD203c. SSC^{low}/CD203c+ is an alternative basophil identification strategy that has the advantage of serving also as an activation marker, enabling BAT to be performed as a two-colour (preferred) or even as a single colour BAT, which would make BAT easier and less expensive to perform.

This is the largest study looking at different strategies for identifying basophils using CD123 and its clinical implications and it is the first study to report the down-regulation of CD123 with basophil activation. The performance of BAT soon after blood collection and the use of live cells for flow cytometry on the same day contributed to the quality of the results. However, our study population was constituted mostly by highly atopic children enrolled in a study examining the use of BAT in the diagnosis of peanut allergy [6]. Therefore, our results may not apply to other populations, namely of non atopic patients or older patients being assessed for other conditions such as drug allergy. While assessing changes in basophil identification markers, we discovered that in a subset of patients basophils down-regulate CD123, the low affinity subunit of the IL-3 receptor, with basophil activation. This phenomenon seems patient-specific rather than specific for atopic or allergic status. In the patients where this is observed, the down-regulation happens only in conditions where basophils are activated and correlates with the degree of activation, as expressed by CD63 and CD203c. It is possible that the patients who showed higher down-regulation of CD123 after basophil activation are the ones with most severe clinical reactions but this remains to be confirmed. IL-3 is predominantly produced by T cells and is able to induce basophils to release histamine and up-regulate CD203c and CD63 in the absence of allergen [33, 34]. It can also act synergistically with allergen or other stimulants to increase basophil activation and histamine release [4, 18, 33]. The basophil intracellular pathways down-stream of the IL-3 and the IgE receptors seem indeed closely connected [34]. The response to this priming effect is variable between basophil donors and requires different concentrations of IL-3 [35]. Some research groups have used exogenous IL-3 to prime basophils in the BAT [4, 18, 36]. However, basophils secrete IL-3 themselves in response to IgE-mediated activation for autocrine priming, which has been suggested to be a possible mechanism underlying the hyper-reactive nature of the basophils of allergic patients [37]. We hypothesize that the down-regulation of CD123, which is part of the IL-3 receptor, could result from a basophil regulatory mechanism to avoid further cell activation, but this deserves further research.

Conclusions

Basophils down-regulate CD123 with activation in a subset of patients and this can have significant deleterious diagnostic implications. While performing the BAT, the use of gating strategies that depend solely on CD123 may lead to loss-to-analysis of basophils, particularly of the ones that highly express CD63 and CD203c, resulting in a false-negative outcome for the test. To overcome this limitation, additional use of CD203c, both identification and activation marker, prevents the loss-to-analysis of activated basophils and allows accurate assessment of basophil activation and, consequently, a more accurate diagnosis of allergy.

Abbreviations

APC: allophycocyanin; BAT: basophil activation test; DBPCFC: double-blind-placebo-controlled-food-challenge; FITC: fluorescein isothiocyanate; fMLP: formyl-methionyl-leucyl-phenylalanine; LAMP: lysosomal-associated membrane protein; PE: phycoerythrin; PerCP: peridinin chlorophyll protein; ROC: receiver-operating characteristic; RPMI: Rosewell Park Memorial Institute medium; SI: stimulation index; SPT: skin prick test.

Authors' contributions

AFS and GL designed the study; AFS developed the basophil activation assay, performed the statistical analyses and wrote the first draft of the manuscript; AFS and NB performed the laboratory experiments; AS and VT provided laboratory assistance; GL critically reviewed the analyses and edited manuscript; all authors reviewed the manuscript and approved its final version. All authors read and approved the final manuscript.

Author details

[1] Division of Asthma, Allergy and Lung Biology, Department of Pediatric Allergy, St Thomas' Hospital, King's College London, 2nd Floor, Stairwell B, South Wing, Westminster Bridge Road, London SE1 7EH, UK. [2] MRC and Asthma UK Centre in Allergic Mechanisms of Asthma, London, UK. [3] Immunoallergology Department, Coimbra University Hospital, Coimbra, Portugal. [4] Gulbenkian Programme for Advanced Medical Education, Lisbon, Portugal.

Acknowledgements

This work was funded by the Medical Research Council (G0902018) and the Department of Health via the National Institute for Health Research (NIHR) comprehensive Biomedical Research Centre award to Guy's & St Thomas' NHS Foundation Trust in partnership with King's College London and King's College Hospital NHS Foundation Trust. The views expressed are those of the author(s) and not necessarily those of the NHS, the NIHR or the Department of Health. The clinical trials unit is supported by the National Peanut Board, Atlanta, Ga. The authors would like to thank Susanne Heck and Pj Chana (BRC Flow Cytometry Core, NIHR GSTT/KCL Comprehensive Biomedical Research Centre); all the members of the LEAP and the PAS Studies' teams, the Clinical Nurse Specialists at the Children's Allergy Service at St Thomas' Hospital and the study participants and their families. The Programme for Advanced Medical Education is sponsored by Fundação Calouste Gulbenkian, Fundação Champalimaud, Ministério da Saúde and Fundação para a Ciência e Tecnologia, Portugal.

Competing interests

A. F. Santos and her institution have received funding from the Medical Research Council (CRTF No. G0902018, MRC Centenary Early Career Award and MRC Clinician Scientist Fellowship MR/M008517/1), the Immune Tolerance Network/National Institute of Allergy and Infectious Diseases, United States (Grant Nos. ITN032AD and ITN049AD); and the National Peanut Board, United States; she has also received funding from the Gulbenkian Programme for Advanced Medical Education. G. Lack has received research support from the Immune Tolerance Network/National Institute of Allergy and Infectious Diseases, United States (Grant Nos. ITN032AD and ITN049AD); the Food Allergy Initiative, United States (Pronuts study); the National Peanut Board, United States (Project 26); the Food Standards Agency, United Kingdom (Grant Nos. T07049 and T07051); the Food Allergy and Anaphylaxis Network, United States; Medical Research Council & AsthmaUK Centre (Grant No. G1100090); Goldman Sachs Gives; and the Department of Health through the National Institute for Health Research Comprehensive Biomedical Research Centre award to the Guy's & St Thomas' NHS Foundation Trust in partnership with King's College London and King's College Hospital NHS Foundation Trust; is on the DBV Technologies advisory board; is a voluntary scientific advisor for the Anaphylaxis Campaign and the National Peanut Board; has received lecture fees from Sodilac; Novartis, Switzerland; Nestl_e Nutrition; GlaxoSmithKline, United Kingdom; and the Serono Symposia International Foundation; and has stock/stock options in DBV Technologies. The rest of the authors declare that they have no relevant competing interests.

References

1. Ebo DG, Bridts CH, Hagendorens MM, Aerts NE, De Clerck LS, Stevens WJ. Basophil activation test by flow cytometry: present and future applications in allergology. Cytom B Clin Cytom. 2008;74:201–10.
2. Chirumbolo S, Vella A, Ortolani R, et al. Differential response of human basophil activation markers: a multi-parameter flow cytometry approach. Clin Mol Allergy. 2008;6:12.
3. Hauswirth AW, Natter S, Ghannadan M, et al. Recombinant allergens promote expression of CD203c on basophils in sensitized individuals. J Allergy Clin Immunol. 2002;110:102–9.
4. Sturm EM, Kranzelbinder B, Heinemann A, Groselj-Strele A, Aberer W, Sturm GJ. CD203c-based basophil activation test in allergy diagnosis: characteristics and differences to CD63 upregulation. Cytom B Clin Cytom. 2010;78:308–18.
5. MacGlashan D Jr. Expression of CD203c and CD63 in human basophils: relationship to differential regulation of piecemeal and anaphylactic degranulation processes. Clin Exp Allergy. 2010;40:1365–77.
6. Santos AF, Douiri A, Becares N, et al. Basophil activation test discriminates between allergy and tolerance in peanut-sensitized children. J Allergy Clin Immunol. 2014;134:645–52.
7. Rubio A, Vivinus-Nebot M, Bourrier T, Saggio B, Albertini M, Bernard A. Benefit of the basophil activation test in deciding when to reintroduce cow's milk in allergic children. Allergy. 2011;66:92–100.
8. Wanich N, Nowak-Wegrzyn A, Sampson HA, Shreffler WG. Allergen-specific basophil suppression associated with clinical tolerance in patients with milk allergy. J Allergy Clin Immunol. 2009;123(789–94):e20.
9. Ford LS, Bloom KA, Nowak-Wegrzyn AH, Shreffler WG, Masilamani M, Sampson HA. Basophil reactivity, wheal size, and immunoglobulin levels distinguish degrees of cow's milk tolerance. J Allergy Clin Immunol. 2013;131(180–6):e3.
10. Santos AF, Douiri A, Bécares N, et al. Basophil activation test discriminates between allergy and tolerance in peanut-sensitized children. J Allergy Clin Immunol. 2014;134:645-52.
11. Jones SM, Pons L, Roberts JL, et al. Clinical efficacy and immune regulation with peanut oral immunotherapy. J Allergy Clin Immunol. 2009;124:292–300.
12. Kim EH, Bird JA, Kulis M, et al. Sublingual immunotherapy for peanut allergy: clinical and immunologic evidence of desensitization. J Allergy Clin Immunol. 2011;127(640–6):e1.
13. Thyagarajan A, Jones SM, Calatroni A, et al. Evidence of pathway-specific basophil anergy induced by peanut oral immunotherapy in peanut-allergic children. Clin Exp Allergy. 2012;42:1197–205.
14. Nopp A, Johansson SG, Ankerst J, et al. Basophil allergen threshold sensitivity: a useful approach to anti-IgE treatment efficacy evaluation. Allergy. 2006;61:298–302.
15. Nopp A, Johansson SG, Ankerst J, Palmqvist M, Oman H. CD-sens and clinical changes during withdrawal of Xolair after 6 years of treatment. Allergy. 2007;62:1175–81.
16. Nopp A, Johansson SG, Adedoyin J, Ankerst J, Palmqvist M, Oman H. After 6 years with Xolair: a 3-year withdrawal follow-up. Allergy. 2010;65:56–60.
17. Hausmann OV, Gentinetta T, Fux M, Ducrest S, Pichler WJ, Dahinden CA. Robust expression of CCR3 as a single basophil selection marker in flow cytometry. Allergy. 2011;66:85–91.
18. Ocmant A, Peignois Y, Mulier S, Hanssens L, Michils A, Schandene L. Flow cytometry for basophil activation markers: the measurement of CD203c up-regulation is as reliable as CD63 expression in the diagnosis of cat allergy. J Immunol Methods. 2007;320:40–8.
19. Wynn TA. Basophils trump dendritic cells as APCs for T(H)2 responses. Nat Immunol. 2009;10:679–81.
20. Tang H, Cao W, Kasturi SP, et al. The T helper type 2 response to cysteine proteases requires dendritic cell-basophil cooperation via ROS-mediated signaling. Nat Immunol. 2010;11:608–17.
21. Charles N, Hardwick D, Daugas E, Illei GG, Rivera J. Basophils and the T helper 2 environment can promote the development of lupus nephritis. Nat Med. 2010;16:701–7.
22. Roberts G, Lack G. Diagnosing peanut allergy with skin prick and specific IgE testing. J Allergy Clin Immunol. 2005;115:1291–6.
23. Fox AT, Sasieni P, du Toit G, Syed H, Lack G. Household peanut consumption as a risk factor for the development of peanut allergy. J Allergy Clin Immunol. 2009;123:417–23.
24. Dijkstra D, Hennig C, Hansen G, Biller H, Krug N, Hohlfeld JM. Identification and quantification of basophils in the airways of asthmatics following segmental allergen challenge. Cytom A. 2014;85:580–7.
25. Chirumbolo S, Ortolani R, Vella A. CCR3 as a single selection marker compared to CD123/HLADR to isolate basophils in flow cytometry: some comments. Cytom A. 2011;79:102–6.
26. Dvorak AM. Ultrastructural studies of human basophils and mast cells. J Histochem Cytochem. 2005;53:1043–70.

27. Kitzmuller C, Nagl B, Deifl S, et al. Human blood basophils do not act as antigen-presenting cells for the major birch pollen allergen Bet v 1. Allergy. 2012;67:593–600.
28. Eckl-Dorna J, Ellinger A, Blatt K, et al. Basophils are not the key antigen-presenting cells in allergic patients. Allergy. 2012;67:601–8.
29. Ford LS, Bloom KA, Nowak-Wegrzyn AH, Shreffler WG, Masilamani M, Sampson HA. Basophil reactivity, wheal size, and immunoglobulin levels distinguish degrees of cow's milk tolerance. J Allergy Clin Immunol. 2013;131(180–6):e1–3.
30. Shreffler WG. Evaluation of basophil activation in food allergy: present and future applications. Curr Opin Allergy Clin Immunol. 2006;6:226–33.
31. Ford LS, Bloom KA, Nowak-Wegrzyn AH, Shreffler WG, Masilamani M, Sampson HA. Basophil reactivity, wheal size, and immunoglobulin levels distinguish degrees of cow's milk tolerance. J Allergy Clin Immunol. 2013;131:180-6.
32. Sampson HA, Broadbent KR, Bernhisel-Broadbent J. Spontaneous release of histamine from basophils and histamine-releasing factor in patients with atopic dermatitis and food hypersensitivity. N Engl J Med. 1989;321:228–32.
33. Okayama Y, Begishvili TB, Church MK. Comparison of mechanisms of IL-3 induced histamine release and IL-3 priming effect on human basophils. Clin Exp Allergy. 1993;23:901–10.
34. Verweij MM, Sabato V, Nullens S, et al. STAT5 in human basophils: IL-3 is required for its FcepsilonRI-mediated phosphorylation. Cytom B Clin Cytom. 2012;82:101–6.
35. Gentinetta T, Pecaric-Petkovic T, Wan D, et al. Individual IL-3 priming is crucial for consistent in vitro activation of donor basophils in patients with chronic urticaria. J Allergy Clin Immunol. 2011;128:1227e5–1234e5.
36. Chirumbolo S. The use of IL-3 in basophil activation tests is the real pitfall. Cytom B Clin Cytom. 2011;80:137–8 **; author reply 9**.
37. Schroeder JT, Chichester KL, Bieneman AP. Human basophils secrete IL-3: evidence of autocrine priming for phenotypic and functional responses in allergic disease. J Immunol. 2009;182:2432–8.
38. Herzenberg LA, Tung J, Moore WA, Parks DR. Interpreting flow cytometry data: a guide for the perplexed. Nat Immunol. 2006;7:681–5.

6

Food allergy in the Netherlands: differences in clinical severity, causative foods, sensitization and DBPCFC between community and outpatients

Thuy-My Le[1*], Els van Hoffen[1,10], Ischa Kummeling[1,2], James Potts[2], Barbara K Ballmer-Weber[3], Carla AFM Bruijnzeel-Koomen[1], Ans FM Lebens[1], Jonas Lidholm[4], Titia M Lindner[1], Alan Mackie[5], EN Clare Mills[6], Ronald van Ree[7], Stefan Vieths[8], Montserrat Fernández-Rivas[9], Peter G Burney[2] and André C Knulst[1]

Abstract

Background: It is unknown whether food allergy (FA) in an unselected population is comparable to those from an outpatient clinic population.

Objective: To discover if FA in a random sample from the Dutch community is comparable to that of outpatients.

Methods: This study was part of the Europrevall-project. A random sample of 6600 adults received a questionnaire. Those with symptoms to one of 24 defined priority foods were tested for sIgE. Participants with a positive case history and elevated sIgE were evaluated by double-blind placebo-controlled food challenge (DBPCFC). Outpatients with a suspicion of FA were evaluated by questionnaire, sIgE and DBPCFC.

Results: In the community, severe symptoms were reported less often than in outpatients (39.3% *vs.* 54.3%). Participants in the community were less commonly sensitized to any of the foods. When selecting only those with a probable FA (i.e. symptoms of priority food and elevation of sIgE to the respective food), no major differences were observed with respect to severity, causative foods, sensitization and DBPCFC between the groups.

Conclusion: In the Netherlands, there are large differences in self-reported FA between community and outpatients. However, Dutch community and outpatients with a probable FA do not differ with respect to severity, causative foods, sensitization and DBPCFC-outcome.

Keywords: Adults, Community, DBPCFC, Food allergy, sIgE

Background

A recent meta-analysis showed that self-reported prevalence of food allergy (FA) ranged from 3% to 35% in adults [1]. However, the prevalence of FA as diagnosed by double-blind placebo-controlled food challenge (DBPCFC) is estimated to be around 2% to 4% for adults [2-7]. A study from a regional allergy center in the UK, serving a population of 1.6 million, reported a population prevalence of 0.03%, being a factor of 100 less than in population-based studies. This suggests that a minority of FA patients present to their GP and are subsequently referred [8].

* Correspondence: t.t.m.le-2@umcutrecht.nl
[1]Department of Dermatology/Allergology, University Medical Center Utrecht, PO Box 855003508 GA Utrecht, The Netherlands
Full list of author information is available at the end of the article

Most studies investigating the clinical aspects of FA involve patients from a (tertiary) allergy clinic. Since only a fraction of food allergic individuals from the general population visit a doctor, [8] it is not clear how representative results from such studies are for the general population. However, studies comparing FA between the community and outpatients are lacking.

The aim of this study was to investigate to what extent FA in a random sample of the Dutch community is comparable to FA in outpatients.

Methods

This study was part of the EuroPrevall-project, a multidisciplinary European project investigating several aspects of FA [9]. It consisted, among many different, of an epidemiological element investigating the prevalence of FA in the community and an outpatient clinical element. This study was approved by the local medical ethical committee (METC) of the University Medical Center Utrecht.

Community

The epidemiological study consisted of three stages and is described in detail elsewhere [10]. In short, the study took place from October 2006 until March 2009. The 1st stage was a population-based study in which a short questionnaire to screen for FA was sent out to a random sample of 6600 adults aged 20–54 years living in the city of Utrecht, The Netherlands.

In the 2nd stage, all those who in the screening questionnaire reported to have experienced adverse reactions to one of the 24 preselected priority foods (hen's egg, cow's milk, peanut, soy, hazelnut, walnut, celery, kiwi, apple, peach, sesame, mustard, wheat, fish and shrimp, buckwheat, corn, carrot, tomato, melon, banana, lentils, sunflower, poppy seeds) were invited to come to the hospital for a detailed questionnaire and serum IgE testing .

In the 3rd stage, participants with self-reported symptoms and sIgE to at least one of the priority foods were called in for DBPCFC and a full clinical evaluation, identical to that of the outpatients (see below).

Outpatients

The outpatient study took place from January 2006 until June 2009. All adult patients (age 18 years and older) who were referred to our tertiary allergy centre with a suspected FA, were asked to participate in the EuroPrevall outpatient clinic study. Inclusion criteria were symptoms developing within 2 hours after ingestion of a food. Participating outpatients underwent a clinical evaluation comprising a thorough medical history using a standardized questionnaire, sIgE testing and DBPCFC.

Clinical evaluation

All clinical information was collected following a standardized questionnaire which was specifically developed for the Europrevall-study. Symptoms were classified into mild (symptoms of the oral cavity), moderate (gastro-intestinal symptoms and symptoms of the skin and mucous membranes) and severe (respiratory or cardiovascular symptoms).

A probable FA was defined as symptoms within 2 hours and sIgE ≥0.35 kU_A/L to a priority food. Although DBPCFC is the gold standard for diagnosis of FA, diagnosis of FA in majority of patients in clinical practice is based on medical history and sIgE. Therefore, in this study we chose a pragmatical approach using a suggestive history (i.e. symptoms <2 hours of ingestion) together with IgE sensitization to define a probable FA.

In vitro diagnosis

sIgE testing for all priority foods were performed in a single laboratory using the ImmunoCAP system and reagents from Phadia (Thermo Fisher Scientific, Uppsala, Sweden). sIgE values of ≥0.35 kU_A/L were regarded as positive.

DBPCFC

All participants with symptoms to hen's egg, cow's milk, peanut, hazelnut, celery, apple, peach, fish or shrimp were asked to participate in DBPCFC. A detailed protocol of the EuroPrevall DBFCFC is described elsewhere [11]. Briefly, active and placebo provocations were randomly performed on two different days with eight increasing doses. The single doses were administered at an interval of at least 20 minutes up to the top dose. The interval could be extended at the request of the patient, according to the case history of the patient, or in case of severe persisting subjective symptoms. Challenges were discontinued after the dose leading to the first objective allergic symptoms or ingestion of the whole meal. Objective symptoms considered for discontinuation of the provocation were blisters of the oral mucosa, skin symptoms such as flush, urticaria, angioedema, rhinitis, conjunctivitis, drop of blood pressure of at least 20 mmHg, drop of FEV1 > 12% or PEF ≥ 20%, laryngeal oedema, diarrhoea, emesis or in case of severe persistent subjective symptoms lasting for more than 45 minutes such as severe itching of palms, soles, head or severe gastric/abdominal pain. If all DBPCFC doses were negative, patients underwent an open food challenge. Patients that had a reaction of any type and any duration on the active day and no reaction on the placebo were classified as reactors, patients that did not react on the active nor the placebo day were tolerant and patients that reacted on the placebo day were placebo responders.

Statistics

Chi-square tests and, where appropriate, Fisher's exact tests were used to test the differences in several clinical characteristics (i.e. gender, severity of symptoms, causative foods, atopic diseases, sensitization and DBPCFC outcome) between the community and outpatients. Differences in age and the number of causative foods between the two groups were calculated using Student's T-test and, where appropriate, Mann–Whitney U test. Statistical analysis was performed using SPSS version 20 (SPSS Inc., Chicago, Illinois, USA) for Windows.

Results

Study population

Of the screening questionnaires that were sent out to a random sample of 6600 adults, 3864 responded, of whom 967 (25.0%) reported adverse food reactions to any food and 416 (10.8%) to at least one priority food (Figure 1). 154 of these 416 (37.0%) were willing to come to our clinic for the second stage consisting of a detailed questionnaire and sIgE testing. In 37.7% (58/154) sIgE was positive for the respective food. Of these 58 cases, 46 entered the 3rd stage for a full clinical evaluation.

In the outpatient clinical part of the study, all outpatients that met the inclusion criteria agreed to participate in the study. In total, 133 outpatients that were referred to our allergy center were included during the study period. Symptoms to at least one priority food were reported by 127 outpatients, in 102 of which sIgE to the same food(s) was detected.

Reported adverse food reactions to any food in the community

Adverse reactions to any food were reported by 25.0% of the responders in the community. Cow's milk (10.7%), nuts (9.5%), apple (9.4%) and fish (6.3%) were the most commonly reported causative foods. Mild symptoms (consisting of only oral allergy symptoms) were reported by 10.1%, moderate symptoms by 58.4% and severe symptoms by 21.4% of participants. In the group with moderate symptoms, gastro-intestinal symptoms dominated (60.2%).

Of the 967 participants reporting adverse reactions to any food, 416 reported symptoms to priority food and 551 reported symptoms to other foods. These two groups were compared and showed that the group with symptoms to priority food significantly more often reported oral allergy symptoms (51.5% vs. 24%), difficulty with swallowing (15.9% vs. 6.3%) and breathlessness (11.3% vs. 6.8%). In the group with symptoms other than priority food gastro-intestinal symptoms dominated and was significantly higher than in the priority food group (47.7% vs. 38.6%). Furthermore, the group without symptoms of priority food significantly more often reported that the symptoms to the culprit food took place once only (26.8%).

Reported adverse reactions to priority foods in community and outpatients

Of the participants reporting adverse reactions to any food (n = 967), 43.0% reported symptoms to at least one of the priority foods. Walnut, apple, cow's milk, hazelnut and kiwi were the most commonly reported priority foods in the community (Table 1, 2nd stage). The frequency of severe symptoms rose from 21.4% in the 1st stage to 39.3% in the 2nd stage in participants from the community. Remarkably, only a small percentage of participants from the community who reported symptoms to priority foods also had a positive sIgE for the respective food (Figure 2).

When comparing the community to outpatients, using reported symptoms to priority food as selection in both groups, it appeared that severe symptoms were significantly more common in outpatients (54.3% *vs.* 39.3%, p = 0.008). The frequency in which the different priority foods were reported, differed significantly for some foods: in the community the frequency of allergy to cow's milk, fish and shrimp was significantly higher, whereas outpatients reported symptoms to peanut,

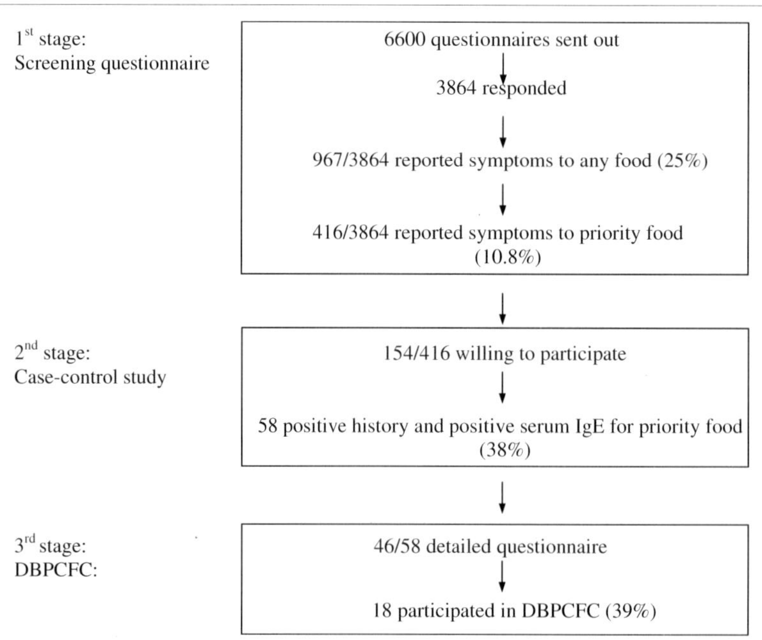

Figure 1 Flow-diagram of the epidemiological part of the study in the community.

Table 1 Patient characteristics of the three different stages

	1st stage (possible FA to any food)[‖]	2nd stage (possible FA to priority food)[‡]			3rd stage: (probable FA to priority food)[§]		
	Community (n = 967) %	Community (n = 154) %	Outpatients (n = 127) %	p-value	Community (n = 46) %	Outpatients (n = 102) %	p-value
Male gender	32.0	31.2	35.4	0.52	30.4	38.2	0.36
Age (mean ± SD)	34.7 (±9.3)	34.1 (±9.2)	32.2 (±12.3)	0.16	35.3	30.4	0.01*
Number of foods causing symptoms (median (range))		4 (1-17)	5 (1-18)	0.40	6 (1-14)	6 (1-18)	0.96
Symptom[¡]:							
-mild	10.1	14.0	26.0	0.01*	26.1	21.0	0.50
-moderate	58.4	46.7	19.7	<0.001*	28.3	19.0	0.21
-severe	21.4	39.3	54.3	0.008*	45.7	60.0	0.11
Atopy:							
-pollen allergy		70.8	94.5	<0.001*	97.8	94.1	0.44
-dermatitis		36.4	33.3	0.61	25.6	37.8	0.18
Symptoms of plant food							
-Hazelnut	2.4	31.2	32.3	0.84	71.7	37.3	<0.001*
-Peanut	2.7	16.2	32.3	0.002*	18.6	34.3	0.04*
-Walnut	2.5	36.4	36.2	0.98	52.2	41.2	0.21
-Apple	9.4	33.1	53.5	0.001*	82.6	57.8	0.003*
-Peach	1.0	18.8	29.1	0.04*	50.0	34.3	0.07
-Kiwi	4.8	29.2	43.3	0.01*	34.8	40.2	0.53
-Melon	1.2	14.9	15.0	1.00	21.7	16.7	0.46
-Banana	1.4	11.0	17.3	0.17	17.4	18.6	0.86
-Tomato	2.8	13.0	17.3	0.31	13.0	18.6	0.40
-Carrot	1.8	8.4	11.8	0.42	19.6	14.7	0.46
Symptoms of animal food							
-Cow's milk	10.7	31.8	8.7	<0.001*	4.3	6.9	0.72
-Hen's egg	2.4	7.8	8.7	0.79	2.2	8.8	0.17
-Fish	6.3	18.2	5.5	0.001*	6.5	5.9	1.00
-Shrimp	3.7	20.8	10.2	0.02*	8.7	10.8	0.78

FA = food allergy.
[¡]mild = oral allergy symptoms, moderate = gastro-intestinal symptoms or symptoms of the skin and mucous membranes, severe = respiratory or cardiovascular symptoms.
[‖]reported adverse food reaction to any food.
[‡]positive history for priority food.
[§]positive history and serum IgE for priority food.
*p-value < 0.05.

apple, peach and kiwi at a significantly higher frequency (Table 1, 2nd stage). Outpatients had significantly more clinically relevant sIgE sensitisation compared to the community for all foods, except for hazelnut and apple, where no difference was seen between both groups (Figure 2).

In summary, causative foods, severity and relevant food sensitization differed between the community and outpatients when only selecting on self-reported symptoms to priority foods.

Probable FA in community and outpatients

Of the participants from the community that reported symptoms to a priority food, 58/154 (37.7%) also had a positive sIgE for that food. These participants were considered to have a probable FA. When comparing the community participants and outpatients, using symptoms and sIgE to priority food as selection in both groups (i.e. probable FA), the differences in causative foods as seen in the 2nd stage disappeared largely. Only hazelnut and apple were significantly more frequently reported as a causative food in the community, whereas peanut was more commonly reported in outpatients (Table 1). In contrast to the 2nd stage, no differences were seen in the severity of symptoms between the community and outpatients (Table 1). Whereas in the 2nd stage major differences were observed between the two

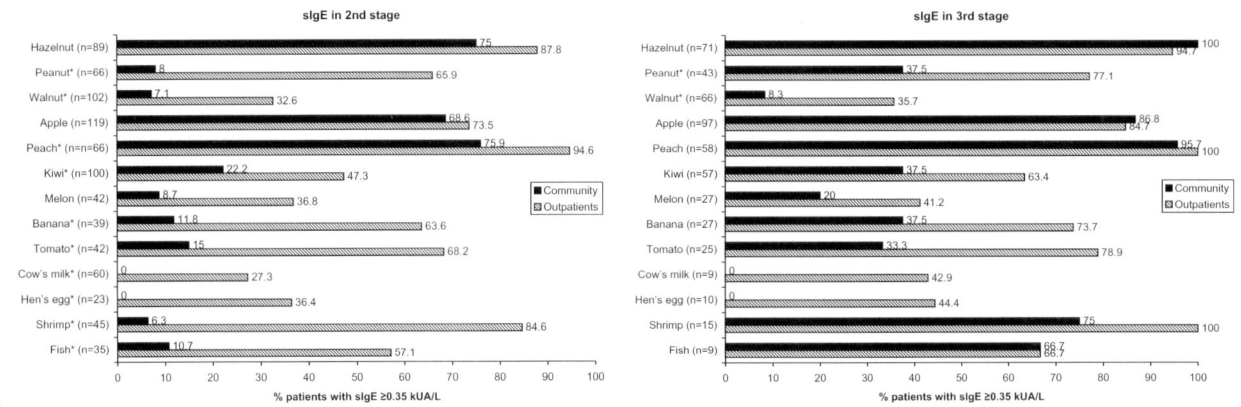

Figure 2 Percentage of positive sIgE in the community and outpatients with symptoms to the food in the 2nd stage (reported symptoms) and 3rd stage (reported symptoms and positive sIgE for at least 1 food) of the study. The number (n = ..) between brackets indicates the total number of the community and outpatients that reported symptoms to that respective priority food. *p-value <0.05.

groups in sensitization to most priority foods, these differences disappeared largely when selecting on FA (Figure 2). Table 2 shows the clinical characteristics in more detail for the main foods. The majority with a probable food allergy were birch pollen sensitized, had symptoms within a few minutes after ingestion of the culprit food and oral allergy symptoms was the most common symptom. A probable cow's milk en hen's egg allergy was rare in our adult population. In those with a cow's milk and hen's egg allergy anaphylaxis was relatively frequent (25%).

In total 18 participants from the community and 30 outpatients underwent DBPCFC. There were no significant differences in the severity of symptoms for the individual foods between those who agreed to participate in DBPCFC and those who declined ($p > 0.05$, data not shown). The percentage of positive DPBCFC did not differ between community and outpatients (77.8% *vs.* 63.3%, $p = 0.47$). Of the patients with a positive DBPCFC, 35.7% of the community and 31.6% of outpatients ($p = 0.80$) had objective signs. In both groups, the percentage of placebo reactors was high: 16.7% in the community and 20% in the outpatients. All placebo reactors reported subjective symptoms and not objective signs on placebo day. The outcome of the challenges per food are shown in Table 3.

In conclusion, when focusing on a probable FA, no difference could be demonstrated between the community participants and the outpatients with regard to severity, causative foods, relevant food sensitization and DBPCFC-outcome.

Discussion

Since most studies investigating FA use outpatients as a study population, the question arises whether such study results are applicable to food allergic persons in the community.

To our knowledge this is the first study to compare FA in the community and outpatients. In this study we found that, when focusing on self-reported symptoms to priority foods, there are large differences in causative foods, severity and relevant food sensitization between community and outpatients. However, when selecting those with a probable FA, as defined by reported symptoms to priority food together with a positive sIgE to the respective food, it became evident that the differences in the community and outpatients disappeared. This indicates that patients with a probable FA seen in a tertiary outpatient allergy center are not different from those with a probable FA in the community.

Previous population based studies showed that the prevalence of self-reported FA to any food varied from 3% to as high as 35%, whereas the prevalence of true FA is estimated to be 2-4% [1-7,12-14]. In our study we confirmed for the Dutch population the discrepancy between the prevalence of self-reported adverse food reactions (10.8%), a FA as defined by a suggestive history and supported by sIgE (4.1%) and a FA confirmed by DBPCFC (3.2%).

Since non-response bias could play a role in the community survey, we performed a non-response analysis. The response rate in the 1st stage of the community survey was 61%. We calculated the cumulative prevalence of adverse food reaction at the time of response to extrapolate the prevalence to non-responders [15]. This showed that the cumulative prevalence of adverse food reaction stabilized after a response rate of 40%, indicating that non-response bias does not play a major role in the 1st stage of the study. For the 2nd stage, we compared age, gender, doctor-diagnosed FA and the symptoms between responders and non-responders. Only the

Table 2 Clinical characteristerics per food in patients with a probable food allergy (i.e. symptoms and specific IgE)

	Community													Outpatients												
		Symptoms						Time interval				sIgE food	Birch IgE*		Symptoms						Time interval				sIgE food	Birch IgE*
	N	OAS (%)	skin (%)	GI (%)	Resp (%)	Cardio (%)	Anaph (%)	<5 min	5-30 min	30-120 min	> 2 hrs	Median (Range)	(%)	N	OAS (%)	skin (%)	GI (%)	Resp (%)	Cardio (%)	Anaph (%)	<5 min	5-30 min	30-120 min	> 2 hrs	Median (range)	(%)
Hazelnut	33	90.9	27.3	6.1	42.4	0	0	84.8	9.4	6.3	0	12.5 (0.47-74.99)	72.7	36	97.2	27.8	27.8	47.2	2.8	5.6	86.1	13.9	0	0	23.37 (0.65-196.54)	97.2
Peanut	3	66.7	33.3	33.3	33.3	0	0	50	50	0	0	2.63 (0.60-5.58)	100	27	88.9	59.3	29.6	48.1	0	0	77.8	22.2	0	0	2.21 (0.35-321.78)	85.2
Walnut	2	100	50	50	50	0	0	100	0	0	0	1.04 (0.51-1.58)	100	15	93.3	60	20	26.7	6.7	6.7	93.3	0	6.7	0	5.53 (0.36-27.56)	93.3
Apple	33	97	24.2	21.2	24.2	0	0	75.8	21.2	3	0	1.49 (0.37-21.18)	69.7	51	100	28	16	30	0	0	77.6	22.4	0	0	2.03 (0.42-31.19)	100
Peach	22	95.5	31.8	13.6	27.3	0	0	77.3	18.2	4.5	0	2.00 (0.53-12.91)	72.7	36	97.1	31.4	17.1	37.1	0	0	77.1	22.9	0	0	3.79 (0.59-44.56)	100
Kiwi	6	100	33.3	16.7	16.7	0	0	100	0	0	0	1.07 (0.40-11.21)	83.3	26	96.2	19.2	19.2	26.9	0	0	80	20	0	0	1.67 (0.35-152.57)	88.5
Cow's milk	0	-	-	-	-	-	-	-	-	-	-	-	-	4	50	50	50	25	25	25	50	25	0	0	10.05 (0.43-34.12)	50
Hen's egg	0	-	-	-	-	-	-	-	-	-	-	-	-	4	75	50	50	25	0	25	25	50	25	0	1.68 (0.40-3.04)	75

OAS = oral allergy symptoms, GI = gastro-intestinal, Resp = respiratory, cardio = cardiovascular, anaph = anaphylaxis.
*Birch sIgE = sIgE birch ≥0.35.

Table 3 Double-blind placebo-controlled food challenge (DBPCFC) in community and outpatients

	Community						Outpatients					
	N	Positive DBPCFC (%)	Negative DBPCFC (%)	Placebo reactor (%)	Objective signs* (%)	Subjective symptoms* (%)	N	Positive DBPCFC (%)	Negative DBPCFC (%)	Placebo reactor (%)	Objective signs* (%)	Subjective symptoms* (%)
Hazelnut	9	77.8	11.1	11.1	42.9	100	10	60	20	20	50	100
Peanut	1	100	0	0	0	100	9	66.7	22.2	11.1	50	100
Apple	5	60	0	40	33.3	66.7	8	50	12.5	37.5	0	100
Peach	2	100	0	0	0	100	1	100	0	0	0	100
Celery	1	100	0	0	100	100	0	-	-	-	-	-
Cow's milk	0	-	-	-	-	-	1	100	0	0	0	100
Hen's egg	0	-	-	-	-	-	1	100	0	0	0	100

* This is calculated as a percentage from those with a positive DBPCFC.

frequency of oral allergy symptoms differed, being higher in the responders (61% *vs* 49%, p = 0.02*)*, which could indicate that responders from the 2nd stage of the study were more likely to have a probable food allergy compared to non-responders. This would mean that the differences found between community and outpatients in the 2nd stage would even be larger. For the 3rd stage, no differences were seen between responders and non-responders with regard to age, sex and symptoms (data not shown).

Although the response rate was low, the profile of responders and non-responders were largely similar, and therefore it is thought that a possible non-response bias would not play a major role. Low response rates are not unusual in population based studies investigating the prevalence of food allergy [3,5].

The gold standard for the diagnosis of FA is DBPCFC [16]. However, DBPCFC is time-consuming, expensive, subjects patients to potential severe allergic reactions, requires the need for well equipped facilities and may not be able to reproduce the conditions that occurred when the reported allergic reaction took place [17,18]. Due to these practical problems, in normal clinical settings FA is often diagnosed by a thorough medical history and a test for sensitization [17,19]. In our study, medical history and sIgE was used to define a probable FA since this could be performed in all participants and outpatients. Certain participants in the community and outpatient studies agreed to undergo DBPCFC and, whilst a relatively small sample, no differences were seen in the rates of either positive DBPCFC (78% and 64%, respectively) or the objective signs between the two groups. These data indicate that the clinical characteristics of individuals with a probable FA in this population were similar between the two populations and that the estimates of prevalence relying only on clinical history and sIgE will over-estimate rates of confirmed food allergy by around 22-37%. A low participation rate in DBPCFC is also reported in other studies [5,7]. The main reason for refusal to participate in DBPCFC in our patients was the lack of time.

In general, it might be expected that the frequency of severe FA in outpatients referred to a tertiary allergy center is higher compared to the community. In this study we observed no significant difference in the frequency of severe symptoms between both groups. Of the participants with a probable FA in the community, 40.4% had never sought medical care for their symptoms to food and of these, 46.4% had severe symptoms upon ingestion of the causative food (data not shown). Thus, severe symptoms are not always a trigger for FA-patients to seek medical care.

Conclusions

In the Netherlands, there are large differences in self-reported FA between community and outpatients. However, Dutch community and outpatients with a probable FA do not differ with respect to severity, causative foods, sensitization and DBPCFC-outcome.

Abbreviations

DBPCFC: Double-blind placebo-controlled food challenge; FA: Food allergy; OR: Odds ratio.

Competing interests

Prof. Dr. S. Vieths reports personal fees from Food Allergy Resource and Research Program, Lincoln, NE USA, personal fees from Medical University of Vienna, Austria, grants from Monsanto Company, personal fees from American Academy of Asthma, Allergy and Immunology, personal fees from Deutsche Dermatologische Gesellschaft, personal fees from Spanish Society of Allergy and Clinical Immunology, personal fees from Westdeutsche Arbeitsgemeinschaft für pädiatrische Pneumologie und Allergologie e.V., Köln, Germany, personal fees from Gesellschaft für pädiatrische Allergologie und Umweltmedizin, personal fees from Ärzteverband Deutscher Allergologen, personal fees from Schattauer Allergologie Handbuch, personal fees from Elsevier Nahrungsmittelallergien und Intoleranzen, non-financial support from German Research Foundation, non-financial support from Federal Institute for Risk Assessment, non-financial support from Austrian Society for Allergology and Immunology, non-financial support from European Directorate for the Quality of Medicines and Health Care, non-financial support from European Academy of Allergy and Clinical Immunology , non-financial support from World

Allergy Organization, non-financial support from Association Monégasque pour le Perfectionnement des Connaissances des Médicins, non-financial support from Federal Office of Consumer Protection and Food Safety , non-financial support from German Chemical Society (GDCh), non-financial support from Austrian Society for Dermatology and Venerology, non-financial support from AKM Allergiekongress, non-financial support from Austrian Food Chemical Society, outside the submitted work. E. N. Clare Mills has received research support from the European Union, the Biological and Biotechnological Sciences Research Council, the UK Food Standards Agency; is a board member for Novartis, the UK Food Standards Agency, PepsiCo International, the UK Biological and Biotechnological Sciences Research Council, the European Food Safety Authority, the European Academy of Allergy and Clinical Immunology; is consultant for Reacta Biotech Ltd; is employed by the University of Manchester and the Institute of Food Research; has stock/stock options in Reacta Biotech Lts; received grants/pending grants from The Biological and Biotechnological Sciences Research Council, the European union, the UK Food Standards Agency, DBV Technology, Reacta Biotech Ltd, North West Lung Centre Charity, Medical Research Council; has received travel support from ILSI, EAACI, Europa Bio, the British High Commission, the Iceland Allergy Society, Fresenius, EuroFood Tox 2013, Campden BRI, Food Matters Live and the IUNS Annual Meeting (Granada, Spain September 2013); and was paid as a lecturer and supervisor of masters students at Imperial College and as an external examiner at the University of Birmingham.
The rest of the authors declare that they have no relevant conflicts of interest.

Authors' contributions

The study was designed by TL, EvH, IK and ACK. Data was collected by AFML and TL. Analysis of the data and preparing a first draft was performed by TL. Interpretation of data, drafting and revising the manuscript was done by TL, EvH, IK, JP, BKB, CAFMB, JL, AFML, TML, AM, ENCM, RvR, SV, MF, PGB and ACK. All authors read and approved the final manuscript.

Acknowledgement

This work was funded by the EU through EuroPrevall (FP6- FOOD-CT-2005-514000).
We would like to thank Lucía Jimeno and Domingo Barber, f0072om ALK-Abelló, Spain, for providing the skin prick tests materials.

Funding

This work was funded by the EU through EuroPrevall (FP6- FOOD-CT-2005-514000).

Author details

[1]Department of Dermatology/Allergology, University Medical Center Utrecht, PO Box 855003508 GA Utrecht, The Netherlands. [2]Department of Respiratory Epidemiology, Occupational Medicine and Public Health, National Heart and Lung Institute, Imperial College London, London, UK. [3]Allergy Unit, Department of Dermatology, University Hospital Zürich, Zürich, Switzerland. [4]Thermo Fisher Scientific, Uppsala, Sweden. [5]Institute of Food Research, Norwich Research Park, Colney, Norwich NR4 7UA, UK. [6]Institute of Inflammation and Repair, Manchester Academic Health Sciences Centre, Manchester Institute of Biotechnology, The University of Manchester, Manchester, UK. [7]Department of Experimental Immunology and Department of Otorhinolaryngology, Academic Medical Center of the University of Amsterdam, Amsterdam, The Netherlands. [8]Division of Allergology, Paul-Ehrlich-Institut, Federal Institute for Vaccines and Biomedicines, Langen, Germany. [9]Allergy Department, Hospital Clinico San Carlos, IdISSC, Madrid, Spain. [10]Current affiliation: NIZO food research, Ede, The Netherlands.

References

1. Rona RJ, Keil T, Summers C, Gislason D, Zuidmeer L, Sodergren E, et al. The prevalence of food allergy: a meta-analysis. J Allergy Clin Immunol. 2007;120(3):638–46.
2. Madsen C. Prevalence of food allergy: an overview. Proc Nutr Soc. 2005;64(4):413–7.
3. Zuberbier T, Edenharter G, Worm M, Ehlers I, Reimann S, Hantke T, et al. Prevalence of adverse reactions to food in Germany - a population study. Allergy. 2004;59(3):338–45.
4. Kanny G, Moneret-Vautrin DA, Flabbee J, Beaudouin E, Morisset M, Thevenin F. Population study of food allergy in France. J Allergy Clin Immunol. 2001;108(1):133–40.
5. Young E, Stoneham MD, Petruckevitch A, Barton J, Rona R. A population study of food intolerance. Lancet. 1994;343(8906):1127–30.
6. Osterballe M, Hansen TK, Mortz CG, Host A, Bindslev-Jensen C. The prevalence of food hypersensitivity in an unselected population of children and adults. Pediatr Allergy Immunol. 2005;16(7):567–73.
7. Jansen JJ, Kardinaal AF, Huijbers G, Vlieg-Boerstra BJ, Martens BP, Ockhuizen T. Prevalence of food allergy and intolerance in the adult Dutch population. J Allergy Clin Immunol. 1994;93(2):446–56.
8. Jones RB, Hewson P, Kaminski ER. Referrals to a regional allergy clinic - an eleven year audit. BMC Public Health. 2010;10:790.
9. Mills EN, Mackie AR, Burney P, Beyer K, Frewer L, Madsen C, et al. The prevalence, cost and basis of food allergy across Europe. Allergy. 2007;62(7):717–22.
10. Kummeling I, Mills EN, Clausen M, Dubakiene R, Perez CF, Fernandez-Rivas M, et al. The EuroPrevall surveys on the prevalence of food allergies in children and adults: background and study methodology. Allergy. 2009;64(10):1493–7.
11. Cochrane SA, Salt LJ, Wantling E, Rogers A, Coutts J, Ballmer-Weber BK, et al. Development of a standardized low-dose double-blind placebo-controlled challenge vehicle for the EuroPrevall project. Allergy. 2012;67(1):107–13.
12. Zuidmeer L, Goldhahn K, Rona RJ, Gislason D, Madsen C, Summers C, et al. The prevalence of plant food allergies: a systematic review. J Allergy Clin Immunol. 2008;121(5):1210–8.
13. Emmett SE, Angus FJ, Fry JS, Lee PN. Perceived prevalence of peanut allergy in Great Britain and its association with other atopic conditions and with peanut allergy in other household members. Allergy. 1999;54(4):380–5.
14. Woods RK, Abramson M, Bailey M, Walters EH. International prevalences of reported food allergies and intolerances. Comparisons arising from the European Community Respiratory Health Survey (ECRHS) 1991–1994. Eur J Clin Nutr. 2001;55(4):298–304.
15. Lessler JT, Kalsbeek WD. Nonsampling error in surveys. New York: Wiley; 1992.
16. Boyce JA, Assa'ad A, Burks AW, Jones SM, Sampson HA, Wood RA, et al. Guidelines for the diagnosis and management of food allergy in the United States: report of the NIAID-sponsored expert panel. J Allergy Clin Immunol. 2010;126(6 Suppl):S1–58.
17. Asero R, Fernandez-Rivas M, Knulst AC, Bruijnzeel-Koomen CA. Double-blind, placebo-controlled food challenge in adults in everyday clinical practice: a reappraisal of their limitations and real indications. Curr Opin Allergy Clin Immunol. 2009;9(4):379–85.
18. Sampson HA. Immunologically mediated food allergy: the importance of food challenge procedures. Ann Allergy. 1988;60(3):262–9.
19. Seitz CS, Pfeuffer P, Raith P, Brocker EB, Trautmann A. Food allergy in adults: an over- or underrated problem? Dtsch Arztebl Int. 2008;105(42):715–23.

7

Milk: a postnatal imprinting system stabilizing FoxP3 expression and regulatory T cell differentiation

Bodo C. Melnik[1*], Swen Malte John[1], Pedro Carrera-Bastos[2] and Gerd Schmitz[3]

Abstract

Background: Breastfeeding has protective effects for the development of allergies and atopy. Recent evidence underlines that consumption of unboiled farm milk in early life is a key factor preventing the development of atopic diseases. Farm milk intake has been associated with increased demethylation of *FOXP3* and increased numbers of regulatory T cells (Tregs). Thus, the questions arose which components of farm milk control the differentiation and function of Tregs, critical T cell subsets that promote tolerance induction and inhibit the development of allergy and autoimmunity.

Findings: Based on translational research we identified at least six major signalling pathways that could explain milk's biological role controlling stable FoxP3 expression and Treg differentiation: (1) via maintaining appropriate magnitudes of Akt-mTORC1 signalling, (2) via transfer of milk fat-derived long-chain ω-3 fatty acids, (3) via transfer of milk-derived exosomal microRNAs that apparently decrease *FOXP3* promoter methylation, (4) via transfer of exosomal transforming growth factor-β, which induces SMAD2/SMAD3-dependent FoxP3 expression, (5) via milk-derived *Bifidobacterium* and *Lactobacillus* species that induce interleukin-10 (IL-10)-mediated differentiation of Tregs, and (6) via milk-derived oligosaccharides that serve as selected nutrients for the growth of bifidobacteria in the intestine of the new born infant.

Conclusion: Accumulating evidence underlines that milk is a complex signalling and epigenetic imprinting network that promotes stable FoxP3 expression and long-lasting Treg differentiation, crucial postnatal events preventing atopic and autoimmune diseases.

Keywords: Epigenetic, Exosome, FoxO1, FoxP3, Milk, MicroRNA, mTORC1, Probiotics, TGF-β, Treg

Background

Children who grow up on traditional farms are protected from atopic diseases [1]. Early-life consumption of unboiled cow's milk has been identified as the most protective factor for the development of atopy [2–10]. Farm milk exposure has been associated with increased numbers of $CD4^{+}CD25^{+}FoxP3^{+}$ regulatory T cells (Tregs), lower atopic sensitization and asthma in 4.5-year-old children [11]. Treg cell numbers are negatively associated with asthma and perennial immunoglobulin E serum levels [11]. However, the allergy-preventive effectors of milk, which stimulate the development of Tregs remain elusive. Based on translational research we provide six potential milk-derived signalling pathways that could promote appropriate differentiation and maturation of Tregs.

Findings

Amino acids

Milk is the postnatal nutritional environment of all mammals that mediates immune stimulatory functions, especially long-term stable expression of FoxP3, the key transcription factor of Tregs. Milk protein provides appropriate amounts of certain insulinotropic amino

*Correspondence: melnik@t-online.de
[1] Department of Dermatology, Environmental Medicine and Health Theory, University of Osnabrück, Sedanstrasse 115, 49090 Osnabrück, Germany
Full list of author information is available at the end of the article

acids such as essential branched-chain amino acids that induce the secretion of insulin as well as amino acids such as tryptophan that increase hepatic insulin-like growth factor-1 (IGF-1) secretion [12–21]. Both growth hormones synergistically activate the phosphoinosite-3 kinase (PI3K)-Akt pathway. Control of PI3K in Treg cells is essential for Treg lineage homeostasis and stability [22, 23]. Diminished control of PI3K activity in Treg cells reduces expression of the interleukin-2 (IL-2) receptor α subunit CD25, accumulation of $FoxP3^{+}CD25^{-}$ cells and, ultimately, loss of expression of the transcription factor FoxP3 in these cells [23]. Excessive postnatal protein intake via infant formula feeding has been demonstrated to increase infant's serum levels of insulin and IGF-1 accelerating growth and weight gain (early protein hypothesis) [24–26]. Rapid weight gain in infancy has been linked to an increased risk of asthma [27–29].

Tregs are a developmentally and functionally distinct T cell subpopulation that is engaged in sustaining immunological self-tolerance and homeostasis. The transcription factor FoxP3 plays a key role in Treg development and function [30–33]. There is accumulating evidence that insufficient maturation and differentiation of Tregs play a key role in the development of common allergic diseases and autoimmunity [34–39].

Notably, FoxP3 expression is linked to nutrient signalling via Akt-mediated phosphorylation of the transcription factors FoxO1 and FoxO3. Increased insulin/IGF-1 signalling leads to inactivation of FoxO1 and FoxO3a by their phosphorylation-dependent extrusion form the nucleus into the cytoplasm. Both FoxO1 and FoxO3a exert stimulatory effects on FoxP3 expression [40] (Fig. 1). A FoxO3a-binding motif is present in the proximal region of the *FOXP3* promoter [40]. The absence of FoxO1 severely curtails the development of $FoxP3^{+}$ Tregs. In addition, the absence of FoxO3 exacerbates the effects of the loss of FoxO1 [41]. Thus, there is compelling evidence that increased PI3K-Akt-signalling blocks FoxP3 expression by sequestering FoxO factors [42]. FoxO transcription factors cooperatively control the differentiation of $FoxP3^{+}$ Tregs [43]. FoxO proteins function in a Treg-intrinsic manner to regulate thymic and TGF-β-induced FoxP3 expression, in line with the ability of FoxO proteins to bind to *FOXP3* locus and control *FOXP3* promoter activity [43]. FoxO proteins are considered to play crucial roles in specifying the Treg cell lineage [43]. Genome-wide analysis of FoxO1 binding sites reveals ~300 FoxO1-bound target genes that do not seem to be directly regulated by FoxP3. These findings show that the evolutionarily ancient Akt-FoxO1 signalling module controls a genetic program indispensable for Treg cell function [44].

Upregulated PI3K-Akt signalling in the presence of sufficient amounts of branched-chain amino acids and

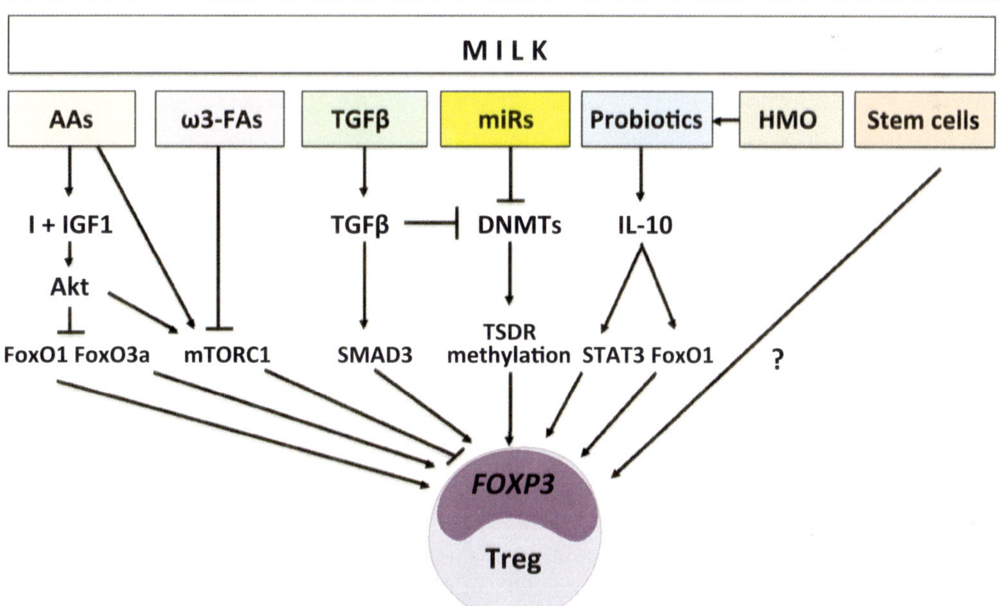

Fig. 1 Synoptic working model for milk-induced FoxP3 expression and regulatory T cell (Treg) differentiation. The transcription factors FoxO1, FoxO3a, SMAD3 and STAT3 all enhance FoxP3 expression. Milk exosomal microRNAs and TGFβ attenuate DNA methyltransferase (DNMT) expression promoting TSDR demethylation (AAs: amino acids; ω3-FAs; ω-3 fatty acids; HMO: human milk oligosaccharides; I: insulin; IGF1: insulin-like growth factor-1; miRs: microRNA-148a, microRNA-29, microRNA-21; mTORC1: mechanistic target of rapamycin complex 1; TGFβ: transforming growth factor-β; STAT3: signal transducer and activator of transcription 3; TSDR: Treg-specific demethylated region)

glutamine increases the activity of the nutrient-sensitive kinase mechanistic target of rapamycin complex 1 (mTORC1) [45–47]. Milk has recently been identified as a signalling system of mammalian evolution controlling mTORC1-dependent translation [48, 49]. Enhanced mTORC1 activity was found in the brain and ileum of mice with cow's milk allergy (CMA) [50]. Treatment with the mTORC1 inhibitor rapamycin significantly increased the mRNA expression of FoxP3 in the ileum and Peyer's patches of CMA mice. A correlation between the extent of mTORC1-mediated S6K1 phosphorylation and FoxP3 mRNA expression in the ileum was demonstrated [50].

Taken together, the Akt-mTORC1 axis controls FoxP3 expression and differentially regulates effector and Treg cell linage commitment [43, 51–53]. It is thus conceivable that a well-balanced transfer of critical amino acids via breastfeeding controls Akt-mTORC1-mediated Treg differentiation, which may be disturbed by artificial formula feeding with high protein content [54, 55].

Long-chain ω-3-fatty acids

Part of the asthma-protective effect is associated with the intake of raw cow's milk and was explained by higher levels of polyunsaturated ω-3 fatty acids of farm milk [56]. Remarkably, it has been demonstrated in a mouse model of atopic dermatitis that administration of the ω-3 fatty acid docosahexaenoic acid upregulates the generation of TGF-β-dependent $CD4^+$ $Foxp3^+$ Tregs [57, 58]. Furthermore, fatty acids play a role in mTORC1 activation. Whereas the saturated fatty acid palmitate activates mTORC1, the ω-3 fatty acid eicosopentaenoic acid inhibits mTORC1 activation [59]. Thus, ω-3-fatty acids may not only attenuate pro-inflammatory eicosanoid biosynthesis but may exert direct effects on FoxP3 Treg activity. In fact, it has been demonstrated that Tregs transfer ω-3 long chain polyunsaturated fatty acids-induced tolerance in mice allergic to cow's milk protein [60].

MicroRNAs

Extracellular RNAs and especially exosomal microRNAs are regarded as most important factors involved in the regulation of the immune system [61, 62]. Human breast milk is a body fluid that is highly enriched in mRNAs and microRNAs [63]. MicroRNAs are either packaged with proteins (i.e. Ago2, HDL, and other RNA-binding proteins or wrapped in small membranous particles (i.e. exosomes, microvesicles, and apoptotic bodies) [64–67]. Human, bovine and porcine milk transfer high numbers of exosomes that contain microRNAs [68–70]. Recent evidence indicates that human milk microRNAs primarily originate from the mammary gland resulting in unique microRNA profiles of fractionated milk [71]. Recently, we hypothesized that milk transmits microRNAs (microRNA-155, microRNA-148a, microRNA-29b, microRNA-21) that may induce thymic $FoxP3^+$ Treg differentiation thereby preventing the development of allergy [72]. Indeed, farm milk consumption is associated with higher *FOXP3* demethylation and higher Treg cell numbers [11]. Stable expression of FoxP3 in Tregs depends on DNA demethylation at the Treg-specific demethylated region (TSDR), a conserved CpG-rich region within the *FOXP3* locus [73–75]. In contrast, hypermethylation of the *FOXP3* gene has been associated with reduced Treg function and allergy [76, 77]. Notably, atopic individuals express lower numbers of demethylated $FoxP3^+$ Tregs [78].

There are two potential mechanisms of DNA demethylation: (1) passive demethylation through inhibition of DNA methyltransferases (DNMTs) and (2) active demethylation mediated by ten-eleven-translocation (TET) 2 and 3 [79]. TET2 binding to CpG-rich regions requires the interaction of TET2 with the protein IDAX (also known as CXXC4) [80]. Intriguingly, the CXXC DNA-binding domains can bind unmethylated DNA and recruit TET2 via IDAX [81]. Thus, DNMT inhibition may favour active TET2-mediated TSDR demethylation.

Both DNMT1 and DNMT3b are associated with the *FOXP3* locus in $CD4^+$ cells [82, 83]. Remarkably, DNMT1 deficiency resulted in highly efficient FoxP3 induction following TCR stimulation [82]. Importantly, DNMT1 is a direct target of microRNA-148a [84], which is abundant in bovine colostrum, mature cow's milk, and human breast milk [68, 85, 86]. MicroRNA-148a is highly expressed in bovine milk fat and milk fat globules of human breast milk [87, 88]. MicroRNA-148a directly downregulates the expression DNMT1 and DNMT3b, whereas microRNA-21, another abundant microRNA of cow's milk, indirectly inhibits DNMT1 expression by targeting RASGRP1 [84]. MicroRNA-29b increases dose-dependently in human serum after intake of pasteurized cow's milk [89]. MicroRNA-29 targets DNMT3a and DNMT3b [90]. Remarkably, nucleotide sequences of microRNA-148a-3p, microRNA-29b and microRNA-21 of *Homo sapiens* and *Bos taurus* are identical (mirbase.org). Kirchner et al. [87] recently suggested that microRNAs of unprocessed cow's milk mediate the allergy preventive farm milk effect. It is of functional importance that most milk-derived microRNAs are transported either in exosomes or milk fat globules [48, 49, 69, 70, 88–93].

It has recently been demonstrated that bovine milk microRNAs (microRNA-29b, microRNA-200c) are taken up in reasonable amounts by healthy human subjects after consumption of pasteurized cow's milk [88]. Further evidence underlines that bovine milk exosomes are able to cross human intestinal cells and vascular endothelial cells via endocytosis [94, 95].

Notably, boiling of raw cow's milk abolishes the allergy-preventive farm milk effect [3] and results in substantial loss of microRNA-148a-3p [87]. MicroRNA-155, another important immune regulatory microRNA of milk [72], targets suppressor of cytokine signalling 1 (SOCS1), which maintains STAT5 activity further enhancing Treg differentiation [96]. Boiling of milk may disrupt the protective lipid bilayer of milk exosomes accelerating the degradation of critical milk microRNAs. Furthermore, heat-induced alterations of exosomal membrane proteins may disturb intestinal exosome uptake. Thus, native milk-derived exosomal microRNAs via suppressing DNMTs may provide pivotal epigenetic signals stabilizing FoxP3 expression and Treg differentiation.

Exosomal transforming growth factor-β

It has been demonstrated that exosomes of cow's milk not only transfer microRNAs but also transforming growth factor-β (TGF-β) [97]. The TGF-β signalling pathway activates the transcription factors SMAD2 and SMAD3 [98, 99]. SMAD3 is a crucial transcription factor enhancing FoxP3 expression via binding to the conserved non-coding sequence 1 (CNS1) of *FOXP3* [100] (Fig. 1). Experimental evidence reveals that TGF-β in the context of T cell receptor (TCR) stimulation induces FoxP3 gene transcription in thymic Treg precursors, $CD4^+$ $CD8^-$ $CD25^-$ semimature and mature single-positive thymocytes [101]. TGF-β also converts naïve T cells into inducible Treg (iTregs) and protects Tregs against apoptosis and destabilization [102]. Importantly, it has been demonstrated that TGF-β-induced expression of FoxP3 in T cells is mediated through inactivation of the kinase ERK [103]. TGF-β via inhibition of ERK activation downregulates the expression of DNMT1, DNMT3a and DNMT3b associated with increased FoxP3 expression [97]. Recently, Arntz et al. [104] confirmed that bovine milk exosomes induce FoxP3 expression and Treg differentiation in murine splenocytes. Thymus-derived exosomes as well are able to induce $FoxP3^+$ Tregs in peripheral tissues [105]. Moreover, the incubation of peripheral blood mononuclear cells with isolated human breast milk exosomes increased the number of $FoxP3^+CD4^+CD25^+$ Tregs [106]. Thus, milk-derived exosomal TGF-β acts via transcriptional control and epigenetic regulation of FoxP3 expression. It is noteworthy to mention that deficient TGF-β signalling is associated with activation of the PI3K/Akt pathway [107], which suppresses FoxO signalling.

Bifidobaceria and lactobacilli

Human milk is a source of living bifidobacteria and lactobacilli for the infant gut [108–111]. *Bifidobacterium breve, B. adolescentis, B. bifidum,* and *Lactobacillus plantarum WLPL04* were isolated from human milk samples [108, 110]. There is accumulating evidence that probiotic bacteria generate FoxP3 T-cell responses in the small intestine [112]. *L. plantarum WCFS1, L. salivarius UCC118,* and *L. lactis MG1363* upregulate numbers of $CD11c^+$ $MHCII^+$ dendritic cells in the immune-sampling Peyer's patches [112]. *L. plantarum, L. salivarius,* and *L. lactis* attenuate Th2 responses and increase Treg frequencies in healthy mice in a strain dependent manner [113]. Oral consumption of *Bifidobacterium infantis 35624* enhanced IL-10 secretion and FoxP3 expression in human peripheral blood cells pointing to the immune-stimulatory effect of bifidobacteria on $FoxP3^+$ iTreg induction [114, 115]. Furthermore, it has been demonstrated that bifidobacteria stimulate TGF-β, which contributes to Treg differentiation [116].

Special attention has been paid on the critical role of the anti-inflammatory cytokine IL-10 in probiotica-induced anti-inflammatoy intestinal immune responses [110, 117, 118]. Despite heat-killing, *Lactobacillus pentosus* strain S-PT84 exhibited anti-allergic effects by modulating the Th1/Th2 balance and inducing Tregs [119]. Live and heat-killed *Lactobacillus rhamnosus* suspensions were able to induce the synthesis of different cytokines including IL-10 [120]. Heat-killed *Lactobacillus acidophilus* strain L-92 produced higher levels of Foxp3, IL-10 and TGF-β compared to control mice and suppresses allergic contact dermatitis [121]. In a bovine β-lactoglobulin-sensitized mice model, oral administration of heat-killed *L. acidophilus* exhibited increased mRNA expression of Foxp3 and TGF-β [122]. It should be noticed, that heat-treatment of probiotics may also result in a loss of immune-regulatory functions. However, the majority of studies using either native or heat-treated bifididobacteria or lactobacilli exhibits an upregulation of IL-10, TGFβ and FoxP3 [116, 119–122]. Remarkably, IL-10 potentiates differentiation of human induced Tregs via STAT3 and FoxO1 [123]. Hsu et al. [123] demonstrated that the presence of IL-10, in addition to TGF-β, leads to increased expansion of $Foxp3^+$ iTregs with enhanced CTLA-4 expression and suppressive capability, comparable to that of natural Tregs. This process is dependent on IL-10R-mediated STAT3 signalling. Additionally, IL-10-induced inhibition of Akt phosphorylation and subsequent preservation of FoxO1 function are critical. In contrast to formula feeding, the presence of maternal milk in β-lactoglobulin-sensitized rat pups exhibited an immune response profile similar to that of unchallenged dam-reared rats but with greater FoxP3 mRNA expression and $CD4^+$ $FoxP3^+$ cells [124]. These data may explain the preventive effect of probiotics for sensitization to common food allergens associated with a reduced incidence of atopic eczema in early childhood [125]. However, due to a lack of well-designed studies convincing evidence for the prevention of allergic asthma by probiotic treatment is still missing [126, 127]. The time of onset of probiotic exposure, which is physiologically natural birth and the period of breastfeeding, may play critical roles for probiotica-induced Treg maturation.

Milk oligosaccharides

Human milk contains large amounts of free oligosaccharides (HMOs). HMOs have been shown to exert anti-inflammatory properties, and evidence for their immune-modulatory effects is increasing [128–130]. A growing literature suggests that human milk contains viable bacteria [131]. McGuire et al. [131] postulated that human milk should be regarded as a probiotic food. Human milk oligosaccharides (HMOs) are minimally digested by the infant and are utilized by bifidobacteria [132]. One postulated function for these oligosaccharides is to enrich a specific "healthy" microbiota containing bifidobacteria, a genus commonly observed in the faeces of breastfed infants [133]. Recent studies show that some species of bifidobacteria are equipped with genetic and enzymatic sets dedicated to the utilization of HMOs promoting HMO-dependent growth of bifidobacteria [134]. Among gut microbes, the presence of enzymes required for degrading HMOs with type-1 chains is essentially limited to infant-gut-associated bifidobacteria, suggesting HMOs serve as selected nutrients for the bacteria pointing to a co-evolution between bifidobacteria and human beings mediated by HMOs [135]. Formula feeding in comparison to breastfeeding compromises the development of the physiological gut microbiome. In breastfed Rhesus infants *Bifidobacteria* and *Lactobacillus* predominated, whereas in formula-fed infants *Ruminococcus* was predominant [26]. Breastfed human infants harbour a faecal microbiota more than twice increased in *Bifidobacterium* numbers compared to formula-fed infants [136]. After formula feeding, *Atopobium* was found in significant counts and the numbers of *Bifidobacteria* dropped followed by increasing numbers of *Bacteroides* population [136]. Infant formulas containing non-digestible oligosaccharides similar to the composition in breast milk or a combination of lactic acid bacteria have been shown to harbour preventive effects towards immune-regulatory disorders [137, 138]. In fact, recent studies with whey and casein-sensitised mice showed that $CD25^+$ Treg contribute to the suppression of the allergic effector response in sensitised mice induced by dietary intervention with non-digestible carbohydrates [139, 140]. Thus, it appears that milk is mammal's early life probiotic nutrient system supporting and maintaining *Bifidobacteria* and *Lactobacillus* species that induce Tregs and control immune responses.

Conclusions

Compelling evidence underlines that milk is not a simple food for infants but represents a sophisticated signalling network that promotes the differentiation and long-lasting maintenance of Tregs, the central players suppressing the development of allergy and autoimmunity. Milk provides an intricate metabolic, epigenetic, probiotic and stem cell-derived system that induces stable expression of FoxP3, the master transcription factor of Tregs. The critical allergy-preventive factor in cow's milk appears to be heat-sensitive and is abolished by boiling of milk. As amino acids and the majority of long-chain ω-3 fatty acids withstand the boiling process, heat-sensitive compounds such as milk exosomes, probiotic bacteria and stem cells are the potential candidates for long-lasting Treg differentiation. In more than 200,000 million years of lactation [141, 142] the evolution of milk had plenty of time to create a sophisticated regulatory network optimizing the infant's Treg differentiation allowing appropriate tolerance development during the postnatal period of mammalian life. In this regard, unprocessed milk should be regarded as a conditioner for tolerance development. After birth, the newborn's immune system encounters foreign environmental antigens such as nutrients, pollens and house dust mite allergens, which via antigen-specific TCR-mediated activation induce antigen-specific Tregs. The milk-related signalling pathways presented here, may in a synergistic manner enhance antigen-specific Treg generation associated with the induction of allergen-specific immune tolerance (Fig. 1).

Most recent data underline that developing natural Treg (nTreg) cells in the thymus acquire a Treg-specific and stable hypomethylation pattern in a limited number of genes, which encode key molecules including FoxP3, essential for Treg cell function. This epigenetic change is acquired via TCR stimulation, beginning prior to FoxP3 expression. The Treg-specific DNA hypomethylated regions generally act as gene enhancers in steady state nTreg cells, contributing to the stable expression of Treg function-associated key genes including Ctla4, Il2ra, and Ikzf4 in addition to FoxP3 [143, 144]. Recent work suggests that the establishment and stability of Tregs is mediated by a number of mechanisms besides FoxP3 expression, such as epigenetic modifications, FoxO1, FoxO3a localization, expression of Eos and signalling via Neuropilin-1 [143]. To understand the pathogenesis of allergy development it is most important to characterize the immune regulatory networking of native milk. Future studies should thus focus on natural unprocessed milk and its regulatory mechanisms that support long-lasting stability of Tregs mediating livelong tolerance induction against harmless environmental antigens and autoantigens [145, 146]. We are at the beginning to understand the complex interplay of milk's regulatory factors inducing and stabilizing the infant's FoxP3 expression. Yet, we have no idea about the functional priority of milk-derived factors involved in Treg lineage commitment. It is thus prudent to rely on the regulatory effectiveness of our own lactation genome, which co-evolved with the lactation-associated microbiome. Therefore, we recommend breastfeeding for adequate Treg maturation and the prevention of allergic diseases of human infants. However, for mothers who are not able to provide breast milk, human donor milk might be an alternative for appropriate Treg differentiation. Countrywide access to operating human milk banks in East Germany before Germany's unification in 1990, may explain the lower prevalence rates of atopic diseases in East versus West Germany [147, 148]. Artificial formulas still substantially differ from human breast milk. If milk exosomal microRNAs play a key role in Treg differentiation, it is of critical concern that current infant formula only contains very few human lactation-specific microRNAs [149]. The addition of bovine milk exosomal microRNAs may represent a future improvement of artificial formula feeding. Due to legal aspects and the risk of pathogen transfer, raw cow's milk can not be recommended as an agent for allergy prevention. However, in the future, it might be possible to prepare sterilized bovine milk exosomes for this purpose. It has already been shown that bovine milk exosomes increased Foxp3 expression and attenuated arthritis in two mouse models [104].

Abbreviations

CMA: cow's milk allergy; CNS: conserved non-coding sequence; DNMT: DNA methyltransferase; FoxO: forkhead box class O; FoxP3: forkhead box P3; HMO: human milk oligosaccharides; IGF-1: insulin-like growth factor-1; IL-2: interleukin 2; IL-10: interleukin 10; microRNA: micro ribonucleic acid; mTORC1: mechanistic target of rapamycin complex 1; PI3K: phosphoinositide-3-kinase; SOCS: suppressor of cytokine signalling; STAT: signal transducer and activator of transcription; TCR: T cell receptor; TSDR: Treg-specific demethylation region; TET: ten-eleven-translocation; Treg: regulatory T-cell.

Authors' contributions

BCM performed translational research and wrote the manuscript. SMJ and PCB screened the literature and proved the data on atopy epidemiology. GS analyzed the data on exosome microRNA biology. All authors read and approved the final manuscript.

Author details

[1] Department of Dermatology, Environmental Medicine and Health Theory, University of Osnabrück, Sedanstrasse 115, 49090 Osnabrück, Germany.
[2] Center for Primary Health Care Research, Lund University, Lund, Sweden.
[3] Institute for Clinical Chemistry and Laboratory Medicine, University Hospital Regensburg, University of Regensburg, Josef-Strauss-Allee 11, 93053 Regensburg, Germany.

Competing interests

The authors declare that they have no competing interests.

References

1. von Mutius E, Vercelli D. Farm living: effects on childhood asthma and allergy. Nat Rev Immunol. 2010;10(12):861–8.
2. Perkin MR, Strachan DP. Which aspects of the farming lifestyle explain the inverse association with childhood allergy? J Allergy Clin Immunol. 2006;117(6):1374–81.
3. Loss G, Apprich S, Waser M, Kneifel W, Genuneit J, Büchele G, et al. The protective effect of farm milk consumption on childhood asthma and atopy: the GABRIELA study. J Allergy Clin Immmunol. 2011;128(4):766–73.
4. Braun-Fahrländer C, von Mutius E. Can farm milk consumption prevent allergic diseases? Clin Exp Allergy. 2011;41(1):29–35.
5. Illi S, Depner M, Genuneit J, Horak E, Loss G, Strunz-Lehner C, et al. Protection from childhood asthma and allergy in Alpine farm environments—the GABRIEL Advanced Studies. J Allergy Clin Immunol. 2012;129(6):1470–7.
6. Loss G, Bitter S, Wohlgensinger J, Frei R, Roduit C, Genuneit J, et al. Prenatal and early-life exposures alter expression of innate immunity genes: the PASTURE cohort study. J Allergy Clin Immunol. 2012;130(2):523–30.
7. von Mutius E. Maternal farm exposure/ingestion of unpasteurized cow's milk and allergic disease. Curr Opin Gastroenterol. 2012;28(6):570–6.
8. Wlasiuk G, Vercelli D. The farm effect, or: when, what and how a farming environment protects from asthma and allergic disease. Curr Opin Allergy Clin Immunol. 2012;12(5):461–6.
9. Lluis A, Schaub B. Lessons from the farm environment. Curr Opin Allergy Clin Immunol. 2012;12(2):158–63.
10. Sozanska B, Pearce N, Dudek K, Cullinan P. Consumption of unpasteurized milk and its effects on atopy and asthma in children and adult inhabitants in rural Poland. Allergy. 2013;68(5):644–50.
11. Lluis A, Depner M, Gaugler B, Saas P, Casaca VI, Raedler D, et al. Increased regulatory T-cell numbers are associated with farm milk exposure and lower atopic sensitization and asthma in childhood. J Allergy Clin Immunol. 2014;133(2):551–9.
12. Hoyt G, Hickey MS, Cordain L. Dissociation of the glycaemic and insulinaemic responses to whole and skimmed milk. Br J Nutr. 2005;93(2):175–7.
13. Hoppe C, Mølgaard C, Dalum C, Vaag A, Michaelsen KF. Differential effects of casein versus whey on fasting plasma levels of insulin, IGF-1 and IGF-1/IGFBP-3: results from a randomized 7-day supplementation study in prepubertal boys. Eur J Clin Nutr. 2009;63(9):1076–83.
14. Nilsson M, Stenberg M, Frid AH, Holst JJ, Björck IM. Glycemia and insulinemia in healthy subjects after lactose-equivalent meals of milk and other food proteins: the role of plasma amino acids and incretins. Am J Clin Nutr. 2004;80(5):1246–53.
15. Nilsson M, Holst JJ, Björck IM. Metabolic effects of amino acid mixtures and whey protein in healthy subjects: studies using glucose-equivalent drinks. Am J Clin Nutr. 2007;85(4):996–1004.
16. Salehi A, Gunnerud U, Muhammed SJ, Ostman E, Holst JJ, Björck I, et al. The insulinogenic effects of whey protein is partially mediated by a direct effect of amino acids and GIP on β-cells. Nutr Metab (Lond). 2012;9(1):48.
17. Wheelhouse NM, Stubbs AK, Lomax MA, MacRae JC, Hazlerigg DG. Growth hormone and amino acid supply interact synergistically to control insulin-like growth factor-I production and gene expression in cultured ovine hepatocytes. J Endocrinol. 1999;163(2):353–61.
18. Stubbs AK, Wheelhouse NM, Lomax MA, Hazlerigg DG. Nutrient–hormone interaction in the ovine liver: methionine supply selectively modulates growth hormone-induced IGF-I gene expression. J Endocrinol. 2002;174(2):335–41.
19. Rich-Edwards JW, Ganmaa D, Pollak MN, Nakamoto EK, Kleinman K, Tserendolgor U, et al. Milk consumption and the prepubertal somatotropic axis. Nutr J. 2007;6:28.
20. Rzehak P, Grote V, Lattka E, Weber M, Gruszfeld D, Socha P, et al. Associations of IGF-1 gene variants and milk protein intake with IGF-I concentrations in infants at age 6 months—results from a randomized clinical trial. Growth Horm IGF Res. 2013;23(5):149–58.
21. Fleddermann M, Demmelmair H, Grote V, Bidlingmaier M, Grimminger P, Bielohuby M, et al. Role of selected amino acids on plasma IGF-I concentration in infants. Eur J Nutr. 2015; **[Epub ahead of print]**.

22. Huynh A, Zhang R, Turka LA. Signals and pathways controlling regulatory T cells. Immunol Rev. 2014;258(1):117–31.
23. Huynh A, DuPage M, Priyadharshini B, Sage PT, Quiros J, Borges CM, et al. Control of PI(3) kinase in Treg cells maintains homeostasis and lineage stability. Nat Immunol. 2015;16(2):188–96.
24. Axelsson IE, Ivarsson SA, Räihä NC. Protein intake in early infancy: effects on plasma amino acid concentrations, insulin metabolism, and growth. Pediatr Res. 1989;26(6):614–7.
25. Socha P, Grote V, Gruszfeld D, Janas R, Demmelmair H, Closa-Monasterolo R, et al. Milk protein intake, the metabolic-endocrine response, and growth in infancy: data from a randomized clinical trial. Am J Clin Nutr. 2011;94(6 Suppl):1776S–84S.
26. O'Sullivan A, He X, McNiven EM, Haggarty NW, Lönnerdal B, Slupsky CM. Early diet impacts infant Rhesus gut microbiome, immunity, and metabolism. J Proteome Res. 2013;12(6):2833–45.
27. Litonjua AA, Gold DR. Asthma and obesity: common early-life influences in the inception of disease. J Allergy Clin Immunol. 2008;121(5):1075–84.
28. Paul IM, Camera L, Zeiger RS, Guilbert TW, Bacharier LB, Taussig LM, et al. Relationship between infant weight gain and later asthma. Pediatr Allergy Immunol. 2010;21(1 Pt 1):82–9.
29. Brüske I, Flexeder C, Heinrich J. Body mass index and the incidence of asthma in children. Curr Opin Allergy Clin Immunol. 2014;14(2):155–60.
30. Haque R, Lei F, Xiong X, Song J. The regulation of FoxP3-expressing regulatory T cells. Endocr Metab Immune Disord Drug Targets. 2011;11(4):334–46.
31. Ohkura N, Kitagawa Y, Sakaguchi S. Development and maintenance of regulatory T cells. Immunity. 2013;38(3):414–23.
32. Passerini L, Santoni de Sio FR, Roncarolo MG, Bacchetta R. Forkhead box P3: the peacekeeper of the immune system. Int Rev Immunol. 2014;33(2):129–45.
33. van Nieuwenhuijze A, Liston A. The molecular control of regulatory T cell induction. Prog Mol Biol Transl Sci. 2015;136:69–97.
34. Elkord E. Role of regulatory T cells in allergy: implications for therapeutic strategy. Inflamm Allergy Drug Targets. 2006;5(4):211–7.
35. Nouri-Aria KT, Durham SR. Regulatory T cells and allergic disease. Inflamm Allergy Drug Targets. 2008;7(4):237–52.
36. Zhang H, Kong H, Zeng X, Guo L, Sun X, He S. Subsets of regulatory T cells and their roles in allergy. J Transl Med. 2014;12:125.
37. Palomares O, Yaman G, Azkur A, Akkoc T, Akdis M, Akdis CA. Role of Treg in immune regulation of allergic diseases. Eur J Immunol. 2010;40(5):1232–40.
38. Pellerin L, Jenks JA, Bégin P, Bacchetta R, Nadeau KC. Regulatory T cells and their roles in immune dysregulation and allergy. Immunol Res. 2014;58(2–3):358–68.
39. Robinson DS. Regulatory T cells and asthma. Clin Exp Allergy. 2009;39(9):1314–23.
40. Harada Y, Harada Y, Elly C, Ying G, Paik JH, DePinho RA, et al. Transcription factors Foxo3a and Foxo1 couple the E3 ligase Cbl-b to the induction of Foxp3 expression in induced regulatory T cells. J Exp Med. 2010;207(7):1381–91.
41. Kerdiles YM, Stone EL, Beisner DR, McGargill MA, Ch'en IL, Stockmann C, et al. Foxo transcription factors control regulatory T cell development and function. Immunity. 2010;33(6):890–904.
42. Merkenschlager M, von Boehmer H. PI3 kinase signalling blocks Foxp3 expression by sequestering Foxo factors. J Exp Med. 2010;207(7):1347–50.
43. Ouyang W, Beckett O, Ma Q, Paik JH, DePinho RA, Li MO. Foxo proteins cooperatively control the differentiation of Foxp3$^+$ regulatory T cells. Nat Immunol. 2010;11(7):618–27.
44. Ouyang W, Liao W, Luo CT, Yin N, Huse M, Kim MV, et al. Novel Foxo1-dependent transcriptional programs control T(reg) cell function. Nature. 2012;491(7425):554–9.
45. Efeyan A, Zoncu R, Sabatini DM. Amino acids and mTORC1: from lysosomes to disease. Trends Mol Med. 2012;18(9):524–33.
46. Jewell JL, Russell RC, Guan KL. Amino acid signalling upstream of mTOR. Nat Rev Mol Cell Biol. 2013;14(3):133–9.
47. Bar-Peled L, Sabatini DM. Regulation of mTORC1 by amino acids. Trends Cell Biol. 2014;24(7):400–6.
48. Melnik BC, John SM, Schmitz G. Milk is not just food but most likely a genetic transfection system activating mTORC1 signaling for postnatal growth. Nutr J. 2013;12:103.
49. Melnik BC. Milk—a nutrient system of mammalian evolution promoting mTORC1- dependent translation. Int J Mol Sci. 2015;16(8):17048–87.
50. Wu J, de Theije CG, da Silva SL, van der Horst H, Reinders MT, Broersen LM, et al. mTOR plays an important role in cow's milk allergy-associated behavioral and immunological deficits. Neuropharmacology. 2015;97:220–32.
51. Haxhinasto S, Mathis D, Benoist C. The AKT-mTOR axis regulates de novo differentiation of CD4$^+$FoxP3$^+$ cells. J Exp Med. 2008;205(3):565–74.
52. Sauer S, Bruno L, Hertweck A, Finlay D, Leleu M, Spivakov M, Knight ZA, et al. T cell receptor signaling controls FoxP3 expression via PI3K, Akt, and mTOR. Proc Natl Acad Sci USA. 2008;105(22):7797–802.
53. Delgoffe GM, Kole TP, Zheng Y, Zarek PE, Matthews KL, Xiao B, Worley PF, et al. The mTOR kinase differentially regulates effector and regulatory T cell lineage commitment. Immunity. 2009;30(6):832–44.
54. Melnik BC. Excessive leucine-mTORC1-signalling of cow milk-based infant formula: the missing link to understand early childhood obesity. J Obes. 2012;2012:197653.
55. Melnik BC. The potential mechanistic link between allergy and obesity development and infant formula feeding. Allergy Asthma Clin Immunol. 2014;10(1):37.
56. Brick T, Schober Y, Böcking C, Pekkanen J, Genuneit J, Loss G, et al. ω-3 fatty acids contribute to the asthma-protective effect of unprocessed cow's milk. J Allergy Clin Immunol. 2016. doi:10.1016/j.jaci.2015.10.042 **[Epub ahead of print]**.
57. Haitz KA, Anandasabapathy N. Docosahexaenoic acid alleviates atopic dermatitis in mice by generating T regulatory cells and m2 macrophages. J Invest Dermatol. 2015;135(6):1472–4.
58. Han SC, Koo DH, Kang NJ, Yoon WJ, Kang GJ, Kang HK, et al. Docosahexaenoic acid alleviates atopic dermatitis by generating Tregs and IL-10/TGF-β-modified macrophages via a TGF-β-dependent mechanism. J Invest Dermatol. 2015;135(6):1556–64.
59. Yasuda M, Tanaka Y, Kume S, Morita Y, Chin-Kanasaki M, Araki H, et al. Fatty acids are novel nutrient factors to regulate mTORC1 lysosomal localization and apoptosis in podocytes. Biochim Biophys Acta. 2014;1842(7):1097–108.
60. van den Elsen LW, Meulenbroek LA, van Esch BC, Hofman GA, Boon L, Garssen J, et al. CD25$^+$ regulatory T cells transfer n-3 long chain polyunsaturated fatty acids-induced tolerance in mice allergic to cow's milk protein. Allergy. 2013;68(12):1562–70.
61. de Candia P, De Rosa V, Casiraghi M, Matarese G. Extracellular RNAs: a secret arm of immune system regulation. J Biol Chem. 2016;291(14):7221–8.
62. McCoy-Simandle K, Hanna SJ, Cox D. Exosomes and nanotubes: control of immune cell communication. Int J Biochem Cell Biol. 2016;71:44–54.
63. Weber JA, Baxter DH, Zhang S, Huang DY, Huang KH, Lee MJ, et al. The microRNA spectrum in 12 body fluids. Clin Chem. 2010;56(11):1733–41.
64. Zhu H, Fan GC. Extracellular/circulating microRNAs and their potential role in cardiovascular disease. Am J Cardiovasc Dis. 2011;1(2):138–49.
65. Chen X, Liang H, Zhang J, Zen K, Zhang CY. Horizontal transfer of microRNAs: molecular mechanisms and clinical applications. Protein Cell. 2012;3(1):28–37.
66. Rayner KJ, Hennessy EJ. Extracellular communication via microRNA: lipid particles have a new message. J Lipid Res. 2013;54(5):1174–81.
67. Boon RA, Vickers KC. Intercellular transport of microRNAs. Arterioscler Thromb Vasc Biol. 2013;33(2):186–92.
68. Zhou Q, Li M, Wang X, Li Q, Wang T, Zhu Q, et al. Immune-related microRNAs are abundant in breast milk exosomes. Int J Biol Sci. 2012;8(1):118–23.
69. Izumi H, Tsuda M, Sato Y, Kosaka N, Ochiya T, Iwamoto H, et al. Bovine milk exosomes contain microRNA and mRNA and are taken up by human macrophages. J Dairy Sci. 2015;98(5):2920–33.
70. Gu Y, Li M, Wang T, Liang Y, Zhong Z, Wang X, et al. Lactation-related microRNA expression profiles of porcine breast milk exosomes. PLoS One. 2012;7(8):e43691.
71. Alsaweed M, Lai CT, Hartmann PE, Geddes DT, Kakulas F. Human milk miRNAs primarily originate from the mammary gland resulting in unique miRNA profiles of fractionated milk. Sci Rep. 2016;6:20680.

72. Melnik BC, John SM, Schmitz G. Milk: an exosomal microRNA transmitter promoting thymic regulatory T cell maturation preventing the development of atopy. J Transl Med. 2014;12:43.
73. Polansky JK, Kretschmer K, Freyer J, Floess S, Garbe A, Baron U, et al. DNA methylation controls Foxp3 gene expression. Eur J Immunol. 2008;38(6):1654–63.
74. Polansky JK, Schreiber L, Thelemann C, Ludwig L, Krüger M, Baumgrass R, et al. Methylation matters: binding of Ets-1 to the demethylated Foxp3 gene contributes to the stabilization of Foxp3 expression in regulatory T cells. J Mol Med (Berl). 2010;88(10):1029–40.
75. Toker A, Engelbert D, Garg G, Polansky JK, Floess S, Miyao T, et al. Active demethylation of the Foxp3 locus leads to the generation of stable regulatory T cells within the thymus. J Immunol. 2013;190(7):3180–8.
76. Bacchetta R, Gambineri E, Roncarolo MG. Role of regulatory T cells and FOXP3 in human diseases. J Allergy Clin Immunol. 2007;120(2):227–35.
77. Nadeau K, McDonald-Hyman C, Noth EM, Pratt B, Hammond SK, Balmes J, et al. Ambient air pollution impairs regulatory T-cell function in asthma. J Allergy Clin Immunol. 2010;126(4):845–52.
78. Hinz D, Bauer M, Röder S, Olek S, Huehn J, Sack U, et al. Cord blood Tregs with stable FOXP3 expression are influenced by prenatal environment and associated with atopic dermatitis at the age of one year. Allergy. 2012;67(3):380–9.
79. Koh KP, Rao A. DNA methylation and methylcytosine oxidation in cell fate decisions. Curr Opin Cell Biol. 2013;25(2):152–61.
80. Ko M, Bandukwala HS, Chavez L, Aijö T, Pastor WA, Segal MF, et al. Modulation of TET2 expression and 5-methylcytosine oxidation by the CXXC domain protein IDAX. Nature. 2013;497(7447):122–6.
81. Dunican DD, Pennings S, Meeha RR. The CXXC-TET bridge—mind the methylation gap! Cell Res. 2013;23(8):973–4.
82. Josefowicz SZ, Wilson CB, Rudensky AY. Cutting edge: TCR stimulation is sufficient for induction of Foxp3 expression in the absence of DNA methyltransferase 1. J Immunol. 2009;182(11):6648–52.
83. Lal G, Bromberg JS. Epigenetic mechanisms of regulation of Foxp3 expression. Blood. 2009;114(18):3727–35.
84. Pan W, Zhu S, Yuan M, Cui H, Wang L, Luo X, et al. MicroRNA-21 and microRNA-148a contribute to DNA hypomethylation in Lupus $CD4^+$ T cells by directly and indirectly targeting DNA methyltransferase 1. J Immunol. 2010;184(12):6773–81.
85. Chen X, Gao C, Li H, Huang L, Sun Q, Dong Y, et al. Identification and characterization of microRNAs in raw milk during different periods of lactation, commercial fluid, and powdered milk products. Cell Res. 2010;20(10):1128–37.
86. Izumi H, Kosaka N, Shimizu T, Sekine K, Ochiya T, Takase M. Bovine milk contains microRNA and messenger RNA that are stable under degradative conditions. J Dairy Sci. 2012;95(9):4831–41.
87. Kirchner B, Pfaffl MW, Dumpler J, von Mutius E, Ege MJ. microRNA in native and processed cow's milk and ist implication fort he farm milk effect on asthma. J Allergy Clin Immunol. 2015. doi:10.1016/j.jaci.2015.10.028 **[Epub ahead of print]**.
88. Munch EM, Harris RA, Mohammad M, Benham AL, Pejerrey SM, Showalter L, et al. Transcriptome profiling of microRNA by Next-Gen deep sequencing reveals known and novel miRNA species in the lipid fraction of human breast milk. PLoS One. 2013;8(2):e50564.
89. Baier SR, Nguyen C, Xie F, Wood JR, Zempleni J. MicroRNAs are absorbed in biologically meaningful amounts from nutritionally relevant doses of cow milk and affect gene expression in peripheral blood mononuclear cells, HEK-293 kidney cell cultures, and mouse livers. J Nutr. 2014;144(10):1495–500.
90. Fabbri M, Garzon R, Cimmino A, Liu Z, Zanesi N, Callegari E, et al. MicroRNA-29 family reverts aberrant methylation in lung cancer by targeting DNA methyltransferases 3A and 3B. Proc Natl Acad Sci USA. 2007;104(40):15805–10.
91. Reinhardt TA, Lippolis JD, Nonnecke BJ, Sacco RE. Bovine milk exosome proteome. J Proteomics. 2012;75(5):1486–92.
92. Zhang J, Li S, Li L, Li M, Guo C, Yao J, et al. Exosome and exosomal microRNA: trafficking, sorting, and function. Genomics Proteomics Bioinform. 2015;13(1):17–24.
93. Alsaweed M, Hartmann PE, Geddes DT, Kakulas F. MicroRNAs in breastmilk and the lactating breast: potential immunoprotectors and developmental regulators for the infant and the mother. Int J Environ Res Public Health. 2015;12(11):13981–4020.
94. Wolf T, Baier SR, Zempleni J. The intestinal transport of bovine milk exosomes is mediated by endocytosis in human colon carcinoma Caco-2 cells and rat small intestinal IEC-6 cells. J Nutr. 2015;145(10):2201–6.
95. Kusuma RJ, Manca S, Friemel T, Sukreet S, Nguyen C, Zempleni J. Human vascular endothelial cells transport foreign exosomes from cow's milk by endocytosis. Am J Physiol Cell Physiol. 2016. doi:10.1152/ajpcell.00169.2015 **[Epub ahead of print]**.
96. Yao R, Ma YL, Liang W, Li HH, Ma ZJ, Yu X, et al. MicroRNA-155 modulates Treg and Th17 cells differentiation and Th17 cell function by targeting SOCS1. PLoS One. 2012;7(10):e46082.
97. Pieters BC, Arntz OJ, Bennink MB, Broeren MG, van Caam AP, Koenders MI, et al. Commercial cow milk contains physically stable extracellular vesicles expressing immunoregulatory TGF-β. PLoS One. 2015;10(3):e0121123.
98. Moustakas A, Heldin CH. The regulation of TGFbeta signal transduction. Development. 2009;136(22):3699–714.
99. Heldin CH, Moustakas A. Role of Smads in TGFβ signaling. Cell Tissue Res. 2012;347(1):21–36.
100. Huehn J, Beyer M. Epigenetic and transcriptional control of $Foxp3^+$ regulatory T cells. Semin Immunol. 2015;27(1):10–8.
101. Chen W, Konkel JE. Development of thymic Foxp3(+) regulatory T cells: TGF-β matters. Eur J Immunol. 2015;45(4):958–65.
102. Tran DQ. TGF-β: the sword, the wand, and the shield of FOXP3(+) regulatory T cells. J Mol Cell Biol. 2012;4(1):29–37.
103. Luo X, Zhang Q, Liu V, Xia Z, Pothoven KL, Lee C. Cutting edge: TGF-beta-induced expression of Foxp3 in T cells is mediated through inactivation of ERK. J Immunol. 2008;180(5):2757–61.
104. Arntz OJ, Pieters BC, Oliveira MC, Broeren MG, Bennink MB, de Vries M, et al. Oral administration of bovine milk derived extracellular vesicles attenuates arthritis in two mouse models. Mol Nutr Food Res. 2015;59(9):1701–12.
105. Wang GJ, Liu Y, Qin A, Shah SV, Deng ZB, Xiang X, et al. Thymus exosomes-like particles induce regulatory T cells. J Immunol. 2008;181(8):5242–8.
106. Admyre C, Johansson SM, Qazi KR, Filén JJ, Lahesmaa R, Norman M, et al. Exosomes with immune modulatory features are present in human breast milk. J Immunol. 2007;179(3):1969–78.
107. Bian Y, Terse A, Du J, Hall B, Molinolo A, Zhang P, et al. Progressive tumor formation in mice with conditional deletion of TGF-beta signaling in head and neck epithelia is associated with activation of the PI3K/Akt pathway. Cancer Res. 2009;69(14):5918–26.
108. Martín R, Jiménez E, Heilig H, Fernández L, Marín ML, Zoetendal EG, et al. Isolation of bifidobacteria from breast milk and assessment of the bifidobacterial population by PCR-denaturing gradient gel electrophoresis and quantitative real-time PCR. Appl Environ Microbiol. 2009;75(4):965–9.
109. Urbaniak C, Angelini M, Gloor GB, Reid G. Human milk microbiota profiles in relation to birthing method, gestation and infant gender. Microbiome. 2016;4(1):1.
110. Jiang M, Zhang F, Wan C, Xiong Y, Shah NP, Wei H, et al. Evaluation of probiotic properties of Lactobacillus plantarum WLPL04 isolated from human breast milk. J Dairy Sci. 2016. doi:10.3168/jds.2015-10434 **[Epub ahead of print]**.
111. Urbaniak C, Burton JP, Reid G. Breast, milk and microbes: a complex relationship that does not end with lactation. Womens Health (Lond Engl). 2012;8(4):385–98.
112. Smelt MJ, de Haan BJ, Bron PA, van Swam I, Meijerink M, Wells JM, et al. Probiotics can generate FoxP3 T-cell responses in the small intestine and simultaneously inducing CD4 and CD8 T cell activation in the large intestine. PLoS One. 2013;8(7):e68952.
113. Smelt MJ, de Haan BJ, Bron PA, van Swam I, Meijerink M, Wells JM, et al. *L. plantarum*, *L. salivarius*, and *L. lactis* attenuate Th2 responses and increase Treg frequencies in healthy mice in a strain dependent manner. PLoS One. 2012;7(10):e47244.
114. Konieczna P, Akdis CA, Quigley EM, Shanahan F, O'Mahony L. Portrait of an immunoregulatory Bifidobacterium. Gut Microbes. 2012;3(3):261–6.
115. Konieczna P, Groeger D, Ziegler M, Frei R, Ferstl R, Shanahan F, et al. Bifidobacterium infantis 35624 administration induces Foxp3 T regulatory cells in human peripheral blood: potential role for myeloid and plasmacytoid dendritic cells. Gut. 2012;61(3):354–66.

116. Donkor ON, Ravikumar M, Proudfoot O, Day SL, Apostolopoulos V, Paukovics G, et al. Cytokine profile and induction of T helper type 17 and regulatory T cells by human peripheral mononuclear cells after microbial exposure. Clin Exp Immunol. 2012;167(2):282–95.
117. de Moreno de Leblanc A, Del Carmen S, Zurita-Turk M, Santos Rocha C, van de Guchte M, Azevedo V, et al. Importance of IL-10 modulation by probiotic microorganisms in gastrointestinal inflammatory diseases. ISRN Gastroenterol. 2011;2011:892971.
118. Demont A, Hacini-Rachinel F, Doucet-Ladevèze R, Ngom-Bru C, Mercenier A, Prioult G, et al. Live and heat-treated probiotics differently modulate IL10 mRNA stabilization and microRNA expression. J Allergy Clin Immunol. 2016;137:1264–7.
119. Nonaka Y, Izumo T, Izumi F, Maekawa T, Shibata H, Nakano A, et al. Antiallergic effects of *Lactobacillus pentosus* strain S-PT84 mediated by modulation of Th1/Th2 immunobalance and induction of IL-10 production. Int Arch Allergy Immunol. 2008;145(3):249–57.
120. Jorjão AL, de Oliveira FE, Leão MV, Carvalho CA, Jorge AO, de Oliveira LD. Live and heat-killed *Lactobacillus rhamnosus* ATCC 7469 may induce modulatory cytokines profiles on macrophages RAW 264.7. ScientificWorldJournal. 2015;2015:716749.
121. Shah MM, Saio M, Yamashita H, Tanaka H, Takami T, Ezaki T, et al. *Lactobacillus acidophilus* strain L-92 induces CD4(+)CD25(+)Foxp3(+) regulatory T cells and suppresses allergic contact dermatitis. Biol Pharm Bull. 2012;35(4):612–6.
122. Li AL, Meng XC, Duan CC, Huo GC, Zheng QL, Li D. Suppressive effects of oral administration of heat-killed *Lactobacillus acidophilus* on T helper-17 immune responses in a bovine β-lactoglobulin-sensitized mice model. Biol Pharm Bull. 2013;36(2):202–7.
123. Hsu P, Santner-Nanan B, Hu M, Skarratt K, Lee CH, Stormon M, et al. IL-10 potentiates differentiation of human induced regulatory T cells via STAT3 and Foxo1. J Immunol. 2015;195(8):3665–74.
124. Tooley KL, El-Merhibi A, Cummins AG, Grose RH, Lymn KA, DeNichilo M, et al. Maternal milk, but not formula, regulates the immune response to beta-lactoglobulin in allergy-prone rat pups. J Nutr. 2009;139(11):2145–51.
125. Allen SJ, Jordan S, Storey M, Thornton CA, Gravenor MB, Garaiova I, et al. Probiotics in the prevention of eczema: a randomised controlled trial. Arch Dis Child. 2014;99(11):1014–9.
126. West CE. Gut microbiota and allergic disease: new findings. Curr Opin Clin Nutr Metab Care. 2014;17(3):261–6.
127. West CE, Jenmalm MC, Kozyrskyj AL, Prescott SL. Probiotics for treatment and primary prevention of allergic diseases and asthma: looking back and moving forward. Expert Rev Clin Immunol. 2016 **[Epub ahead of print]**.
128. Eiwegger T, Stahl B, Schmitt J, Boehm G, Gerstmayr M, Pichler J, et al. Human milk-derived oligosaccharides and plant-derived oligosaccharides stimulate cytokine production of cord blood T-cells in vitro. Pediatr Res. 2004;56(4):536–40.
129. Eiwegger T, Stahl B, Haidl P, Schmitt J, Boehm G, Dehlink E, et al. Prebiotic oligosaccharides: in vitro evidence for gastrointestinal epithelial transfer and immunomodulatory properties. Pediatr Allergy Immunol. 2010;21(8):1179–88.
130. Castanys-Muñoz E, Martin MJ, Vazquez E. Building a beneficial microbiome from birth. Adv Nutr. 2016;7(2):323–30.
131. McGuire MK, McGuire MA. Human milk: mother nature's prototypical probiotic food? Adv Nutr. 2015;6(1):112–23.
132. Sela DA, Mills DA. Nursing our microbiota: molecular linkages between bifidobacteria and milk oligosaccharides. Trends Microbiol. 2010;18(7):298–307.
133. Zivkovic AM, German JB, Lebrilla CB, Mills DA. Human milk glycobiome and its impact on the infant gastrointestinal microbiota. Proc Natl Acad Sci USA. 2011;108(Suppl 1):4653–8.
134. Asakuma S, Hatakeyama E, Urashima T, Yoshida E, Katayama T, Yamamoto K, et al. Physiology of consumption of human milk oligosaccharides by infant gut-associated bifidobacteria. J Biol Chem. 2011;286(40):34583–92.
135. Katayama T. Host-derived glycans serve as selected nutrients for the gut microbe: human milk oligosaccharides and bifidobacteria. Biosci Biotechnol Biochem. 2016;3:1–12.
136. Bezirtzoglou E, Tsiotsias A, Welling GJ. Microbiota profile in feces of breast- and formula-fed newborns by using in situ hybridization (FISH). Anaerobe. 2011;17(6):478–82.
137. Kerperien J, Jeurink PV, Wehkamp T, van der Veer A, van de Kant HJ, Hofman GA, et al. Non-digestible oligosaccharides modulate intestinal immune activation and suppress cow's milk allergic symptoms. Pediatr Allergy Immunol. 2014;25(8):747–54.
138. Lehmann S, Hiller J, van Bergenhenegouwen J, Bergenhenegouwen LM, Garssen J, Traidl-Hoffmann C. In vitro evidence for immune-modulatory properties of non-digestible oligosaccharides: direct effect on human monocyte derived dendritic cells. PLoS One. 2015;10(7):e0132304.
139. Schouten B, van Esch BC, Hofman GA, Boon L, Knippels LM, Willemsen LE, et al. Oligosaccharide-induced whey-specific CD25(+) regulatory T-cells are involved in the suppression of cow milk allergy in mice. J Nutr. 2010;140(4):835–41.
140. Schouten B, van Esch BC, Hofman GA, de Kivit S, Boon L, Knippels LM, et al. A potential role for $CD25^+$ regulatory T-cells in the protection against casein allergy by dietary non-digestible carbohydrates. Br J Nutr. 2012;107(1):96–105.
141. Capuco AV, Akers RM. The origin and evolution of lactation. J Biol. 2009;8(4):37.
142. Lefèvre CM, Sharp JA, Nicholas KR. Evolution of lactation: ancient origin and extreme adaptations of the lactation system. Annu Rev Genomics Hum Genet. 2010;11:219–38.
143. Morikawa H, Sakaguchi S. Genetic and epigenetic basis of Treg cell development and function: from a FoxP3-centered view to an epigenome-defined view of natural Treg cells. Immunol Rev. 2014;259(1):192–205.
144. Kitagawa Y, Ohkura N, Sakaguchi S. Epigenetic control of thymic Treg-cell development. Eur J Immunol. 2015;45(1):11–6.
145. Li X, Zheng Y. Regulatory T cell identity: formation and maintenance. Trends Immunol. 2015;36(6):344–53.
146. Overacre AE, Vignali DA. Treg stability: to be or not to be. Curr Opin Immunol. 2016;39:39–43.
147. Trepka MJ, Heinrich J, Wichmann HE. The epidemiology of atopic diseases in Germany: an east-west comparison. Rev Environ Health. 1996;11(3):119–31.
148. Weiland SK, von Mutius E, Hirsch T, Duhme H, Fritzsch C, Werner B, et al. Prevalence of respiratory and atopic disorders among children in the East and West of Germany five years after unification. Eur Respir J. 1999;14(4):862–70.
149. Alsaweed M, Lai CT, Hartmann PE, Geddes DT, Kakulas F. Human milk miRNAs primarily originate from the mammary gland resulting in unique miRNA profiles of fractionated milk. Sci Rep. 2016;8(6):20680. doi:10.1038/srep20680.

Genetic susceptibility for cow's milk allergy in Dutch children: the start of the allergic march?

Peter Henneman[1*†], Nicole C. M. Petrus[2†], Andrea Venema[1], Femke van Sinderen[1], Karin van der Lip[1], Raoul C. Hennekam[1], Marcel Mannens[1†] and Aline B. Sprikkelman[2†]

Abstract

Background: Cow's milk allergy (CMA) is the most common allergic disease in infancy. It is not clear, whether infants with CMA have an increased risk of developing other allergic diseases later in life, the so-called "allergic march". We aimed to detect genetic associations of CMA using reported single nucleotide polymorphisms (SNP) in other allergic diseases and genetic mutations within the filaggrin (*FLG*) gene. Both to investigate possible causes of CMA, which also suggests an "allergic march".

Methods: Thirty children from the Dutch EuroPrevall birth cohort study with CMA in infancy and twenty-three healthy controls were studied. Six candidate SNPs were selected (minor allele frequency 10–50 % combined with a large effect) based on the literature. Thirteen *FLG* candidate mutations were selected spread over repeats 1, 3, 4, 5, 6, 7, 9 and 10 respectively.

Results: We found two SNP's, rs17616434 ($P = 0.002$) and rs2069772 ($P = 0.038$), significantly associated with CMA. One is located near the toll like receptor 6 (*TLR6*) gene, which functionally interacts with toll-like receptor 2, and is associated with an increased risk of other allergic diseases. One is located at the Interleukin 2 (*IL2*) locus. Twelve *FLG* amplicons were analyzed, but showed no significant enrichment. Nevertheless, we did observe more *FLG* mutations in the CMA-group compared to controls.

Conclusion: We significantly associated two SNPs with CMA, suggesting that variation in the *TLR6* and *IL2* genes contribute to the expression of CMA. In addition, since *TLR6* and *IL2* were earlier associated with other later onset allergies, this also favours the "allergic march" hypothesis. We observed more *FLG* mutations in the CMA-group, albeit we found no statistical significant enrichment of *FLG* mutations. Further studies are necessary to investigate the role of common variants and *FLG* or other skin barrier gene mutations in CMA.

Keywords: Epigenetics, Food allergy, Gender differences, Cow's milk allergy, Genetic susceptibility

Background

Cow's milk allergy

Cow's milk allergy (CMA) is the most common food allergy in young children, although an accurate incidence is difficult to establish because of discrepancies between self-reported and proper diagnosed allergy [1–4]. CMA and other food allergies have a heterogeneous clinical presentation, the estimated heritability of food-specific IgE ranged from 0.15 (cow's milk) to 0.35 (wheat) [5, 6]. Young children are likely to develop tolerance for cow's milk protein within a few years. However, infants who suffered from CMA in their early childhood seem to have an increased risk to develop other allergic diseases like asthma later in life [6–12]. Accumulating evidence suggest involvement of gut-microbiota, maturation of the

*Correspondence: p.henneman@amc.nl
†Peter Henneman and Nicole C.M. Petrus contributed equally to this workMarcel Mannens and Aline B. Sprikkelman contributed equally to this work
[1] Department Clinical Genetics, DNA-diagnostics laboratory, Amsterdam Medical Center, Amsterdam, The Netherlands
Full list of author information is available at the end of the article

immune-system and epicutaneous allergen sensitization [6, 13, 14]. Pre- and postnatal environmental factors, parent-of-origin factor and stress are likely to be involved in the susceptibility and expression of allergy [15]. So far, a clear cause for CMA has not been found.

Genetic component of food allergy

Genetic surveys on food allergy (FA) are to our knowledge still limited to candidate gene studies, and studies investigating CMA solely are not available. GWAS on other atopic diseases like asthma and eczema identified few candidate genes, as presented by Bonnelykke et al. However, these genes were only found in single FA allergy studies, as presented by Tan et al. [16–18]. Recently, it was shown that loss-of-function mutations of filaggrin (*FLG*) are a major risk factor for peanut food allergy [19]. *FLG* has already been described in studies on eczema [16, 20]. The *FLG* protein is an important skin barrier protein, but is not expressed in the gastrointestinal tract [13, 19]. Studies on the sensitizing mechanisms involved in FA, suggest that exposure to food antigens through the skin, i.e. epicutaneous, leads to allergic sensitization while (early) oral administration of food antigens just may prevent the onset of allergy [13]. An impaired skin barrier is however not essential for epicutaneous sensitization. It has been shown that high molecular weight antigens can be taken up by dendritic cells, which are present in hair follicles, which on turn can either initiate a sensitization or repression of immunological responses [13, 21]. During a sensitization period, different immunological processes may lead to the full expression of allergy.

To summarize, susceptibility factors among different types of allergies other than CMA are well investigated. It is known that CMA is an ultimate complex disease involving different immunological pathways and different environmental factors. Here we aim to discover new insight in the genetic susceptibility of CMA by means of: (1) Genetic association of six allergy associated common and high effect genetic variants identified by GWAS and (2) genetic association of rare but high effect genetic mutations in the filaggrin gene.

Methods

Dutch EuroPrevall Birth Cohort Study

In this study only children participating in the Dutch EuroPrevall Birth Cohort Study were investigated. The EuroPrevall study has been described in detail previously [3, 4, 22, 23]. In summary, children were included around birth and standardized measurements were performed by questionnaires. All children with symptoms suggestive of CMA underwent, among others a double blind placebo controlled food challenge (DBPCFC). Age-matched healthy control children were selected from the entire Dutch cohort. In both symptomatic and control children measurements where repeated annually. Controls had no symptoms suggestive of any food allergy nor suffered from atopic dermatitis. In all children undergoing blood drawing an attempt was made to obtain one full blood sample (EDTA KE 2.6 ml Monovette, Sarstedt BV, Etten-Leur, Netherlands) for DNA-isolation too. The Medical Ethics Committee of the Academic Medical Hospital (METC 06/005) approved the Dutch EuroPrevall Birth Cohort Study. Written informed consent, for both the study and genetic sampling, was obtained from both parents of each child, unless only one of them had parental rights.

CMA diagnosis

DBPCFC is the gold standard for diagnosing CMA and the challenge of choice according to the study protocol [22–24]. All children suspected of CMA were challenged according the international gold standard. The DBPCFC procedure was described in detail previously [3]. DBPCFC was repeated annually, in children with CMA, until the child was tolerant for CMP [3, 22]. Tolerance was defined as previously a positive DBPCFC for CMA, but at DNA-sampling a negative DBPCFC and/or eating CMP without experiencing symptoms.

Samples selected for genetic analysis

DNA samples of 20 children with proven CMA were selected, based on the longest possible time between the age of DNA-sampling and the age of CMP-tolerance. Since DNA is generally assumed to be stable throughout life we state that former CMA patients and active CMA patients represent both CMA cases. Also ten samples of children with proven CMA who developed CMP tolerance during the course of the study were selected, called former CMA children. Together these 30 samples are called the CMA-group. Control samples (N = 23), were selected from the group of control children and matched on age at DNA-sampling.

Patient characteristics were analysed with *t* test (Mann–Whitney U test when data was not normally distributed) for continuous parameters. Chi square test was used for categorical variables and Chi square test for trend for multiple categories categorical variables. All characteristics were analysed using SPSS version 20 (IBM SPSS Statistics for Windows, Armonk, NY).

Genetic association analysis

GWAS-studies reporting on SNPs associated with sensitization and/or allergy were selected [25]. SNP Inclusion criteria were based on the minor allele frequency (MAF) of 20–50 % and an odds ratio (OR) >1.2 [26, 27]. Based on the literature and our prior stated selection criteria, six

SNPs were selected for evaluation. A description of the SNPs with regard nearby located genes is described in Table 1. Linkage disequilibrium (LD) was used to identify the most plausible involved gene, using LD plots per SNP on SNAP Broad institute with the following values: $R^2 = 0.8$, distance limit = 500, CEU population [28]. Target reference sequences were downloaded using the database ENSEMBL [29]. These reference sequences were subsequently submitted to the web tool Primer3 in order to obtain a primer set. Primers were M13 tail extended [30]. Primer sequences of all 6 SNPs are described in Additional file 1: Table S1. Final quality control of the primer set was performed using the web tool SNPCheck [31].

The *FLG* gene involves at least ten highly homolog repeat sequences. The primer sequences or primer design for detection of *FLG* mutations was based on the report of Sandilands et al. [32]. In total we selected 13 *FLG* candidate mutations spread over repeats 1, 3, 4, 5, 6, 7, 9 and 10 respectively (Table 2) [32]. Mutations reported only in the Chinese or Japanese population (3321delA and S2554X) were not included in this study. Since for most *FLG* primers specificity is based on not more than three repeat specific bases, the highest possible annealing temperature was used in the PCR in order to obtain the required regional specificity. All mutations were analysed using PCR, followed by Sanger sequencing. *FLG* Primers sequences are described in Additional file 1: Table S2. SNPs and *FLG* mutations were Sanger sequenced using standard protocols (BigDye Terminator® mix, Applied Biosystems) and analysed using an ABI3730® of Applied Biosystems.

Raw sequence data was analysed using CodonCode Aligner® and Alamut® software. Since all tested mutations in the *FLG* gene result in an absent or defective protein, we constructed a cumulative variant score per patient. This cumulative score included a score of zero risk alleles versus one or more risk alleles present in exon 3 repeats of *FLG*. The CMA-group was compared to controls. In population based genetic studies the Hardy–Weinberg equilibrium (HWE) is a golden standard for quality control of the analysed genotypes. Deviation of this equilibrium indicates genotyping errors or the presence of a certain genetic selection bias. Since we did analyze in this study a strongly selected sample of CMA patients, which obviously does not represent the general population, it would be inappropriate to apply the Hardy–Weinberg equilibrium as genotyping quality control in this study. All genetic statistical analyses were performed in SPSS (v20) using a Pearson's Chi square test or Fisher's exact test. P values <0.05 were considered significant.

Table 1 Candidate SNPs

SNP	Chr	Genotype*	HWP	Nearby gene(s): function
rs2155219[a]	11	G/G: 0,30 G/T: 0,43	0.15	***C11orf30***: Regulator, represses transcription, possibly via its interaction with a multiprotein chromatin remodeling complex that modifies the chromatin. ***LRRC32***: Associated with allergic rhinitis and rhinitis
rs17616434[b]	4	C/C: 0,06 C/T: 0,31 T/T: 0,62	0.371	***TLR10***: Toll Like Receptor 10. Pathogen activation, activation innate immunity. ***TLR1***: Toll Like Receptor 1. Specifically recognizes diacylated and triacylated lipopeptide. ***TLR6***: Toll Like Receptor 6. This receptor functionally interacts with toll-like receptor 2. associated with an increased risk of asthma in some populations. ***FAM114A1***: May play a role in neuronal cell development
rs6586513[a]	1	A/A: 0,51 A/C: 0,49	0.15	***CROCC***: Major structural component of the ciliary rootlet. Contributes to centrosome cohesion before mitosis. ***ATP13A2***: ATPase Type 13A2. Transports inorganic cations and other substrates. ***SDHB***: succinate dehydrogenase complex. Complex 2 of respiratory chain. ***MFAP2***: Microfibrillar-associated protein. Major antigen of elastin-associated microfibrils
rs3860069[a]	4	A/A: 0,50 A/C: 0,45 C/C: 0,05	0.343	***TLR6***: Toll Like Receptor 6. This receptor functionally interacts with toll-like receptor 2. associated with an increased risk of asthma in some populations. ***TLR10***: Toll Like Receptor 10. Pathogen activation, activation innate immunity. ***TLR1***: Toll Like Receptor 1. Specifically recognizes diacylated and triacylated lipopeptide. ***FAM114A1***: May play a role in neuronal cell development
rs6898653[a]	5	A/A: 0,59 A/G: 0,36 G/G: 0,05	1	***SEMA6A***: expression in developing neuronal tissue. Is required for proper development of the thalamocortical projection
rs2069772[a]	4	A/A: 0,52 A/G: 0,38 G/G: 0,10	0.527	***IL2***: Interleukin 2. Secreted cytokine for proliferation of T and B lymphocytes. Produced by T cells. ***ADAD1***: binds to RNA. Plays a role in spermatogenesis. ***KIAA1109***: associated with celiac disease

Chr chromosome

* CEU genotype, NCBI database, *HWP* Hardy–Weinberg p value, NCBI database

[a] candidate SNP earlier reported by Ramasamy. A. 2011

[b] candidate SNP earlier reported by Bønnelykke K. 2013

Table 2 Selected filaggrin mutations according Sandilands et al.

FLG mutation	Amplicon	Repeat	g. (H19)	c.	ATG	bp	p.	Ethnicity[b]
R501X	FLG-1	1	152285861	1501	2072	C>T	501	EUR/AM
2282del4	FLG-2	1	152285080	2282	2853	del4 (CAGT-2286)	761/762	EUR/AM
3702delG	FLG-3	3	152283660	3702	4273	delG	1234	IR
R1474X	FLG-4	4	152282942	4420	4991	C>T	1474	IR
5360delG	FLG-5	5	152282002	5360	5931	delG	1787	NL
6867delAG	FLG-6	6	152280495	6867	7438	delAG (AG-2268)	2289/2290	AUS
E2422X	FLG-7	7	152280098	7264	7835	G>T	2422	NL
7267delCA	FLG-7	7	152280095	7267	7838	delCA (CA-7268)	2423	NL
R2447X	FLG-7	7	152280023	7339	7910	C>G	2447	IR
S3247X	FLG-8	9	152277622	9740	10311	C>A	3247	IR
11029delCA	FLG-9	10	152276333	11029	11600	delCA (CA-11030)	3677	IR
11033del4	FLG-9	10	152276329	11033	11604	Del4(CAGT-11036)	3678/3679	NL
Q3683X	FLG-9	10	152276312	11050	11050	C>T	3684[a]	Ir

[a] Sandilands reported p. 3683. *FLG* filaggrin, *g* genomic position, *c* coding postion, *ATG* distance from transcription start site, *bp* basepair change(s), *p.* affected amino acid

[b] Ethnic group were mutations were first reported, adapted from Sandilands et al. EUR (European), AM (American.), IR (Irish), AUS (Austrian), NL (Dutch)

Results

Patient and control characteristics are shown in Table 3. Controls and children with CMA were well matched except for age at DNA-sampling. Children with CMA were significantly younger ($P = 0.008$) compared to controls. Our CMA group consists of both IgE as well as non-IgE mediated CMA, with slightly more IgE positive children (specific IgE >0.35 kU/L, $P = 0.044$) in the CMA group compared to controls. Comparison of the former CMA group, showed no significant difference in age at DNA-sampling ($P = 0.71$) nor IgE status ($P = 0.49$).

Table 3 Characteristics of Dutch allergy study population; cow's milk allergy (CMA), former CMA and controls

	CMA	Control	P
N (♀)	20 (8)	20 (10)	*NS*
Age diagnosis CMA ± SD[a]	6.5 ± 2.5	*NA*	*NA*
Age at Sampling ± SD[a]	11.8 ± 4.9	17.2 ± 7.1	0.008
N of children with CMP specific sIgE >0.35 kU/L[b]	7	1	0.044
Mean CMP specific sIgE value ± SD (kU/L)	1.15 ± 3.6	0.16 ± 0.64	*NS*
Range IgE value (kU/L)	16.4	2.9	*NA*
	Former CMA	Control	P
N (♀)	10 (0)	13 (0)	*NA*
Age diagnosis CMA ± SD[a]	5.8 ± 2.2	*NA*	*NA*
Age at Sampling ± SD[a]	18.0 ± 5.6	17.2 ± 4.3	*NS*
Age at Tolerance ± SD[a]	17.2 ± 3.9	*NA*	*NA*
N sIgE >0.35 kU/L[b]	*0*	*0*	*NA*

CMA cow's milk allergy, *N* number, *CMP* cow's milk protein, *SD* standard deviation, *NA* not applicable, *NS* not significant, *sIgE* serum specific IgE

[a] age in months ANOVA

[b] Fisher's exact test, 2-sided

Genetic contribution of common variants to CMA

For two SNPs we observed significant enrichment of risk genotypes in the CMA-group compared to controls, illustrated in Table 4. For rs17616434, located on chromosome 4; *TLR10/1/6* and *FAM114A1* locus, C/C risk alleles were absent in the control group while 9 CMA/former CMA subjects showed this genotype ($P = 0.002$). The rs17616434 C/T and T/T genotypes were both enriched in the controls. For rs2069772 located on chromosome 4 as well, the T/T genotype was enriched in the CMA-group compared to the controls (80 vs. 46.7 % respectively), while the heterozygotes (C/T) and common genotype (C/C) was enriched in the controls ($P = 0.038$). Analysis based on the genotype frequencies within the CMA-group vs. controls was insignificant associated ($P > 0.05$) for rs2155219 (*LRRC32* locus), rs6586513 (*CROCC/ATP13A2/SDHB/MFAP2* locus), rs3860069 (*TLR6/10/1* and *FAM114A1* locus) and rs6898653 (*SEMA6A* locus).

Genetic contribution of rare FLG mutations to CMA

The investigated FLG-mutations were covered by 9 amplicons of which we successfully optimized PCR conditions for 8 amplicons. The 4th amplicon, covering the R1474X mutation in *FLG* repeat 4, did not show consistent results and was therefore excluded from analysis (data not shown). The latter mutation is extremely rare and was only reported in the Irish population [32].

Figure 1 illustrates the percentage of present risk alleles per group. According to the report of

Table 4 Comparison of SNPs between cow's milk allergy (CMA), former CMA and controls

SNP	Group	Genotype details				P value
rs2155219		GG	GT	TT	Total	0.548
	CMA + former CMA	6 (24 %)	11 (44 %)	8 (32 %)	25 (100 %)	
	Control	7 (23.3 %)	17 (56.7 %)	6 (20 %)	30 (100 %)	
rs17616434		CC	CT	TT	Total	0.002
	CMA + former CMA	9 (36 %)	5 (20 %)	11 (44 %)	25 (100 %)	
	Control	0 (0 %)	10 (33.3 %)	20 (66.7 %)	30 (100 %)	
rs6586513		AC	AA		Total	0.456
	CMA + former CMA	12 (48 %)	13 (52 %)		25 (100 %)	
	Control	11 (37.9 %)	18 (62.1 %)		29 (100 %)	
rs3860069		CC	AC	AA	Total	0.336
	CMA + former CMA	4 (16 %)	8 (32 %)	13 (52 %)	25 (100 %)	
	Control	2 (6.7 %)	7 (23.3 %)	21 (70 %)	30 (100 %)	
rs6898653		GG	AG	AA	Total	0.951
	CMA + former CMA	1 (4 %)	13 (52 %)	11 (44 %)	25 (100 %)	
	Control	1 (3.4 %)	14 (48.3 %)	14 (48.3 %)	29 (100 %)	
rs2069772		CC	CT	TT	Total	0.038
	CMA + former CMA	1 (4 %)	4 (16 %)	20 (80 %)	25 (100 %)	
	Control	2 (6.7 %)	14 (46.7 %)	14 (46.7 %)	30 (100 %)	

CMA cow's milk allergy

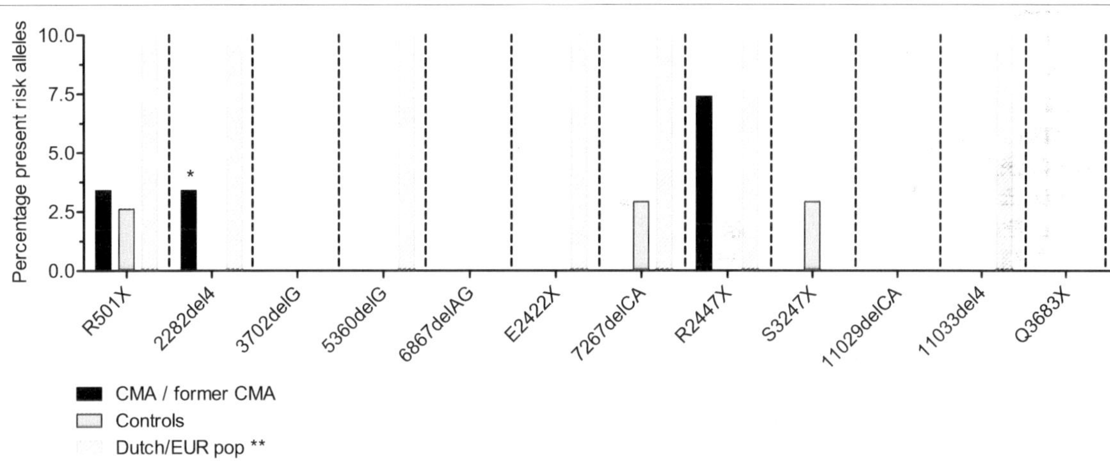

Fig. 1 Enrichment analysis of filaggrin risk alleles in cow's milk allergy patients vs. controls. Percent present risk alleles: total number of alleles/number of risk alleles per group [cow's milk allergy (CMA) patients, former CMA patients and controls]. Dutch/EUR *pop column* indicates for every FLG mutation the discovery population according Sandilands et al. only and *does not* represent an actual percentage

Sandilands et al. [32] some mutations were, so far, only observed in European and/or Dutch populations annotated as dashed bars in this figure. One sample, homozygote for the 2282del4 mutation involved a CMA patient. Geographic origin/ethnicity are known confounders in genetic surveys. Therefore, we evaluated the ethnic distribution (Fig. 2) and observed no difference between the two groups. All *FLG* mutations are rare, and in combination with a relative small sample, this implies extremely low statistical power. In order to diminish this power problem we counted per sample the number of present mutations yielding a cumulative *FLG* risk allele score. Samples who carried 1 or more risk alleles were annotated as 1. Figure 3 illustrates the scores in the CMA-group and controls. Although insignificant (Chi square test), more risk alleles carriers were present in the CMA-group compared to controls.

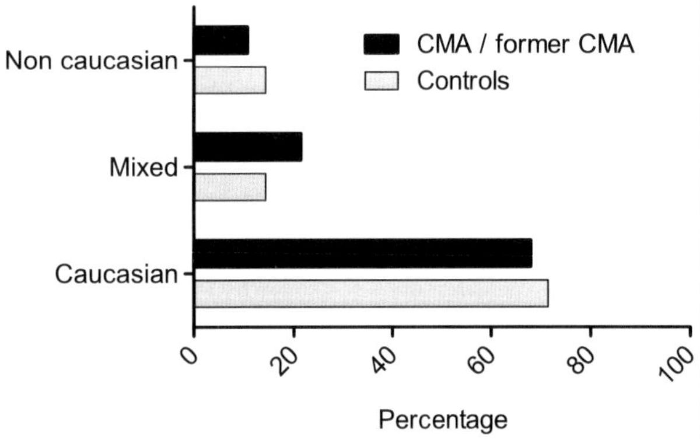

Fig. 2 Ethnicity distribution among cow's milk allergy (CMA), former CMA patients and controls Caucasian: both parents are of Caucasian background. Mixed: one parent is of Caucasian and one parent of non-Caucasian background. Non-Caucasian: both parents are of non-Caucasian background

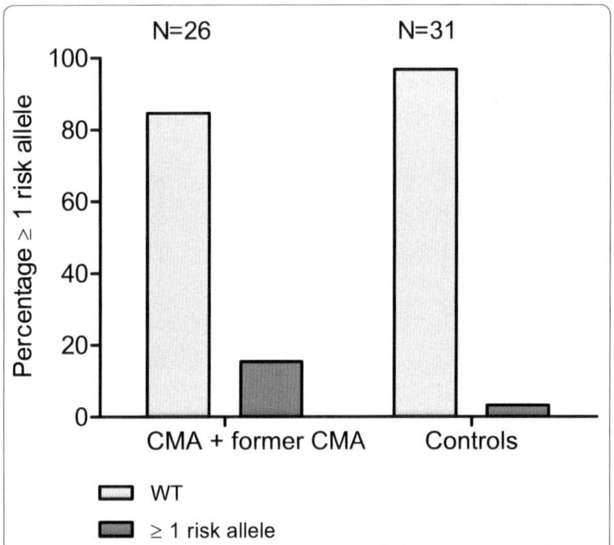

Fig. 3 Enrichment analysis of filaggrin risk alleles in cow's milk allergy patients vs. controls Percentage ≥1 risk alleles represents a cumulative score of all filaggrin (FLG) mutations within cow's milk allergy (CMA) + former CMA and control groups. *WT* Wild type

Discussion

In this study we observed association of two earlier reported non-CMA allergies and/or allergy sensitization associated SNPs with CMA. Although insignificant, we observed more *FLG* mutations in the CMA-group compared to controls which suggest that a role of the *FLG*-gene in CMA cannot be excluded. Since our candidates were earlier reported to be associated with other types of late(r) onset allergic diseases, our data suggest not only that rs17616434, rs2069772 and *FLG* mutations are involved in CMA, but also suggest that these genetic variations might contribute to the so-called "allergic march".

Genetic analysis

We analysed six SNPs which have been described previously in relation to allergic diseases [26, 27]. Out of these six, two SNPs showed significantly different genotypic distribution between CMA and controls. First, rs17616434 ($P = 0.002$) was associated with CMA and is located near a cluster of toll like receptor (*TLR1, 6, 10*) genes, which has earlier been associated with allergic disease [33]. Secondly, rs2069772 ($P = 0.038$), was earlier described to be associated with allergic rhinitis, and is located near the *IL2* and *KIAA1109* genes [27]. *IL2* is known to be involved in cytokine secretion that stimulates proliferation of B and T -cells. The other gene, *KIAA1109*, is known to be involved in celiac disease, a disease characterized by a strong immunological response to food proteins (gluten), found in wheat, rye and barley [34]. Moreover, the *KIAA1109/Tenr/IL2/IL21* locus was also earlier associated with another immunological disorder, namely rheumatoid arthritis [35]. Therefore, both *IL2* and *KIAA1109* are good candidates to be involved in CMA. Earlier reports involving allergic diseases have shown that a defective *FLG*-gene was involved, albeit the prevalence of these mutations is ethnicity specific [32]. In our cohort we constructed a cumulative score of *FLG*-mutations. Although, the absolute number of mutations was higher in the CMA-group this difference was not statistical significant. The presence of ethnic specific mutations in our sample of mainly Dutch children was in concordance with the report of Sandilands et al., with exception of S3247X mutation, which was reported only in the Irish population [32]. Since *FLG* mutations are rare and our study sample is small we cannot state that *FLG* is not involved in CMA. To our knowledge, *FLG* has not been studied in CMA before. Therefore, studies involving a larger sample size are necessary to conclusively rule out or rule in the involvement of *FLG* in CMA.

Allergic march

The allergic march hypothesize that children who suffered from food allergy or atopic dermatitis in early childhood have an increased risk of developing other allergic diseases, e.g. asthma and allergic rhinitis, in later in life. However, evidence for the existence of the allergic march is still very limited [6–12]. Recent reports describe pathways involved in allergic diseases and implied common genetic variation behind these affected pathways, among others, defects involving the skin barrier. The filaggrin protein is involved in maintaining a healthy skin barrier [18, 36]. Although in our study rare *FLG* mutations were not significantly enriched in CMA patients, we did observe more *FLG* mutations in our CMA group. The function of regulatory T-cells and the Th2 responses have been previously reported in relation to allergic diseases as well. These pathways have been associated with several other allergic diseases, which might favour the allergic march hypothesis, since the onset of these different types of allergies seem to manifest at specific ages [18, 36]. In our small sample study, we found a significant associated locus located close to the *IL2* gene which is involved in the Th2 response. Both our observations on *FLG* mutations and the *IL2* locus favour the allergic march hypothesis but have to be confirmed in a prospective study design.

Strength and weaknesses of the study

The main strength of the studied samples is that CMA is diagnosed according to the current available, internationally recommended, gold standard [24]. Furthermore, clinical data are well documented due to the setup of the study with regular questionnaires [22]. Unfortunately, it was not possible to obtain DNA-samples in all children. Furthermore, the amount of blood drawing for research purposes in infants is in the Netherlands limited to 2.5 ml. These are both limiting the sample size of this study. This resulted in missing values for statistical analysis, however there were no significant differences in distribution between valid and missing cases between CMA-infants and controls (data not shown). Since this is only a very small sample size study in a very heterogeneous disease, further studies in larger cohorts are necessary. Obviously, many more genetic and environmental factors are involved in the development of CMA. With respect to an epidemiological approach unravelling mechanisms involved in CMA, large cohorts are essential. On the other hand, using well characterized small cohorts or even single cases might be essential to elucidate distinct mechanisms, that underlie at the basis of the complex character of CMA.

Conclusion

Current studies indicates that genetic variation of *TLR6* and *IL2*, which were earlier reported to be associated with non-CMA allergies and/or allergy sensitization, contribute to the expression of CMA in young children. In addition, this favours the "allergic march" hypothesis. Furthermore, we cannot exclude a possible role for *FLG*-mutations being involved in CMA or the sensitization process prior to the establishment of CMA. Follow-up studies are necessary before definite conclusions about a link between early onset CMA and expression of later onset other allergic diseases can be drawn.

Abbreviations

CMA: cow's milk allergy; CMP: cow's milk protein; DBPCFC: double blind placebo controlled food challenge; DNA: deoxyribonucleic acid; FA: food allergy; *FLG*: filaggrin; GWAS: genome wide association studies; HWE: Hardy–Weinberg Equilibrium; LD: linkage disequilibrium; MAF: minor allele frequency; OR: odds ratio; SNP: single nucleotide polymorphism.

Authors' contributions

PH supervised laboratory experiments, analysed data and drafted the manuscript. NP collected clinical data, analysed data and drafted the manuscript. AV, FS and KL performed laboratory experiments and critically revised the manuscript. RH interpreted the data and critically revised the manuscript. MM and AS supervised the studies (MM laboratory; AS clinical studies) and critically revised the manuscript. All authors read and approved the final version of the manuscript.

Author details

[1] Department Clinical Genetics, DNA-diagnostics laboratory, Amsterdam Medical Center, Amsterdam, The Netherlands. [2] Department of Paediatric Respiratory Medicine and Allergy, Emma Children's Hospital, Amsterdam Medical Center, Amsterdam, The Netherlands.

Acknowledgements

The authors would like to thank all children and their parents for participating in the Dutch EuroPrevall Birth Cohort Study. Furthermore the authors would like to thank everyone involved in collecting clinical data. The employees of the department Department of Parasitology, Leiden University Medical Center, for storing blood samples.

Competing interests

This study was supported by an unrestricted grant from the "Stichting Steun Emma", Emma Children's Hospital, Academic Medical Center, The Netherlands. The EuroPrevall study is funded by the European Commission (FOOD-CT_2005-514000). The Dutch cohort received unrestricted grants from Nutricia, the Netherlands, Nutricia Advanced Medical Nutrition, the Netherlands, AstraZeneca, the Netherlands, TEVA, the Netherlands and GlaxoSmithKline, the Netherlands.
The authors declare that they have no competing interests.

References

1. Chafen JJ, Newberry SJ, Riedl MA, Bravata DM, Maglione M, Suttorp MJ, et al. Diagnosing and managing common food allergies: a systematic review. JAMA. 2010;303(18):1848.
2. Rona RJ, Keil T, Summers C, Gislason D, Zuidmeer L, Sodergren E, et al. The prevalence of food allergy: a meta-analysis. J Allergy Clin Immunol. 2007;120(3):638.
3. Petrus NC, Schoemaker AF, van Hoek MW, Jansen L, Jansen-van der Weide MC, van Aalderen WM, Sprikkelman AB. Remaining symptoms in half the children treated for milk allergy. Eur J Pediatr. 2015;174(6):759.
4. Schoemaker AA, Sprikkelman AB, Grimshaw KE, Roberts G, Grabenhenrich L, Rosenfeld L, et al. Incidence and natural history of challenge-proven cow's milk allergy in European children—EuroPrevall birth cohort. Allergy. 2015;70:963.
5. Tsai HJ, Kumar R, Pongracic J, Liu X, Story R, Yu Y, et al. Familial aggregation of food allergy and sensitization to food allergens: a family-based study. Clin Exp Allergy. 2009;39(1):101.
6. Benhamou AH, Schappi Tempia MG, Belli DC, Eigenmann PA. An overview of cow's milk allergy in children. Swiss Med Wkly. 2009;139(21–22):300.
7. Host A, Halken S. A prospective study of cow milk allergy in Danish infants during the first 3 years of life. Clinical course in relation to clinical and immunological type of hypersensitivity reaction. Allergy. 1990;45(8):587.

8. Host A, Halken S, Jacobsen HP, Christensen AE, Herskind AM, Plesner K. Clinical course of cow's milk protein allergy/intolerance and atopic diseases in childhood. Pediatr Allergy Immunol. 2002;13(Suppl):15.
9. Longo G, Berti I, Burks AW, Krauss B, Barbi E. IgE-mediated food allergy in children. Lancet. 2013;382:1656.
10. Morita H, Nomura I, Matsuda A, Saito H, Matsumoto K. Gastrointestinal food allergy in infants. Allergol Int. 2013;62(3):297.
11. Saarinen KM, Pelkonen AS, Makela MJ, Savilahti E. Clinical course and prognosis of cow's milk allergy are dependent on milk-specific IgE status. J Allergy Clin Immunol. 2005;116(4):869.
12. Aldurаywish SA, Lodge CJ, Campbell B, Allen KJ, Erbas B, Lowe AJ, Dharmage SC. The march from early life food sensitisation to allergic disease: a systematic review and meta-analyses of birth cohort studies. Allergy. 2015;71:77.
13. Matsumoto K, Saito H. Epicutaneous immunity and onset of allergic diseases—per-"eczema"tous sensitization drives the allergy march. Allergol Int. 2013;62(3):291.
14. Noverr MC, Huffnagle GB. The 'microflora hypothesis' of allergic diseases. Clin Exp Allergy. 2005;35(12):1511.
15. Chen W, Mempel M, Schober W, Behrendt H, Ring J. Gender difference, sex hormones, and immediate type hypersensitivity reactions. Allergy. 2008;63(11):1418.
16. Tan TH, Ellis JA, Saffery R, Allen KJ. The role of genetics and environment in the rise of childhood food allergy. Clin Exp Allergy. 2012;42(1):20.
17. Lockett GA, Holloway JW. Genome-wide association studies in asthma; perhaps, the end of the beginning. Curr Opin Allergy Clin Immunol. 2013;13(5):463.
18. Bonnelykke K, Sparks R, Waage J, Milner JD. Genetics of allergy and allergic sensitization: common variants, rare mutations. Curr Opin Immunol. 2015;36:115.
19. Asai Y, Greenwood C, Hull PR, Alizadehfar R, Ben-Shoshan M, Brown SJ, et al. Filaggrin gene mutation associations with peanut allergy persist despite variations in peanut allergy diagnostic criteria or asthma status. J Allergy Clin Immunol. 2013;132(1):239.
20. van den Oord RA, Sheikh A. Filaggrin gene defects and risk of developing allergic sensitisation and allergic disorders: systematic review and meta-analysis. BMJ. 2009;339:b2433.
21. Dioszeghy V, Mondoulet L, Dhelft V, Ligouis M, Puteaux E, Benhamou PH, Dupont C. Epicutaneous immunotherapy results in rapid allergen uptake by dendritic cells through intact skin and downregulates the allergen-specific response in sensitized mice. J Immunol. 2011;186(10):5629.
22. Keil T, McBride D, Grimshaw K, Niggemann B, Xepapadaki P, Zannikos K, et al. The multinational birth cohort of EuroPrevall: background, aims and methods. Allergy. 2010;65(4):482.
23. McBride D, Keil T, Grabenhenrich L, Dubakiene R, Drasutiene G, Fiocchi A, et al. The EuroPrevall birth cohort study on food allergy: baseline characteristics of 12,000 newborns and their families from nine European countries. Pediatr Allergy Immunol. 2012;23(3):230.
24. Boyce JA, Assa'ad A, Burks AW, Jones SM, Sampson HA, Wood RA, et al. Guidelines for the diagnosis and management of food allergy in the United States: summary of the NIAID-sponsored expert panel report. J Allergy Clin Immunol. 2010;126(6):1105.
25. National Human Genome Research Institute. http://www.genome.gov/gwastudies. Catalog Data Update: 20 Feb 2015.
26. Bonnelykke K, Matheson MC, Pers TH, Granell R, Strachan DP, Alves AC, et al. Meta-analysis of genome-wide association studies identifies ten loci influencing allergic sensitization. Nat Genet. 2013;45(8):902.
27. Ramasamy A, Curjuric I, Coin LJ, Kumar A, McArdle WL, Imboden M, et al. A genome-wide meta-analysis of genetic variants associated with allergic rhinitis and grass sensitization and their interaction with birth order. J Allergy Clin Immunol. 2011;128(5):996.
28. SNP Annotation and Proxy Search Broad Institute. Version 2.2. http://www.broadinstitute.org/mpg/snap.
29. Ensembl. http://www.ensembl.org/index.html. Accessed Dec 2014.
30. Koressaar T, Remm M. Enhancements and modifications of primer design program Primer3. Bioinformatics. 2007;23(10):1289.
31. National Genetics Refence Laboratory. SNPCheck version 3.1.1, 2013. http://www.ngrl.org.uk/Manchester/projects/informatics/snpcheck.
32. Sandilands A, Terron-Kwiatkowski A, Hull PR, O'Regan GM, Clayton TH, Watson RM, et al. Comprehensive analysis of the gene encoding filaggrin uncovers prevalent and rare mutations in ichthyosis vulgaris and atopic eczema. Nat Genet. 2007;39(5):650.
33. Reijmerink NE, Kerkhof M, Bottema RW, Gerritsen J, Stelma FF, Thijs C, et al. Toll-like receptors and microbial exposure: gene-gene and gene-environment interaction in the development of atopy. Eur Respir J. 2011;38(4):833.
34. van Heel DA, Franke L, Hunt KA, Gwilliam R, Zhernakova A, Inouye M, et al. A genome-wide association study for celiac disease identifies risk variants in the region harboring IL2 and IL21. Nat Genet. 2007;39(7):827.
35. Teixeira VH, Pierlot C, Migliorini P, Balsa A, Westhovens R, Barrera P, et al. Testing for the association of the KIAA1109/Tenr/IL2/IL21 gene region with rheumatoid arthritis in a European family-based study. Arthritis Res Ther. 2009;11(2):R45.
36. Pellerin L, Jenks JA, Begin P, Bacchetta R, Nadeau KC. Regulatory T cells and their roles in immune dysregulation and allergy. Immunol Res. 2014;58(2–3):358.

9

Current challenges facing the assessment of the allergenic capacity of food allergens in animal models

Katrine Lindholm Bøgh[1], Jolanda van Bilsen[2], Robert Głogowski[3], Iván López-Expósito[4], Grégory Bouchaud[5], Carine Blanchard[6], Marie Bodinier[5], Joost Smit[7], Raymond Pieters[7], Shanna Bastiaan-Net[8], Nicole de Wit[8], Eva Untersmayr[9], Karine Adel-Patient[10], Leon Knippels[11,12], Michelle M. Epstein[13], Mario Noti[14], Unni Cecilie Nygaard[15], Ian Kimber[16], Kitty Verhoeckx[2] and Liam O'Mahony[17*]

Abstract

Food allergy is a major health problem of increasing concern. The insufficiency of protein sources for human nutrition in a world with a growing population is also a significant problem. The introduction of new protein sources into the diet, such as newly developed innovative foods or foods produced using new technologies and production processes, insects, algae, duckweed, or agricultural products from third countries, creates the opportunity for development of new food allergies, and this in turn has driven the need to develop test methods capable of characterizing the allergenic potential of novel food proteins. There is no doubt that robust and reliable animal models for the identification and characterization of food allergens would be valuable tools for safety assessment. However, although various animal models have been proposed for this purpose, to date, none have been formally validated as predictive and none are currently suitable to test the allergenic potential of new foods. Here, the design of various animal models are reviewed, including among others considerations of species and strain, diet, route of administration, dose and formulation of the test protein, relevant controls and endpoints measured.

Keywords: Food allergy, Animal models, Novel allergens, Hazard identification

Background

Food allergy affects a significant proportion of the population and is associated with important health effects. In addition, food allergy has an impact on quality of life and represents a substantial economic burden [1, 2]. The exponential growth of the human population means that existing protein sources, such as soy, are being consumed by a wider population, while novel protein sources, such as insect and algae, are currently being examined for inclusion in human foodstuffs. The introduction of new proteins into the diet inevitably creates a potential opportunity for the development of new food allergies. There is a need, therefore, for the development and application of appropriate strategies for evaluating the allergenic potential of existing and new food proteins as an important component of safety assessment. A crucial question in food allergy research is what characteristics confer on proteins the ability to cause sensitization and allergy. Current understanding of this is incomplete and this has limited the development of predictive methods based on in silico analysis of protein sequence and structure, and in vitro methods most often based on the measurement of a single parameter. For this reason, there is a continued interest in the development of suitable animal models that provide a more holistic approach to the assessment of the allergic potential of proteins. Although there is a variety of animal models for evaluating allergenicity, none of the existing models has been validated, is predictive, or widely accepted [3]. Because the choice of animal

*Correspondence: liam.omahony@siaf.uzh.ch
[17] Swiss Institute of Allergy and Asthma Research, University of Zürich, Obere Strasse 22, 7270 Davos Platz, Switzerland
Full list of author information is available at the end of the article

experimental design as well as the selection of appropriate endpoints and evaluation parameters may lead to contradictory results, there is an enormous impact on performance and predictive accuracy of animal models. Here, we review the experimental design and interpretation of animal models for the assessment of the allergenic potential of novel food proteins (Fig. 1).

Reference proteins

To assess the relative allergenicity of novel proteins, it is essential to use known allergens in humans as reference proteins. It is unknown why certain proteins are allergenic, compared to the large majority of non-allergenic food proteins. As reviewed extensively elsewhere [4], most plant allergens belong to the prolamin superfamily, including the lipid transfer proteins (LTP) and 2S albumins or to the cupin superfamily, which include the 11S and 7S globulins. Animal food allergens predominately belong to the parvalbumin, tropomysin and casein protein families. The shared conserved structure and biological activity among proteins in these families contribute to their allergenicity. However, protein homology alone does not guarantee allergenicity [5]. Sensitizing rats with 7S globulins from peanut, hazelnut, soy or pea induced IgE with different biological activities [6]. In addition, patients allergic to goat's milk, but who tolerate cow's milk, show an absence IgE-binding to bovine b-casein by IgE specific to caprine b-casein, despite a sequence identity of 91 % between the respective proteins [7]. This suggests that subtle differences in physical or biological properties are modulators of allergic responses even to well-described food allergens.

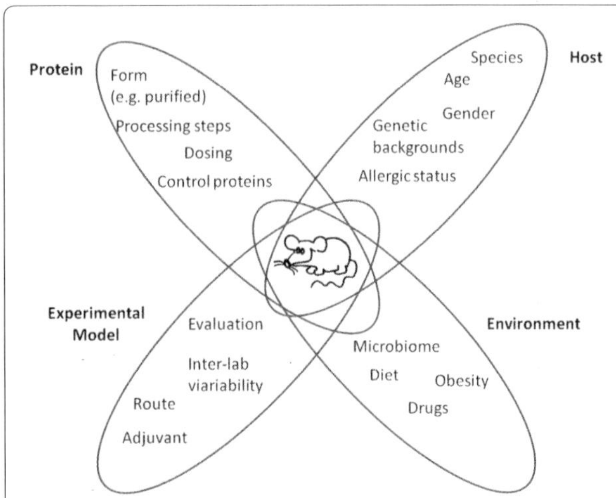

Fig. 1 Factors which influence animal model design. Important considerations in the design, conduct and interpretation of animal models for assessment of the allergenic potential of food proteins are shown

Initial studies by Astwood et al. [8] proposed that stability of proteins to in vitro gastric digestion significantly discriminated known allergens from non/low-allergens. However, subsequent studies with a wider range of proteins did not support these findings [9, 10]. Thus, additional tests, including those in animal models, may be useful in the assessment of the allergenic potential of novel proteins. Dearman and Kimber [11] showed that known allergenic proteins (peanut agglutinin and ovalbumin (OVA)) induced specific IgE upon intraperitoneal (i.p.) injection of mice, while presumed non/low-allergenic proteins (potato agglutinin, potato acid phosphatase) were immunogenic, but induced only low IgE titer responses. In contrast, a multi-laboratory study was unable to accurately differentiate between known allergens and putative non/low-allergens, including spinach rubisco and soy lipoxygenase [12]. Oral exposure to allergens under specific experimental conditions was able to distinguish allergenic from non/low-allergenic food extracts, while systemic exposure did not [13].

There is a significant need to validate a toolbox of reference proteins, which contain potent allergenic, weak and non/low-allergenic proteins. Published data, to date, demonstrate a lack of reproducible and predictive measurements, which emphasizes the need for in vivo models, that are thoroughly tested with a wide range of well-characterized, purified, and endotoxin-free potent, weak or non/low-allergenic proteins.

Animal species and strain

The species most commonly employed in food allergy research is the mouse. In addition to their small size and short breeding cycle, the sequence of immunological events involved in the development of sensitization and the elicitation of allergic reactions is similar, although not identical to humans [14]. Moreover, the availability of various immunological and molecular reagents and transgenic animals makes them a powerful tool for investigating immunological mechanisms related to food allergies and evaluating the sensitizing potential of new food proteins.

As for humans, genetic predisposition in mice is important for measuring in vivo sensitization to novel food proteins. Smit et al. [15] examined three different murine strains following oral administration of peanut extract. Higher concentrations of peanut-specific IgE were found in BALB/c mice compared with other strains. In contrast, Berin et al. [16] reported no differences between BALB/c and C3H/HeOuJ mice in their IgE response to β-lactoglubulin (BLG) and C3H/HeOuJ mice produced higher peanut protein-specific IgE levels. These disparate results were attributed to the use of different protocols for inducing sensitization. Both Berin et al. [16] and Smit et al. [15] reported that spleen cells from peanut sensitized BALB/c mice secreted more IL-4, IL-5, IL-13 and IFN-γ than those from C3H/HeOuJ mice, suggesting that BALB/c mice might be the preferable strain.

As an alternative to the mouse, Brown Norway (BN) rats mount strong IgE antibody responses and due to their size, it is possible to monitor kinetics of serum specific antibody responses within individual animals. Another advantage is that the test protein can be delivered by daily gavage over a period of weeks in the absence of adjuvant [17]. On the downside, oral dosing of rats requires a larger amount of protein, compared to mice, which influences the cost of the experiment and fewer immunological reagents are available than for mouse.

In contrast to murine models, dogs spontaneously develop allergies [18]. Thus, it is a good species for evaluating food allergy. Moreover, it is also possible to immunize the same animal with multiple allergens. Furthermore, it is possible to do repeated endoscopy of the gut, to identify high IgE responder animals and their larger organ size and blood volume allows for more analyses and longitudinal studies. Although dogs are well suited for mechanistic studies, it is not feasible to use them for routine testing for safety assessment. They are expensive to maintain, there are a limited number of strains, they have greater inter-animal variation than rodents, and commercially available immunological reagents are lacking [17]. Similar drawbacks are present in swine with the addition of long dosing times needed for sensitization [12].

Other potential animal species are guinea pigs and rabbits. However, guinea pigs do not produce IgE. Allergic responses in guinea pigs are IgG1a mediated and possibly other mechanisms are also involved, thereby making the translation to humans more difficult. Rabbits generate high levels of IgE after subcutaneous sensitization, but are poorly characterized and thereby rarely used as a model species for food allergy [19].

In conclusion, mice are currently the most commonly used in vivo model for evaluating potential sensitizing capacities of food proteins. Notably, when using mouse models, it is important to wisely select an optimal strain and sensitization protocol, depending on the allergen source and specific research question.

Route of sensitization

There are multiple routes used to induce allergic sensitization to food allergens including i.p., oral, intranasal (i.n.) and cutaneous administration [20, 21]. However, the route of administration may alter the resulting immune response. For example, i.p. sensitization with wheat proteins induced a specific IgE response with similar IgE-binding epitopes to humans [22], whereas i.p. sensitization with OVA led to more OVA-specific IgE-binding epitopes compared to oral sensitization [23].

Sensitization to food allergens such as peanut or cow's milk (CM) may occur in the gut with oral sensitization. Over the last few years, several oral food allergy models were established in rodents [24, 25] and are useful for investigating the mechanisms underlying sensitization and clinical reactions to food proteins. For example, Li et al. [26] demonstrated that oral exposure of C3H/HeJ mice to peanut extract (PE) in combination with cholera toxin (CT) induced PE-specific IgE in serum and systemic anaphylactic symptoms upon oral challenge. Alternatively, the skin may also be a route for sensitization to food allergens [27]. For example, in a human study it was found that cutaneous exposure, rather than maternal or infant allergen consumption, led to peanut sensitization [28]. Recently, Spergel et al. [29] started to decipher cutaneous sensitization mechanisms with food allergens in mice. These authors found that epicutaneous (e.p.) sensitization with OVA, in the absence of aluminum hydroxide, resulted in higher antibody levels compared to i.p. administration of OVA with aluminum hydroxide [29], suggesting that e.p. sensitization is a robust sensitization route. Furthermore, Strid et al. [30] reported that an aqueous solution of either peanut allergen or OVA, when applied to abraded skin of mice, induced the production of antigen-specific IgE. Notably, the most effective route of food allergen sensitization varies significantly between mouse strains [15, 31].

Therefore, the route of allergen sensitization is an important and necessary consideration for the use of any relevant animal model of food allergy. Oral sensitization may be required to mimic the effect of digestion and the gut epithelium on sensitization to food proteins. However, it is not yet known which route of sensitization is best to predict the allergenic potency of food proteins in the human population.

Dose–sensitization relationships

Risk assessment for food allergens does not fundamentally differ from assessing the risk of chemical substances or microbiological agents as they often include similar methodologies [32–34]. In the hazard characterization of food allergens, a qualitative, and, wherever possible, quantitative description of the sensitizing property of a food allergen is made, together with its relationship to dose, where possible. These dose–sensitization data are helpful to classify food allergens by creating threshold values below which the risk of inducing a new food allergy is considered to be negligible or acceptable.

In humans, knowledge on dose–sensitization relationships to food allergens is extremely limited. Probably both low- and high- dose tolerance induction may be relevant mechanisms for explaining the fact that just a small percentage of the human population develops food allergy [35]. Since many variables (e.g. exposure route and frequency, food-related factors, host-related factors, matrix effects) are likely to be of importance, the doses required for sensitization might prove highly variable.

No animal model has been adopted for use in the generation of dose–sensitization data. Ideally, an appropriate animal model should be (a) validated by dose–response curves with different sensitizations and (b) be sensitive for distinguishing a threshold beyond which significant sensitization would be predicted and (c) potentially be sensitive for producing graded responses comparable to what is known regarding their prevalence and severity of responses in humans, e.g. peanut > egg > spinach [12]. Previously, animal studies demonstrated dose–response relationships within a restricted dose range for only a limited number of proteins [12, 13, 36]. Using these animal studies one can only conclude that there is a hazard connected to a given protein, because the mechanistic knowledge to interpret the dose–sensitization profile in terms of risk assessment is lacking. This was nicely illustrated by Kroghsbo et al. [36] where dose–sensitization data of two related proteins (gluten and enzymatically hydrolysed gluten) were compared to determine which protein is the strongest sensitizer. Enzymatically hydrolysed gluten gave the highest immune response, which was dose-related. Gluten showed no dose-related responses. However, in contrast to the hydrolysed gluten, gluten showed a response at the low dose. Thus, one can conclude that both forms of this protein possess sensitizing capacity and the doses relevant for human exposure should be taken into consideration when qualifying the potential risks for humans.

In conclusion, dose–sensitization studies in animals can be used to enhance our mechanistic knowledge on the sensitization process and characterize the allergenic hazard of novel food proteins. However, the current lack of dose–sensitization data in food allergy makes it difficult to perform a risk assessment. In addition, dose-dependent effects on immunological responses are not always linear, which further complicates interpretation.

Protein preparation

Ideally, an animal model should assess the sensitizing capacity of the individual novel proteins, as well as the novel protein in the context of the whole food. However, the choice of how the proteins are prepared prior to sensitization assessment may have significant implications on the predictive value of the model. Should purified proteins, protein extracts or the complex whole food be used as test materials? Could the use of whole foods predict the sensitizing potential of individual proteins? Will purified proteins fold into the correct structure in the absence of the food matrix? Are there matrix proteins that modify (potentiate or inhibit) sensitizing capacity? These are only a few of the considerations that should be addressed before choosing a predictive animal model. Studying the sensitizing capacity of an allergen, as a constituent of different protein preparations is a major task that requires well-conducted and controlled animal studies [37].

For novel foods where there is no prior knowledge of the potential allergenicity of proteins contained herein, whole food allergenicity assessment might be the only option to identify potential de novo sensitizing proteins. The use of whole foods has the advantage of presenting the proteins to the immune system in the context of lipids, sugars and other proteins, and matrix factors known to influence the sensitizing capacity of a given protein [37, 38].

When using protein extracts, proteins may be lost or the relative amounts may be changed during the extraction process [37], because extraction is dependent on protein solubility and may be influenced by the processing of the foods [39]. This could result in the testing of an incomplete panel of proteins.

Additionally, the purity and quality of purified proteins must be of a high standard, because the predictive value of the animal model may be greatly influenced by contaminants. Both protein and endotoxin contamination can confuse allergenicity assessments. This issue was highlighted following the use of commercially "purified" OVA, where contamination with ovomucoid (OVM) resulted in an overestimation of the intrinsic sensitizing potential of OVA [40],. This indicates that the presence of small amounts of a potent sensitizer may obscure the sensitizing capacity of the intended study protein. Immune-modulating effects occur with endotoxin contamination, which may potentially lead to an overestimation of the protein-specific sensitizing capacity [41]. Thus, purified proteins should ideally be free of all possible modifying contaminants.

Protein processing

Foods are subjected to a wide variety of different processing methods before being consumed. Processing may affect the inherent allergenicity of the proteins contained within the food, by either decreasing or increasing their allergenic properties [39, 42]. However, there are no general rules on how and to what degree different forms of processing impact the allergenic properties of the food [39, 42].

Processing methods that affect the allergenic properties of food include heating, hydrolysis, pH and pressure treatment, which may modify the chemical and structural features of the proteins. The impact of heating on the sensitizing capacity of peanut was described by Ladics et al. [12] who compared the sensitizing capacity of raw and roasted peanut extract and observed no clear differences after oral or i.p. dosing of BN rats. Additionally, Bowman and Selgrade [13] showed similar results after oral administration to C3H/HeJ mice. In contrast, Kroghsbo et al. [37] demonstrated that oral dosing of BN rats with roasted peanut, but not whole blanched peanut, resulted in Ara h 1- and 2-specific IgE responses. These studies show that heating intensity can influence the sensitizing capacity of peanut proteins.

Hydrolysis usually reduces allergenicity, however, a study by Kroghsbo et al. [36] showed that acid hydrolysis of gluten proteins resulted in a significantly higher specific IgE response than unmodified gluten, in contrast to enzymatically hydrolyzed gluten, after i.p. immunization of BN rats. In vitro digestion abolished the sensitizing capacity of the CM protein BLG, but the same procedure did not affect sensitization to the peanut protein Ara h 1, even though Ara h 1 was digested to smaller peptides than BLG [9]. These studies collectively showed that hydrolysis may affect individual proteins differently and that the type of hydrolyses may affect the outcome.

Food matrix

Foods are composed of proteins, fat, carbohydrates, micronutrients and various contaminants, all of which may have various effects on intrinsic allergenicity of proteins by changing protein digestibility, bioaccessibility and/or bioavailability, or due to adjuvant or immune-modulatory effects. These factors should be considered in the in vivo allergenicity assessment of new proteins/protein sources.

Various food constituents can alter the digestibility of proteins, thus affecting the form and the way they will reach the site where immune responses are induced. This can simply result from a buffering effect of the whole food or from the presence of protease inhibitors. Additionally, emulsion of protein with lipids will modify their structure and the accessibility of enzymes to cleavage sites, with various effects on digestibility [43]. Similar effects were observed for added constituents such as stabilizers, thickeners or emulsifiers [44]. Competitive effects of other proteins for enzymatic digestion and active epithelial transport can also impact allergen digestibility and bioavailability [45]. Sequestration of protein in low accessible substructures, such as within protein body organelles as observed in seeds, can delay their release and limit their digestion [46]. High fat food increases gastric residence in humans, thus leading to an increased threshold for the occurrence of objective symptoms [47].

Proteins can co-localize with other food constituents such as pro-Th2 or modulating factors, whereby the corresponding microenvironment will determine the polarization of the specific immune response. Some studies have reported a lack of intrinsic immunogenicity/allergenicity of certain major allergens from milk, peanut or Brazil nuts [48–50]. The immune response was prompted by the adjuvant effect of other food constituents, as demonstrated by (defatted) extract from peanut [48] or with lipids from Brazil nuts that will activate iNKT cells to produce IL-4 [50]. Other proteins (lectins) or contaminants such as aflatoxin present in the food matrix influence sensitization [51], whereas ω-3 PUFA-derived metabolites decrease mast cell activation [52].

Lastly, the quantity of any new protein(s) in food items should be considered. For example, the newly expressed protein Cry1Ab (MON810 maize) was demonstrated to be highly immunogenic when administered as a purified protein, but no Cry1Ab-specific immune response was evident after experimental sensitization with maize flour, probably due to the low levels of Cry1Ab within the flour [50].

Adjuvants

T cell sensitization to allergenic proteins requires fully activated professional antigen presenting cells (APC) that not only present relevant peptides in the context of MHCII, but also express a range of costimulatory signals [53]. Importantly, the lack of appropriate costimulatory signals results in anergy or tolerance. Substances that can induce costimulation are considered adjuvants, being defined as components that are able to potentiate and/or modulate adaptive immune responses.

It is not well understood to what extent adjuvants are needed to promote an allergic response, but adjuvant signals appear crucial at least in a range of animal studies. Adjuvants influence both the activation and subsequent migration of dendritic cells (DCs) to a draining lymph node, which reside in the vicinity of the first exposure site to potential allergens. It is increasingly realized that signals coming from epithelial cells can instruct DC to become activated APC. These epithelium-derived signals together are referred to as a danger associated molecular pattern (DAMP) and include innate cytokines and chemokines or alarmins [54–56]. Together with a range of immune cells such as innate lymphoid cells, intraepithelial lymphocytes (IELs) [57–59], eosinophils and mast cells, DAMPs determine the outcome of the immune response. The importance of the epithelial barrier in controlling Th2 immune responses has been reviewed more extensively elsewhere [56, 60].

In animal models of food allergy, sensitization by the i.p. route with the use of aluminum hydroxide as an adjuvant is common [61]. The mechanisms behind the adjuvant effect of aluminum hydroxide are still not fully understood [62], but stimulation of DC antigen presentation [63] and a IL-4-driven Th2 response have been described [64]. Additionally, changes in specific antibody responses to aluminum hydroxide-adsorbed antigens have been observed [62, 65, 66] and is probably due to the modulation of antibody responses related to structural changes of the antigens [67].

One of the best known mucosal adjuvants used to sensitize animals to food proteins is CT [26]. The adjuvant effect of CT depends on CD11b DCs and cAMP [68]. Importantly, because *Vibrio cholera* infection is relatively rare in humans, CT should be regarded as an experimental model adjuvant and is not relevant for promoting food allergy in man.

Additional modulating substances may influence sensitization to food proteins. *Staphylococcus aureus* enterotoxin B (SEB), a bacterial superantigen relevant to humans, promotes sensitization to OVA [69]. The NSAID diclofenac causes epithelial damage in the intestinal tract and stimulates the allergic response to peanut extract, but only in combination with CT [57, 58]. Medium chain triglyceride (MCT), but not long-chain triglycerides induce sensitization to peanut in mice, without CT [70]. The role of endotoxin as a possible adjuvant remains unclear because data are not consistent across different experimental models and doses [16, 71]. Uric acid is a DAMP produced by epithelial cells and administration of monosodium urate can replace CT as an adjuvant [72].

Occasionally, allergy in test animals can be induced without adjuvant. Birmingham et al. [73] and Gonipeta et al. [74] sensitized mice to hazelnut and milk whey protein, by transdermal application of the allergen, for 6 consecutive weeks. Although they did not add an adjuvant, they clipped the hair from skin and used mild occlusion for 1 day, which may cause mild inflammatory responses and release DAMPs [75]. Others [54, 76], have used tape stripping methods to promote epicutaneous sensitization to food allergens. Noti et al. [54] showed that this route of exposure requires the TSLP-basophil axis, indicating activation of innate immune responses. Guinea pigs have also been used as a model to investigate the allergenicity of specifically CM without adding adjuvant by exposing the guinea pigs to the CM via their drinking water for several weeks [77]. However it is difficult to translate this model to the human setting due to differences in immune physiology and limited knowledge and tools to study their immune system. Lastly, the BN rat model for food allergy is performed without added adjuvant, but in this model the allergen is gavaged for 35 to 42 days [78], again possibly inducing epithelial stress (in the oesophagus) with associated adjuvant effects.

In conclusion, primarily based on mouse data, adjuvants or at least adjuvant-like activation of innate immunity seems to be important for the induction of sensitization to food proteins. However, addition of an adjuvant will not always be necessary in an animal model when testing sensitizing capacity of novel proteins, especially when the novel protein/food has inherent sensitizing capacity.

Environmental factors

Not everyone becomes allergic to foods. This suggests that other factors like lifestyle and environmental factors, interacting with a genetic predisposition, play a role. To accurately predict the allergenic potential of novel food proteins using animal models, it is essential to consider the various environmental factors that could influence sensitization in humans.

Firstly, unintended dietary pre-exposure to the food protein under investigation or to a cross-reactive protein could lead to the induction of allergen-specific oral tolerance, which would prevent further sensitization in the animal model and lead to false negative results. Dietary control in parental generations before mating or during suckling [79, 80] and monitoring other dietary factors such as the quantity of bioactive lipid components or non-digestible fibers in animal diet, which influence the immune response, can help minimize potential bias in sensitization profiles [81–83]. However, other currently unknown dietary factors, may also influence immune responses within the gut and further research is needed to identify these factors.

Protein modifications (e.g. due to environmental pollution or during food processing) have a substantial impact on the elicitation of protein-specific immune responses. In addition, interference with the physiological digestion capacity of the GI tract contributes to food allergy. Pharmacological gastric acid suppression is associated with food allergy development via the oral route in experimental mouse models [84, 85]. While animal age seems to play a minor role in many models [86], the use of newborn/weaned animals can be relevant when using a different experimental approach to induce sensitization or if the protein being investigated is ultimately intended for consumption by human infants [87].

The composition of the gut microbiome may influence the outcome of food allergy models and may contribute to inter-laboratory variation. There is increasing evidence that gut microbiota plays a critical role in allergic sensitization and tolerance induction in humans and rodents [88, 89]. The fetal immune system favors a Th2 response that is related to an increased risk of developing allergic disease. Bacterial colonization after birth provides a microbial stimulus affecting the maturation and modulation of the intestinal and systemic immune system [90]. Commensal bacteria can stimulate tight junction-related proteins thereby reducing epithelial permeability, while also promoting immunoregulatory responses within mucosal tissue which protects against allergic sensitization [91–94]. Germ-free mice display a characteristic increased immune response to allergens with a remarkable Th2 bias. Thus, these animals could represent a highly sensitive model to study allergenicity of new proteins [95, 96], but are difficult to maintain. The gut microbiome of different animal facilities will be influenced by the breeding environment (e.g. specific pathogen free (SPF) versus specific and opportunistic pathogen free (SOPF), diet and water). In particular, microbiome alterations associated with ω-fatty acids and obesity should be controlled. Lastly, there are indications that vitamin A and D deficiencies, which modify intestinal homeostasis, might moderate intestinal immunity via interaction with the microbiome [79, 97].

Breeding environment and experience of the experimenter should be taken into consideration, since stress responses may influence the immune response to the administered protein/food [98]. In conclusion, breeding conditions (parental generations, housing, stress), diet and other environmental factors must be carefully adjusted between different laboratories and standardized whenever possible to develop a reproducible animal model to study protein sensitization. Unfortunately, many published manuscripts still do not describe these parameters in detail and therefore, currently, it is not possible to recommend a specific dietary regimen, other than the protein of interest should not be included in the diet before testing the animals.

In vivo readouts

Common food allergy signs and symptoms in patients include itching, swelling of lips, tongue, face and throat, abdominal pain, diarrhea, nausea, or vomiting, while anaphylactic reactions involve constriction of airways, cardiovascular shock with a severe drop in blood pressure, rapid pulse and/or loss of consciousness [99]. Upon exposure to food allergens, a number of allergy signs that mimic clinical symptoms in patients can be observed in animal model systems [3, 100]. Such in vivo parameters are useful to study allergenicity of food proteins, the impact of genetics or microbial colonization [101]. To model food allergy, animals are typically sensitized with an allergenic food or protein (with or without adjuvant) by feeding or other routes, followed by challenges to the GI tract, circulation (intravenous (i.v.), i.p.), or skin (subcutaneous), which then manifests in an organ-specific distinct readout.

Repeated oral food allergen challenges of previously sensitized animals results in measureable clinical signs including diarrhea, piloerection, changes in activity, mobility and behavior or most often a combination of all signs that can be enumerated in a clinical allergy score [54].

Systemic food allergen challenges often result in severe allergic reactions mimicking anaphylaxis in patients. Such reactions are evaluated using anaphylaxis scoring protocols that assess severity including scratching, diarrhea, piloerection, labored respiration, cyanosis around mouth and tail, reduced activity, tremors, convulsion or death [26]. Measuring hypothermia (rectal temperature or subcutaneously (s.c.) implanted programmable temperature transponder) or vascular leakage (i.p allergen challenge immediately followed by i.v. Evan's blue injection and animals are monitored for blue color accumulation in the extremities) are additional in vivo readouts [102, 103].

To measure airway hyperreactivity (AHR) in the context of food allergen sensitization, allergen challenge may be intranasal, intra-tracheal or via nebulization [104]. Upon allergen challenge, animals are assessed for airway resistance and compliance in response to methacholine and not by allergen exposure using invasive or enhanced pause (PenH) non-invasive techniques [105]. Notably, this read out may be more dependent upon changes in the airways (e.g., inflammation and increased airway smooth muscle) than to the mast cell-IgE-histamine axis.

Passive cutaneous anaphylaxis (PCA) is an immediate dermal response to an allergen-IgE interaction that is typically characterized by increased vascular leakage within the skin that can be assessed by i.v. injection of Evans blue. In vivo PCA readouts include ear swelling (thickening of skin) and skin color [103]. Alternatively animals are injected intradermally (i.d.) in the ear pinnae with the allergen and ear swelling is measured within 1 h. This acute allergic skin response can be used to asses an immediate type hypersensitivity (ITH) [106, 107]. Delayed type hypersensitivity (DTH) represents an additional skin test to assess late-phase cutaneous food allergic reactions, in which animals are injected s.c. with allergen into the hind footpads or in the ear pinnae and edema measured [108].

While in vivo readouts allow for a rapid assessment of allergic responses, a caveat of these readouts is that measures of allergy are often subjective and thus, require blinding of experimental groups. In vivo readouts provide more information than just sensitization potential as allergy effector mechanisms become activated, although not all of these responses are IgE-dependent. Lastly, one should ensure that ethical concerns are considered, particularly when inducing severe allergic reactions. The advantages and disadvantages of the different in vivo readouts are summarized in Table 1.

Table 1 In vivo readouts

Test	Advantages	Disadvantages
Gastrointestinal [54]	Non-invasive, does not harm animals, qualitative and quantitative allergy scoring, blinded scoring possible	No standardized scoring system, lab to lab variations, subjective, diarrhea as only GI specific sign
Systemic		
Anaphylaxis score [76]	Non-invasive, qualitative and quantitative allergy scoring, blinded scoring possible	Subjective, ethical consideration
Hypothermia [109, 110]	Rectal temperature (semi-invasive), quantitative readout, blinded scoring possible	Accuracy of rectal measurements, transplanted responders (invasive), ethical consideration
Vascular leakage [24, 110]	Qualitative readout, blinded scoring possible	Invasive
Airways		
AHR [105]	Qualitative and quantitative, objective readout, blinded measurements are possible, anesthesia not required for non-invasive AHR	Invasive and anesthesia required (only for invasive AHR), usually endpoint measurement, expensive equipment required
Skin [111]		
PCA	Quantitative measurement of skin thickness, qualitative assessement of vascular leakage	Invasive, blinded scoring not possible
ITH	Quantitative measurement of skin swelling	Invasive, blinded scoring not possible
DTH	Quantitative measurement of skin/tissue swelling	Invasive, blinded scoring not possible

Ex vivo readouts

A wide range of ex vivo readouts can be utilized to assess or support the sensitizing capacity of novel proteins. The most common readout consists of measuring specific IgE antibody levels from exposed animals by ELISA [112]. However, allergen-specific IgG may obscure the analysis as allergen-specific IgG generally is present at 100 to 1000-fold higher concentrations than allergen-specific IgE. IgE detection can be improved by depleting IgG or by employing a capture ELISA [48, 113, 114]. In addition, new technologies such as rapid evanescent biosensor technology would be useful to avoid the influence of IgG when measuring allergen-specific IgE [115]. Although total IgE may be correlated with specific IgE in controlled experimental settings [116], identification of allergen-specific IgE is required for allergenic assessment of novel foods. It is also important to assess the biological activity of antigen-specific IgE. For example, functionality of serum IgE may be assessed in vitro as the ability to induce specific degranulation of basophils or mast cells [117].

Allergic sensitization starts with activation of innate cells, including epithelial cells, DCs and ILC2 s, T cells and Th2 cytokines [118, 119]. Cytokine production and immune cell proliferation are typically measured after ex vivo stimulation of cells from the lymph node or spleen with the allergen or with T cell mitogens [113, 120]. While intracellular cytokine production on the single cell level can be determined by flow cytometry, cytokine secretion from cell suspensions is measured as supernatant concentrations by ELISA or multiplex assays. The Th1/Th2/Th17/Treg cytokine balance, rather than the absolute cytokine levels, is thought to be important [121]. Current models suggest that cytokine and proliferation responses during the induction phase of sensitization in the draining lymph node may be useful in predicting sensitizing capacity [122–124]. Measuring TSLP, IL-25 and IL-33, along with ILC2 s, in the intestine during food allergy sensitization may provide additional predictive markers of sensitizing potential [26, 55].

Determination of cell phenotypes, subsets and co-stimulatory molecules on innate and adaptive immune cells in the lymph node, spleen or intestines are readouts possibly useful to support a sensitizing potential. Such measurements can be performed by high throughput flow cytometric or mass spectrometry-based assays. Determination of gene expression (e.g. mRNA) and cytokine gene epigenetics, co-stimulatory molecules or inflammatory markers are also ex vivo endpoints currently applied.

Many animal models for food allergy investigate the anaphylactic response to a food allergy challenge [24, 76, 107, 110]. Ex vivo endpoints for anaphylaxis include serum mast cell proteases (mMCP-1), [125] and histamine release assays.

Future perspectives and conclusions

Considerable progress has been made in using animal models to better understand the basic mechanisms and environmental influences contributing to food allergen sensitization. Researchers intending to utilize animal models of food allergy should be aware of the experimental parameters outlined in this review, which may have

Table 2 Pros and Cons of different food allergy model design parameters

Design parameter	Sub-parameter	Pros	Cons
Reference proteins	Strong, weak and non-allergenic proteins	Confirm reproducibility and predictability	Requires additional groups of animals
Animal species	Mice	Small size, short breeding cycle, availability of many reagents	Usually need adjuvants, low amount of sera can be obtained
	Rats	Small size, short breeding cycle, larger amount of sera can be obtained, no need for use of adjuvant	Restricted availability of reagents, larger amount of protein/food required
	Dogs	Large organ size and increased amount of sera can be obtained, spontaneously develop allergies	Restricted availability of reagents, Very large amount of protein/food required, large animals, prolonged duration of animal studies, expensive and ethical consideration
Route of sensitization	Oral	Relevant route of sensitization	Often needs the use of adjuvant, require large amount of protein
	i.p.	No adjuvant, robust sensitization route, no need for large amount of proteins/food	Non-physiological relevant route
	Cutaneous	Relevant route of sensitization	Usually requires immunological danger signals
Dose–response relationship		Helps in creating threshold levels, helps in hazard identification	Several groups of animals required for each protein
Protein preparation	Whole foods	Ability to study the sensitizing capacity of proteins in their natural matrix, Ability to study the allergenicity of true novel foods, Easy to prepare	Difficult to identify the sensitising proteins
	Purified proteins	Ability to study the inherent sensitizing capacity of the individual protein	Difficult to prepare, need large amounts of high quality purified protein, protein structure may change
	Food Extracts	Easy to prepare	Difficult to identify the sensitizing protein, some proteins may be lost or the relative amounts may change, protein structure may change
Protein processing	Raw protein/food	Ability to study the inherent allergenicity	May not reflect the end use of the protein
	Processed protein/food	Ability to study the sensitizing capacity of the consumed version which cannot be predicted otherwise	May impact the allergenic properties
Adjuvant		Provides a danger signal	Artificially modifies the immune response

an impact on their results. In addition, published reports should include sufficient details concerning all of these parameters, to allow for reproduction in other laboratories. The Pros and Cons of the experimental parameters discussed in this review are summarized in Table 2. The ideal animal model for assessing the potential sensitizing capacity of new proteins has yet to be developed, but the ideal model must predict known strong and weak food allergens. The development of a reference protein toolbox is essential and would revolutionize the use of animal models in the future risk assessment of potential allergens. Ideally, the sensitization route would be oral or via the skin and not only IgE measurements, but also functional or symptomatic responses should be recorded. In addition, more research is required to determine why only some proteins are allergenic in contrast to the majority of proteins. The identification of certain protein characteristics such as structural similarities or intrinsic activities will greatly assist the development of animal models for the screening of allergenic potential. However, even known food allergens do not induce food allergy in all exposed individuals and therefore, host and environmental factors also need to be explored further, which can be achieved through the use of animal models.

Abbreviations

APC: antigen presenting cell; BLG: beta-lactoglubulin; BN: Brown Norway; CM: cow's milk; CT: cholera toxin; DAMP: danger associated molecular pattern; DC: dendritic cells; DTH: delayed type hypersensitivity; e.p.: epicutaneous; i.d.: intradermally; IEL: intraepithelial lymphocytes; IL: interleukin; ILC: innate lymphoid cell; i.n.: intranasal; iNKT: invariant natural killer T cell; i.p.: intraperitoneal; ITH: immediate type hypersensitivity; i.v.: intravenous; LTP: lipid transfer protein; MCT: medium chain triglyceride; OVA: ovalbumin; OVM: ovomucoid; PCA: passive cutaneous anaphylaxis; PE: peanut extract; SEB: staphylococcus aureus enterotoxin B; SOPF: specific and opportunistic pathogen free; SPF: specific pathogen free; Th: T helper cell; TSLP: thymic stromal lymphopoietin.

Authors' contributions

JS wrote the reference proteins section, RG and IL-E wrote the animal species and strains section, MB, GB and CB wrote the route of sensitization section, JB wrote the dose–sensitization relationships section, KLB wrote the protein preparation and processing sections, KAP wrote the food matrix section, RP wrote the adjuvants section, SB-N, KAP and EU wrote the environmental factors section, LK, ME and MN wrote the in vivo readouts section, while IL-E and UCN wrote the ex vivo readouts section. LOM, KLB, IK and KV wrote the introduction and conclusions and coordinated the drafting of the manuscript. All authors read and approved the final manuscript.

Author details

[1] National Food Institute, Technical University of Denmark, Søborg, Denmark. [2] TNO, Zeist, The Netherlands. [3] Warsaw University of Life Sciences, Warsaw, Poland. [4] Department of Bioactivity and Food Analysis, Institute for Food Science Research (CIAL) (CSIC-UAM), Madrid, Spain. [5] INRA, Nantes, France. [6] Nestlé Research Center, Lausanne, Switzerland. [7] Institute for Risk Assessment Sciences, Utrecht University, Utrecht, The Netherlands. [8] Food and Biobased Research, Wageningen University and Research Centre, Wageningen, The Netherlands. [9] Department of Pathophysiology and Allergy Research, Medical University of Vienna, Vienna, Austria. [10] UMR-INRA-CEA, Service de Pharmacologie et d'Immunoanalyse, Université Paris-Saclay, Gif-sur-Yvette, France. [11] Danone Nutricia Research, Utrecht, The Netherlands. [12] Utrecht Institute for Pharmaceutical Sciences, Utrecht University, Utrecht, The Netherlands. [13] Experimental Allergy Laboratory, DIAID, Department of Dermatology, Medical University of Vienna, Vienna, Austria. [14] Institute of Pathology, University of Bern, Bern, Switzerland. [15] Norwegian Institute of Public Health, Oslo, Norway. [16] University of Manchester, Manchester, UK. [17] Swiss Institute of Allergy and Asthma Research, University of Zürich, Obere Strasse 22, 7270 Davos Platz, Switzerland.

Acknowledgements

The authors are all part of the COST Action FA1402 entitled: Improving Allergy Risk Assessment Strategy for New Food Proteins (ImpARAS). LOM is supported by Swiss National Foundation grants (Project Numbers: CRSII3_154488 and 310030-144219) and European Union research grants.

Competing interests

Liam O'Mahony is a consultant to Alimentary Health Ltd and has received research funding from GSK.

References

1. Muraro A, Werfel T, Hoffmann-Sommergruber K, Roberts G, Beyer K, Bindslev-Jensen C, et al. EAACI food allergy and anaphylaxis guidelines: diagnosis and management of food allergy. Allergy. 2014;69:1008–25.
2. Muraro A, Halken S, Arshad SH, Beyer K, Dubois AE, Du TG, et al. EAACI food allergy and anaphylaxis guidelines. Primary prevention of food allergy. Allergy. 2014;69:590–601.
3. McClain S, Bannon GA. Animal models of food allergy: opportunities and barriers. Curr Allergy Asthma Rep. 2006;6:141–4.
4. Radauer C, Bublin M, Wagner S, Mari A, Breiteneder H. Allergens are distributed into few protein families and possess a restricted number of biochemical functions. J Allergy Clin Immunol. 2008;121:847–52.
5. Lin J, Shewry PR, Archer DB, Beyer K, Niggemann B, Haas H, et al. The potential allergenicity of two 2S albumins from soybean (Glycine max): a protein microarray approach. Int Arch Allergy Immunol. 2006;141:91–102.
6. Kroghsbo S, Bøgh KL, Rigby NM, Mills EN, Rogers A, Madsen CB. Sensitization with 7S globulins from peanut, hazelnut, soy or pea induces IgE with different biological activities which are modified by soy tolerance. Int Arch Allergy Immunol. 2011;155:212–24.
7. Hazebrouck S, Ah-Leung S, Bidat E, Paty E, Drumare MF, Tilleul S, et al. Goat's milk allergy without cow's milk allergy: suppression of non-cross-reactive epitopes on caprine β-casein. Clin Exp Allergy. 2014;44:602–10.
8. Astwood JD, Leach JN, Fuchs RL. Stability of food allergens to digestion in vitro. Nat Biotechnol. 1996;14:1269–73.
9. Bøgh KL, Madsen CB. Food allergens: is there a correlation between stability to digestion and allergenicity? Crit Rev Food Sci Nutr. 2015. [Epub ahead of print]
10. Fu TT, Abbott UR, Hatzos C. Digestibility of food allergens and nonallergenic proteins in simulated gastric fluid and simulated intestinal fluid—a comparative study. J Agric Food Chem. 2002;50:7154–60.
11. Dearman RJ, Kimber I. Determination of protein allergenicity: studies in mice. Toxicol Lett. 2001;120:181–6.
12. Ladics GS, Knippels LM, Penninks AH, Bannon GA, Goodman RE, Herouet-Guicheney C. Review of animal models designed to predict the potential allergenicity of novel proteins in genetically modified crops. Regul Toxicol Pharmacol. 2010;56:212–24.
13. Bowman CC, Selgrade MK. Differences in allergenic potential of food extracts following oral exposure in mice reflect differences in digestibility: potential approaches to safety assessment. Toxicol Sci. 2008;102:100–9.
14. Eigenmann PA, Antonella MM, Sampson HA, Wahn U. iPAC: an initiative to fight the burden of allergies in children. Pediatr Allergy Immunol. 2008;19:1–3.
15. Smit JJ, Willemsen K, Hassing I, Fiechter D, Storm G, van Bloois L, et al. Contribution of classic and alternative effector pathways in peanut-induced anaphylactic responses. PLoS One. 2011;6:e28917.
16. Berin MC, Zheng Y, Domaradzki M, Li XM, Sampson HA. Role of TLR4 in allergic sensitization to food proteins in mice. Allergy. 2006;61:64–71.

17. Dearman RJ, Kimber I. Animal models of protein allergenicity: potential benefits, pitfalls and challenges. Clin Exp Allergy. 2009;39:458–68.
18. Teuber SS, Del VG, Morigasaki S, Jung HR, Eisele PH, Frick OL, Buchanan BB. The atopic dog as a model of peanut and tree nut food allergy. J Allergy Clin Immunol. 2002;110:921–7.
19. Vinuesa M, Bassan N, Cases AI, Krumrik G. Montelukast treatment (cysteinyl leukotriene receptor antagonist) in a model of food allergy: modifications in lymphatic cell population from rectal mucosa. Rev Esp Enferm Dig. 2010;102:421–5.
20. Dearman RJ, Kimber I. A mouse model for food allergy using intraperitoneal sensitization. Methods. 2007;41:91–8.
21. Gourbeyre P, Dery-Papini S, Larre C, Gaudin JC, Brossard C, Bodinier M. Wheat gliadins modified by deamidation are more efficient than native gliadins in inducing a Th2 response in Balb/c mice experimentally sensitized to wheat allergens. Mol Nutr Food Res. 2012;56:336–44.
22. Dery-Papini S, Bodinier M, Pineau F, Triballeau S, Tranquet O, Adel-Patient K, et al. Immunoglobulin-E-binding epitopes of wheat allergens in patients with food allergy to wheat and in mice experimentally sensitized to wheat proteins. Clin Exp Allergy. 2011;41:1478–92.
23. Mine Y, Yang M. Epitope characterization of ovalbumin in BALB/c mice using different entry routes. Biochim Biophys Acta. 2007;1774:200–12.
24. Li XM, Schofield BH, Huang CK, Kleiner GI, Sampson HA. A murine model of IgE-mediated cow's milk hypersensitivity. J Allergy Clin Immunol. 1999;103:206–14.
25. Knippels LM, Penninks AH, Spanhaak S, Houben GF. Oral sensitization to food proteins: a Brown Norway rat model. Clin Exp Allergy. 1998;28:368–75.
26. Li XM, Serebrisky D, Lee SY, Huang CK, Bardina L, Schofield BH, et al. A murine model of peanut anaphylaxis: T- and B-cell responses to a major peanut allergen mimic human responses. J Allergy Clin Immunol. 2000;106:150–8.
27. Lack G, Fox D, Northstone K, Golding J. Factors associated with the development of peanut allergy in childhood. N Engl J Med. 2003;348:977–85.
28. Fox AT, Sasieni P, Du TG, Syed H, Lack G. Household peanut consumption as a risk factor for the development of peanut allergy. J Allergy Clin Immunol. 2009;123:417–23.
29. Spergel JM, Mizoguchi E, Brewer JP, Martin TR, Bhan AK, Geha RS. Epicutaneous sensitization with protein antigen induces localized allergic dermatitis and hyperresponsiveness to methacholine after single exposure to aerosolized antigen in mice. J Clin Invest. 1998;101:1614–22.
30. Strid J, Hourihane J, Kimber I, Callard R, Strobel S. Disruption of the stratum corneum allows potent epicutaneous immunization with protein antigens resulting in a dominant systemic Th2 response. Eur J Immunol. 2004;34:2100–9.
31. Morafo V, Srivastava K, Huang CK, Kleiner G, Lee SY, Sampson HA, Li AM. Genetic susceptibility to food allergy is linked to differential TH2-TH1 responses in C3H/HeJ and BALB/c mice. J Allergy Clin Immunol. 2003;111:1122–8.
32. Madsen CB, Hattersley S, Buck J, Gendel SM, Houben GF, Hourihane JO, et al. Approaches to risk assessment in food allergy: report from a workshop "developing a framework for assessing the risk from allergenic foods". Food Chem Toxicol. 2009;47:480–9.
33. Spanjersberg MQ, Lucas Luijckx NB, Houben GF. Risk analysis of food allergens. In: Jedrychowski L, Wichers HJ, editors. Chemical and biological properties of food allergens. CRC Press, Florence, KY, 2009. p. 387–97.
34. Crevel RW, Baumert JL, Baka A, Houben GF, Knulst AC, Kruizinga AG, et al. Development and evolution of risk assessment for food allergens. Food Chem Toxicol. 2014;67:262–76.
35. van Ree R, Hummelshoj L, Plantinga M, Poulsen LK, Swindle E. Allergic sensitization: host-immune factors. Clin Transl Allergy. 2014;4:12.
36. Kroghsbo S, Andersen NB, Rasmussen TF, Jacobsen S, Madsen CB. Acid hydrolysis of wheat gluten induces formation of new epitopes but does not enhance sensitizing capacity by the oral route: a study in "gluten free" Brown Norway rats. PLoS One. 2014;9:e107137.
37. Kroghsbo S, Rigby NM, Johnson PE, Adel-Patient K, Bøgh KL, Salt LJ, et al. Assessment of the sensitizing potential of processed peanut proteins in Brown Norway rats: roasting does not enhance allergenicity. PLoS One. 2014;9:e96475.
38. Madsen JL, Kroghsbo S, Madsen CB, Pozdnyakova I, Barkholt V, Bøgh KL. The impact of structural integrity and route of administration on the antibody specificity against three cow's milk allergens—a study in Brown Norway rats. Clin Transl Allergy. 2014;4:25.
39. Verhoeckx KC, Vissers YM, Baumert JL, Faludi R, Feys M, Flanagan S, et al. Food processing and allergenicity. Food Chem Toxicol. 2015;80:223–40.
40. Bernhisel-Broadbent J, Dintzis HM, Dintzis RZ, Sampson HA. Allergenicity and antigenicity of chicken egg ovomucoid (Gal d III) compared with ovalbumin (Gal d I) in children with egg allergy and in mice. J Allergy Clin Immunol. 1994;93:1047–59.
41. Brix S, Kjaer TM, Barkholt V, Frokiaer H. Lipopolysaccharide contamination of beta-lactoglobulin affects the immune response against intraperitoneally and orally administered antigen. Int Arch Allergy Immunol. 2004;135:216–20.
42. Thomas K, MacIntosh S, Bannon G, Herouet-Guicheney C, Holsapple M, Ladics G, et al. Scientific advancement of novel protein allergenicity evaluation: an overview of work from the HESI Protein Allergenicity Technical Committee (2000–2008). Food Chem Toxicol. 2009;47:1041–50.
43. Benede S, Lopez-Exposito I, Molina E, Lopez-Fandino R. Egg proteins as allergens and the effects of the food matrix and processing. Food Funct. 2015;6:694–713.
44. Mouecoucou J, Sanchez C, Villaume C, Marrion O, Fremont S, Laurent F, Mejean L. Effects of different levels of gum arabic, low methylated pectin and xylan on in vitro digestibility of beta-lactoglobulin. J Dairy Sci. 2003;86:3857–65.
45. Schulten V, Lauer I, Scheurer S, Thalhammer T, Bohle B. A food matrix reduces digestion and absorption of food allergens in vivo. Mol Nutr Food Res. 2011;55:1484–91.
46. Teuber SS. Hypothesis: The protein body effect and other aspects of food matrix effects. Ann N Y Acad Sci. 2002;964:111–6.
47. Mackie A, Knulst A, Le TM, Bures P, Salt L, Mills EN, et al. High fat food increases gastric residence and thus thresholds for objective symptoms in allergic patients. Mol Nutr Food Res. 2012;56:1708–14.
48. van Wijk F, Nierkens S, Hassing I, Feijen M, Koppelman SJ, de Jong GAH, et al. The effect of the food matrix on in vivo immune responses to purified peanut allergens. Toxicol Sci. 2005;86:333–41.
49. Adel-Patient K, Guimaraes VD, Paris A, Drumare MF, Ah-Leung S, Lamourette P, et al. Immunological and metabolomic impacts of administration of Cry1Ab protein and MON 810 maize in mouse. PLoS One. 2011;6:e16346.
50. Mirotti L, Florsheim E, Rundqvist L, Larsson G, Spinozzi F, Leite-de-Moraes M, et al. Lipids are required for the development of Brazil nut allergy: the role of mouse and human iNKT cells. Allergy. 2013;68:74–83.
51. Kocabas CN, Sekerel BE. Does systemic exposure to aflatoxin B(1) cause allergic sensitization? Allergy. 2003;58:363–5.
52. Kunisawa J, Arita M, Hayasaka T, Harada T, Iwamoto R, Nagasawa R, et al. Dietary omega3 fatty acid exerts anti-allergic effect through the conversion to 17,18-epoxyeicosatetraenoic acid in the gut. Sci Rep. 2015;5:9750.
53. Schiavi E, Smolinska S, O'Mahony L. Intestinal dendritic cells. Curr Opin Gastroenterol. 2015;31:98–103.
54. Noti M, Kim BS, Siracusa MC, Rak GD, Kubo M, Moghaddam AE, et al. Exposure to food allergens through inflamed skin promotes intestinal food allergy through the thymic stromal lymphopoietin-basophil axis. J Allergy Clin Immunol. 2014;133:1390–9.
55. Chu DK, Llop-Guevara A, Walker TD, Flader K, Goncharova S, Boudreau JE, et al. IL-33, but not thymic stromal lymphopoietin or IL-25, is central to mite and peanut allergic sensitization. J Allergy Clin Immunol. 2013;131:187–200.
56. Hammad H, Lambrecht BN. Barrier epithelial cells and the control of type 2 immunity. Immunity. 2015;43:29–40.
57. Bol-Schoenmakers M, Bleumink R, Marcondes RM, Mouser E, Hassing I, Ludwig I, et al. Diclofenac enhances allergic responses in a mouse peanut allergy model. Clin Exp Allergy. 2011;41:424–33.
58. Bol-Schoenmakers M, Marcondes RM, Bleumink R, Boon L, Man S, Hassing I, et al. Regulation by intestinal gammadelta T cells during establishment of food allergic sensitization in mice. Allergy. 2011;66:331–40.
59. Frossard CP, Asigbetse KE, Burger D, Eigenmann PA. Gut T cell receptor-gammadelta(+) intraepithelial lymphocytes are activated selectively by cholera toxin to break oral tolerance in mice. Clin Exp Immunol. 2015;180:118–30.
60. Swamy M, Jamora C, Havran W, Hayday A. Epithelial decision makers: in search of the 'epimmunome'. Nat Immunol. 2010;11:656–65.

61. Oyoshi MK, Oettgen HC, Chatila TA, Geha RS, Bryce PJ. Food allergy: insights into etiology, prevention, and treatment provided by murine models. J Allergy Clin Immunol. 2014;133:309–17.
62. Heydenreich B, Bellinghausen I, Lund L, Henmar H, Lund G, Adler WP, Saloga J. Adjuvant effects of aluminium hydroxide-adsorbed allergens and allergoids—differences in vivo and in vitro. Clin Exp Immunol. 2014;176:310–9.
63. Harrison WT. Some observations on the use of alum precipitated diphtheria toxoid. Am J Public Health Nations Health. 1935;25:298–300.
64. Comoy EE, Capron A, Thyphronitis G. In vivo induction of type 1 and 2 immune responses against protein antigens. Int Immunol. 1997;9:523–31.
65. Zlatkovic J, Tsouchnikas G, Jarmer J, Koessl C, Stiasny K, Heinz FX. Aluminum hydroxide influences not only the extent but also the fine specificity and functional activity of antibody responses to tick-borne encephalitis virus in mice. J Virol. 2013;87:12187–95.
66. Bøgh KL, Barkholt V, Madsen CB. Characterization of the immunogenicity and allergenicity of two cow's milk hydrolysates–a study in Brown Norway rats. Scand J Immunol. 2015;81:274–83.
67. Jones LS, Peek LJ, Power J, Markham A, Yazzie B, Middaugh CR. Effects of adsorption to aluminum salt adjuvants on the structure and stability of model protein antigens. J Biol Chem. 2005;280:13406–14.
68. Mattsson J, Schon K, Ekman L, Fahlen-Yrlid L, Yrlid U, Lycke NY. Cholera toxin adjuvant promotes a balanced Th1/Th2/Th17 response independently of IL-12 and IL-17 by acting on Gsalpha in CD11b(+) DCs. Mucosal Immunol. 2015;8:815–27.
69. Ganeshan K, Neilsen CV, Hadsaitong A, Schleimer RP, Luo X, Bryce PJ. Impairing oral tolerance promotes allergy and anaphylaxis: a new murine food allergy model. J Allergy Clin Immunol. 2009;123:231–8.
70. Li J, Wang Y, Tang L, de Villiers WJ, Cohen D, Woodward J, et al. Dietary medium-chain triglycerides promote oral allergic sensitization and orally induced anaphylaxis to peanut protein in mice. J Allergy Clin Immunol. 2013;131:442–50.
71. Torii I, Shimizu S, Daimon T, Shinohara Y, Kudo T, Sato A, Tsujimura T. Exposure to high doses of Lipopolysaccharide during ovalbumin sensitization prevents the development of allergic Th2 responses to a dietary antigen. J Toxicol Pathol. 2014;27:205–15.
72. Kong J, Chalcraft K, Mandur TS, Jimenez-Saiz R, Walker TD, Goncharova S, et al. Comprehensive metabolomics identifies the alarmin uric acid as a critical signal for the induction of peanut allergy. Allergy. 2015;70:495–505.
73. Birmingham NP, Parvataneni S, Hassan HM, Harkema J, Samineni S, Navuluri L, et al. An adjuvant-free mouse model of tree nut allergy using hazelnut as a model tree nut. Int Arch Allergy Immunol. 2007;144:203–10.
74. Gonipeta B, Parvataneni S, Tempelman RJ, Gangur V. An adjuvant-free mouse model to evaluate the allergenicity of milk whey protein. J Dairy Sci. 2009;92:4738–44.
75. Chandra SA, Stokes AH, Hailey R, Merrill CL, Melich DH, DeSmet K, et al. Dermal toxicity studies: factors impacting study interpretation and outcome. Toxicol Pathol. 2015;43:474–81.
76. Bartnikas LM, Gurish MF, Burton OT, Leisten S, Janssen E, Oettgen HC, et al. Epicutaneous sensitization results in IgE-dependent intestinal mast cell expansion and food-induced anaphylaxis. J Allergy Clin Immunol. 2013;131:451–60.
77. Devey ME, Anderson KJ, Coombs RR, Henschel MJ, Coates ME. The modified anaphylaxis hypothesis for cot death. Anaphylactic sensitization in guinea-pigs fed cow's milk. Clin Exp Immunol. 1976;26:542–8.
78. Knippels LM, Houben GF, Spanhaak S, Penninks AH. An oral sensitization model in Brown Norway rats to screen for potential allergenicity of food proteins. Methods. 1999;19:78–82.
79. Knippels LMJ, Penninks AH, Houben GF. Continued expression of anti-soy protein antibodies in rats bred on a soy protein-free diet for one generation: the importance of dietary control in oral sensitization research. J Allergy Clin Immunol. 1998;101:815–20.
80. Bernard H, Ah-Leung S, Drumare MF, Feraudet-Tarisse C, Verhasselt V, Wal JM, et al. Peanut allergens are rapidly transferred in human breast milk and can prevent sensitization in mice. Allergy. 2014;69:888–97.
81. Julia V, Macia L, Dombrowicz D. The impact of diet on asthma and allergic diseases. Nat Rev Immunol. 2015;15:308–22.
82. Merrill AH Jr, Schmelz EM, Wang E, Dillehay DL, Rice LG, Meredith F, et al. Importance of sphingolipids and inhibitors of sphingolipid metabolism as components of animal diets. J Nutr. 1997;127:830S–3S.
83. Hogenkamp A, Knippels LM, Garssen J, van Esch BC. Supplementation of mice with specific nondigestible oligosaccharides during pregnancy or lactation leads to diminished sensitization and allergy in the female offspring. J Nutr. 2015;145:996–1002.
84. Untersmayr E, Jensen-Jarolim E. The role of protein digestibility and antacids on food allergy outcomes. J Allergy Clin Immunol. 2008;121:1301–8.
85. Diesner SC, Knittelfelder R, Krishnamurthy D, Pali-Scholl I, Gajdzik L, Jensen-Jarolim E, Untersmayr E. Dose-dependent food allergy induction against ovalbumin under acid-suppression: a murine food allergy model. Immunol Lett. 2008;121:45–51.
86. Untersmayr E, Diesner SC, Bramswig KH, Knittelfelder R, Bakos N, Gundacker C, et al. Characterization of intrinsic and extrinsic risk factors for celery allergy in immunosenescence. Mech Ageing Dev. 2008;129:120–8.
87. Hanson DG. Ontogeny of orally induced tolerance to soluble proteins in mice. I. Priming and tolerance in newborns. J Immunol. 1981;127:1518–24.
88. Frei R, Lauener RP, Crameri R, O'Mahony L. Microbiota and dietary interactions: an update to the hygiene hypothesis? Allergy. 2012;67:451–61.
89. Konieczna P, Groeger D, Ziegler M, Frei R, Ferstl R, Shanahan F, et al. Bifidobacterium infantis 35624 administration induces Foxp3 T regulatory cells in human peripheral blood: potential role for myeloid and plasmacytoid dendritic cells. Gut. 2012;61:354–66.
90. Kelly D, King T, Aminov R. Importance of microbial colonization of the gut in early life to the development of immunity. Mutat Res. 2007;622:58–69.
91. Frei R, Akdis M, O'Mahony L. Prebiotics, probiotics, synbiotics, and the immune system: experimental data and clinical evidence. Curr Opin Gastroenterol. 2015;31:153–8.
92. Lyons A, O'Mahony D, O'Brien F, MacSharry J, Sheil B, Ceddia M, et al. Bacterial strain-specific induction of Foxp3+ T regulatory cells is protective in murine allergy models. Clin Exp Allergy. 2010;40:811–9.
93. Sibartie S, O'Hara AM, Ryan J, Fanning A, O'Mahony J, O'Neill S, et al. Modulation of pathogen-induced CCL20 secretion from HT-29 human intestinal epithelial cells by commensal bacteria. BMC Immunol. 2009;10:54.
94. O'Mahony C, Scully P, O'Mahony D, Murphy S, O'Brien F, Lyons A, et al. Commensal-induced regulatory T cells mediate protection against pathogen-stimulated NF-kappaB activation. PLoS Pathog. 2008;4:e1000112.
95. Hazebrouck S, Przybylski-Nicaise L, Ah-Leung S, del-Patient K, Corthier G, Wal JM, Rabot S. Allergic sensitization to bovine beta-lactoglobulin: comparison between germ-free and conventional BALB/c mice. Int Arch Allergy Immunol. 2009;148:65–72.
96. Morin S, Bernard H, Przybylski-Nicaise L, Corthier G, Rabot S, Wal JM, Hazebrouck S. Allergenic and immunogenic potential of cow's milk beta-lactoglobulin and caseins evidenced without adjuvant in germ-free mice. Mol Nutr Food Res. 2011;55:1700–7.
97. Konieczna P, Ferstl R, Ziegler M, Frei R, Nehrbass D, Lauener RP, et al. Immunomodulation by Bifidobacterium infantis 35624 in the murine lamina propria requires retinoic acid-dependent and independent mechanisms. PLoS One. 2013;8:e62617.
98. McEwen BS. The neurobiology of stress: from serendipity to clinical relevance. Brain Res. 2000;886:172–89.
99. Perry TT, Pesek RD. Clinical manifestations of food allergy. Pediatr Ann. 2013;42:96–101.
100. Knippels LMJ, van Wijk F, Penninks AH. Food allergy: what do we learn from animal models? Curr Opin Allergy Clin Immunol. 2004;4:205–9.
101. Kimber I, Dearman RJ, Penninks AH, Knippels LMJ, Buchanan RB, Hammerberg B, et al. Assessment of protein allergenicity on the basis of immune reactivity: animal models. Environ Health Perspect. 2003;111:1125–30.
102. Strait RT, Morris SC, Yang M, Qu XW, Finkelman FD. Pathways of anaphylaxis in the mouse. J Allergy Clin Immunol. 2002;109:658–68.
103. Evans H, Killoran KE, Mitre E. Measuring local anaphylaxis in mice. J Vis Exp. 2014;92:e52005.

104. Reiner D, Lee RY, Dekan G, Epstein MM. No adjuvant effect of *Bacillus thuringiensis*-maize on allergic responses in mice. PLoS One. 2014;9:e103979.
105. Cockcroft DW, Davis BE. Mechanisms of airway hyperresponsiveness. J Allergy Clin Immunol. 2006;118:551–9.
106. Schouten B, van Esch BC, Hofman GA, van den Elsen LW, Willemsen LE, Garssen J. Acute allergic skin reactions and intestinal contractility changes in mice orally sensitized against casein or whey. Int Arch Allergy Immunol. 2008;147:125–34.
107. van Esch BC, Schouten B, Hofman GA, van Baalen T, Nijkamp FP, Knippels LM, et al. Acute allergic skin response as a new tool to evaluate the allergenicity of whey hydrolysates in a mouse model of orally induced cow's milk allergy. Pediatr Allergy Immunol. 2010;21:e780–6.
108. Prescott VE, Forbes E, Foster PS, Matthaei K, Hogan SP. Mechanistic analysis of experimental food allergen-induced cutaneous reactions. J Leukoc Biol. 2006;80:258–66.
109. Mathias CB, Hobson SA, Garcia-Lloret M, Lawson G, Poddighe D, Freyschmidt EJ, et al. IgE-mediated systemic anaphylaxis and impaired tolerance to food antigens in mice with enhanced IL-4 receptor signaling. J Allergy Clin Immunol. 2011;127:795–805.
110. Han H, Thelen TD, Comeau MR, Ziegler SF. Thymic stromal lymphopoietin-mediated epicutaneous inflammation promotes acute diarrhea and anaphylaxis. J Clin Invest. 2014;124:5442–52.
111. Zabel BA, Nakae S, Zúñiga L, Kim JY, Ohyama T, Alt C, et al. Mast cell-expressed orphan receptor CCRL2 binds chemerin and is required for optimal induction of IgE-mediated passive cutaneous anaphylaxis. J Exp Med. 2008;205:2207–20.
112. Birmingham N, Payankaulam S, Thanesvorakul S, Stefura B, HayGlass K, Gangur V. An ELISA-based method for measurement of food-specific IgE antibody in mouse serum: an alternative to the passive cutaneous anaphylaxis assay. J Immunol Methods. 2003;275:89–98.
113. Adel-Patient K, Bernard H, Ah-Leung S, Creminon C, Wal JM. Peanut- and cow's milk-specific IgE, Th2 cells and local anaphylactic reaction are induced in Balb/c mice orally sensitized with cholera toxin. Allergy. 2005;60:658–64.
114. Lovik M, Hogseth AK, Gaarder PI, Hagemann R, Eide I. Diesel exhaust particles and carbon black have adjuvant activity on the local lymph node response and systemic IgE production to ovalbumin. Toxicology. 1997;121:165–78.
115. Olzhausen J, Schawaller M, Wiki M, Akdis C, Jutel M, Crameri R, Rhyner C. Evanescent field-based fast measurements of allergen specific antibodies during SIT. Allergy. 2014;69(s99):72.
116. Granum B, Gaarder PI, Groeng E, Leikvold R, Namork E, Lovik M. Fine particles of widely different composition have an adjuvant effect on the production of allergen-specific antibodies. Toxicol Lett. 2001;118:171–81.
117. Bøgh KL, Kroghsbo S, Dahl L, Rigby NM, Barkholt V, Mills EN, Madsen CB. Digested Ara h 1 has sensitizing capacity in Brown Norway rats. Clin Exp Allergy. 2009;39:1611–21.
118. Vercelli D, Jabara HH, Arai K, Geha RS. Induction of human IgE synthesis requires interleukin 4 and T/B cell interactions involving the T cell receptor/CD3 complex and MHC class II antigens. J Exp Med. 1989;169:1295–307.
119. Finkelman FD, Holmes J, Katona IM, Urban JF Jr, Beckmann MP, Park LS, et al. Lymphokine control of in vivo immunoglobulin isotype selection. Annu Rev Immunol. 1990;8:303–33.
120. Nakajima-Adachi H, Kikuchi A, Fujimura Y, Shibahara K, Makino T, Goseki-Sone M, et al. Peyer's patches and mesenteric lymph nodes cooperatively promote enteropathy in a mouse model of food allergy. PLoS One. 2014;9:e107492.
121. Akdis M, Burgler S, Crameri R, Eiwegger T, Fujita H, Gomez E, et al. Interleukins, from 1 to 37, and interferon-γ: receptors, functions, and roles in diseases. J Allergy Clin Immunol. 2011;127:701–21.
122. van Zijverden M, van der Pijl A, Bol M, van Pinxteren FA, de Haar C, Penninks AH, et al. Diesel exhaust, carbon black, and silica particles display distinct Th1/Th2 modulating activity. Toxicol Appl Pharmacol. 2000;168:131–9.
123. Nygaard UC, Ormstad H, Aase A, Lovik M. The IgE adjuvant effect of particles: characterisation of the primary cellular response in the draining lymph node. Toxicology. 2005;206:181–93.
124. Gerberick GF, Ryan CA, Dearman RJ, Kimber I. Local lymph node assay (LLNA) for detection of sensitization capacity of chemicals. Methods. 2007;41:54–60.
125. Vaali K, Puumalainen TJ, Lehto M, Wolff H, Rita H, Alenius H, Palosuo T. Murine model of food allergy after epicutaneous sensitization: role of mucosal mast cell protease-1. Scand J Gastroenterol. 2006;41:1405–13.

Self-reported adverse reactions and IgE sensitization to common foods in adults with asthma

G. Rentzos[1*], L. Johanson[2], S. Sjölander[4], E. Telemo[3] and L. Ekerljung[2]

Abstract

Background: There is very few data available on the prevalence of food hypersensitivity among adults with asthma. The aim of this study was to explore the prevalence of self-reported adverse reactions and IgE sensitization to the different foods and to determine the spectrum and the prevalence of food-related gastrointestinal symptoms in adults with and with no asthma.

Methods: A cross sectional study based on interviews and questionnaire responses from 1527 subjects, aged 18–75 years of age, from Västra Götaland in Sweden, as part of the larger West Sweden Asthma Study. IgE analyses were performed in sera from all subjects.

Results: Fifty three percent of adults with asthma reported adverse reactions to foods compared to 30 % of non-asthmatics. Most asthmatics reported symptoms from eating hazelnut, followed by other nuts, birch-related foods, milk, peanut and shellfish. Furthermore, adults with asthma experienced significantly more often gastrointestinal symptoms from hazelnut, apple and milk and were found to significantly more often be sensitized to the most common foods compared to the non-asthmatic subjects. The asthmatics showed a significant correlation between IgE to both hazelnut and birch and self-reported symptoms after ingestion of hazelnut and to a lesser extent to almonds.

Conclusions: The prevalence of self-reported adverse reactions and sensitization to the most common foods was much higher among the asthmatic subjects. Hazelnut was the food that asthmatics most frequently experienced adverse reactions from, and the strong correlation between IgE to hazelnut and birch indicate that the observed adverse reactions are partly due to sensitization to allergens from the PR-10 family.

Keywords: Asthma, Food allergy, Epidemiology

Background

Determining the prevalence of food hypersensitivity and food allergy is a complex issue due to the different cultures, dietary habits, and geographical and regional differences of allergen distribution. It is still unclear if the prevalence of food allergy is continuously rising although many studies conclude that there is a rising trend at least in western and developing countries [1–3]. Most of the studies concerning the prevalence of food allergy are carried out in children, and therefore it is largely unknown as to what extent the adult population is affected.

* Correspondence: grentzos@gmail.com
[1]Section of Allergology, University Hospital of Sahlgrenska, 413 45 Gothenburg, Sweden
Full list of author information is available at the end of the article

The relationship between asthma and food allergy has also been discussed but the available data demonstrating a common pathogenetic mechanism are still few. In adults this relation was often denoted by case-reports, which claim that food hypersensitivity may trigger or affect asthma symptoms. It has been shown previously that having asthma might be a risk factor for a fatal food reaction and having food allergy might be a risk for complicated or poorly controlled asthma [4–6]. Oehling et al. has previously shown that one third of children with food allergy also have asthma [7] and about 4-8 % of children with asthma have food allergies [8], the prevalence though of food allergy in adults with asthma is still not known. However, it has been demonstrated that adult patients with one or more food allergies had increased hospitalizations for asthma [4], and in a study from Woods et al., it was shown that adults with probable peanut and shrimp allergy often have more frequent asthma episodes and doctor's diagnosed asthma [9]. In addition, it has been also shown that inhalation of aerosolized food particles may lead to the development of asthma in adults [10–12]. The relation between asthma and gastrointestinal symptoms in adults is not extensively studied. A study on children by Cafarrelli et al. found a possible correlation between asthma and gastrointestinal symptoms [13]. In a previous study from Kivity et al., a relation between food allergy and concomitant asymptomatic bronchial hyper-reactivity could be shown [14]. It is still not fully explored though, if adults with asthma experience more often gastrointestinal adverse reactions to different food items in a greater frequency than non-asthmatics. The notion that there is a probable relation between asthma and gastrointestinal symptoms in adults was supported previously in a study by Powel et al. who confirmed that asthmatics generally experienced more gastrointestinal symptoms than the non-asthmatic population [15]. In a recent study, performed in the Netherlands, an association between gastrointestinal symptoms and asthma/COPD was found [16]. In addition, it has been shown that patients with irritable bowel syndrome (IBS) and inflammatory bowel disease (IBD) showed increased frequency of bronchial hyper-reactivity compared to control subjects [17, 18]. These results were further supported in a study on patients who suffered from asthma compared to asymptomatic atopic subjects [19].

The aim of this study was to explore the prevalence of self-reported adverse reactions to foods and to estimate the prevalence of IgE sensitization for the most common food among adults with asthma compared to non-asthmatics. We also wanted to describe the spectrum and the prevalence of gastrointestinal symptoms caused by the most common and different foods in both asthmatics and non-asthmatics.

Materials and methods

A postal questionnaire, which has been described in detail elsewhere [20], was mailed out to 30,000 randomly selected subjects, aged 18–75 years, living in the West of Sweden; 15,000 subjects lived in the urban area of Gothenburg and 15,000 in the remaining region of West Sweden. The total response rate was 62 %, and a non-response study showed no differences in prevalence of asthma symptoms or lung disease between responders and non-responders [20]. Of the responders to the postal questionnaire, 2000 were randomly selected for clinical examination and interviews. In addition, all responders that reported physician diagnosed asthma, or reported ever having asthma and used asthma medication or reported symptoms such as wheeze or attacks of shortness of breath during the last year, were included. In total, 3524 subjects were invited, of which 2006 participated. All participants received a questionnaire containing detailed questions on food hypersensitivity as well as other hypersensitivity symptoms (Additional file 1: Hypersensitivity questionnaire). The questionnaire did not contain specific questions on gluten (coeliac disease) or lactose intolerance. Of the 2006 participants, 1725 responded to the food questionnaire of which 1527 were included in the analyses. A schematic flow chart of the study set up can be seen in Fig. 1. The clinical assessment of the subjects in the study included spirometry, blood samples for specific IgE-tests and a clinical interview performed by a specialist nurse. The clinical interview was used to assess whether the subjects currently suffered from asthma. This was defined as: a) asthma diagnosed by physician, and reported asthma symptoms or asthma medication during the last year, *b)* belief to have suffered from asthma, and currently report asthma symptoms and/or taking asthma medication, *c)* currently suffer from asthma symptoms and have either positive methacholine bronchial challenge test or positive reversibility test.

Specific IgE-tests included three allergen panel tests, Phadiatop Europe (cat, dog, horse, Dermatophagoides pteronyssinus, Dermatophagoides farinae Cladosporium herbarum, timothy grass, birch, mugwort, olive, wall pellitory), fx1 (peanut, hazel nut, brazil nut, almond, coconut) and fx5 (egg white, milk, fish, wheat, peanut, soy bean) (Thermofisher Scientific, Uppsala, Sweden). Subjects with a positive response to a panel were additionally tested specifically for the IgE of the allergens included in this positive panel, according to manufacturer's instructions. The foods tested in panels fx1 and fx5 were characterized as "common foods" since they comprise some of the most frequent food items consumed on a daily basis at least in Sweden and other Western countries.

Collection and encoding of data

The replies from food questionnaire (Additional file 1: Hypersensitivity questionnaire) regarding reactions to different foods were encoded for the different symptoms according to Table 1.

Then, encoded fields for milk, sour milk and cheese were added which were dissociated from the most relevant clinical symptoms for suspicious lactose intolerance as abdominal pain (abd), flatulence (gas) and diarrhea/loose stools (dia), or if lactose intolerance was specified in any free text field. Likewise, encoded fields were added for flour from wheat and flour from other cereal grains, in case of suspicious gluten intolerance (coeliac disease), that were dissociated from the clinical symptoms tiredness (tir), abdominal pain (abd), feeling of illness (gen), diarrhea/loose stools (dia), flatulence (gas) and/or hives, urticaria (urt), or if gluten intolerance was

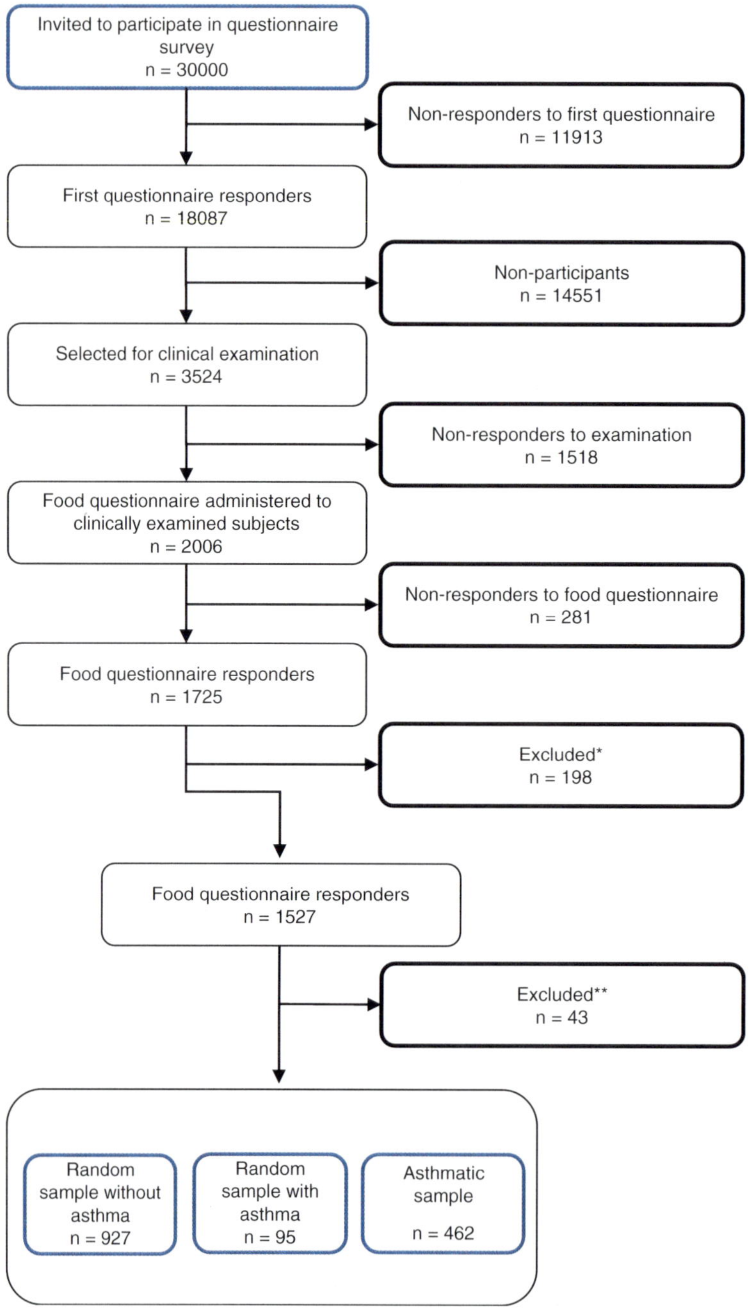

Fig. 1 Flow-chart of the subjects included or excluded from the study and the numbers of responders and non-responders of the selected participants. *198 subjects were excluded from the study since their initial categorization as asthmatics, while considered inappropriate, based on the questionnaire response and inclusion clinical criteria. **43 subjects were excluded from the study since they reported no symptoms from any food item, but did report that they avoided at least one food item in the food questionnaire

specified in any free text field. Three subjects reported that they suffered from gluten intolerance of which two avoided eating gluten strictly. Ten subjects reported that they suffered from lactose intolerance of which five avoided lactose strictly. In total thirty-two subjects suffered from symptoms that were interpreted as intolerance either to gluten or lactose. Using the above described procedure, most cases of suspicious lactose and gluten intolerance could be excluded from the data of the analyses. Subjects with suspected asthma, based on the questionnaire, that could not be verified by the clinical examination as described in the previous section were also excluded from the analyses.

Table 1 Encoding for self-reported hypersensitivity reactions in food hypersensitivity questionnaire

Code	Meaning
Skin	Symptoms from the skin (urticaria, eczema, angioedema, flush, itching, tingling, skin pain, papules, redness etc.)
GI	Abdominal pain, oral symptoms, diarrhea, flatulence, reflux, vomiting, constipation
Airup	Symptoms from the upper airways –nose(rhinitis, nasal congestion, nasal itching, sneezing, red nasal papules), eyes
Airlo	Lower airways –respiratory symptoms(heavy breathing, difficulty getting air, wheezing, cough, chest pressure, bronchospasm, hoarseness, mucus/saliva in the throat)
Circ	Palpation, fainting, dizziness
CNS	Headache, confusion
Oth	Other(e.g., ear itching, gallstone)
Not	Do not eat
Unk	Unknown, uncertain whether intolerant or not
Ana	Anaphylactic reactions
Gen	General symptoms such as tiredness, feeling ill

Statistics

The statistical analyses were performed using SPSS 22.0 and Microsoft Excel 2007. Chi-squared test was used for the prevalence of self-reported symptoms as well as gastrointestinal symptoms to different foods among subjects with and without asthma. A p–value < 0.05 using Fischer's two tailed exact test was considered statistically significant. Correlations between different parameters within the same group were evaluated by using the Pearson's or Spearman's correlation coefficient. Tests were two-tailed and the level of significance was set to $P < 0.05$. Agreement between clinical objective asthma and self-reported asthma was analyzed by calculating the kappa coefficients (κ). κ < 0.00 was considered a poor strength of agreement, κ: 0.00–0.20 a slight strength, κ: 0.21–0.40 a fair strength, κ: 0.41–0.60 a moderate strength, κ: 0.61–0.80 a substantial strength, and κ: 0.81–1.00 an almost perfect agreement [21].

Ethical approval

The regional ethic committee in West Sweden (Central Ethical Review Board in Gothenburg) approved the study (Dnr 593–08).

Results

Of the total 1527 subjects that answered the food questionnaire, 43 reported no symptoms from any food item, but did report that they avoided at least one food item. These subjects were excluded from calculation of food hypersensitivity since the reason for their avoidance was unclear. From the 1527 subjects totally included in the study, 583 (38.2 %) had asthma while 944 (61.8 %) had no asthma ($p < 0.001$). Among the subjects with asthma 192 (32.9 %) were sensitized to birch pollen compared with 119 (12.6 %) among non-asthmatic subjects ($p < 0.001$). When evaluating the level of agreement between clinical objective asthma and self-reported asthma, the kappa-coefficient is equal to 0.94.

Prevalence of food hypersensitivity in adults with asthma compared to adults with no asthma

Of the remaining 1484, when excluding the 43 subjects reporting no symptoms from any food item, subjects with asthma reported a considerably higher prevalence of adverse reactions to food compared to those without asthma 53.1 % (49.0 % - 57.3 %, 95 % CI) vs. 29.8 % (26.8 % - 32.7 %, 95 % CI) with p < 0.001. When symptoms from suspicious lactose and gluten intolerance were excluded, asthmatics still reported more adverse reactions to food compared to non-asthmatics, 51.3 % (47.1 % - 55.4 %, 95 % CI) vs. 28.2 % (25.2 % - 31.1 %, 95 % CI) with $p < 0.001$ (Fig. 2).

Association between adverse reactions from specific foods and asthma

Subjects with asthma most commonly experienced adverse reactions (including all types of symptoms) to hazelnut (20.5 %), apple (17.5 %), kiwi (14.3 %), walnut (12.8 %), milk (11.5 %), peach (10.7 %), brazil nut (9.8 %), almond (9.5 %), nectarine (9.3 %), pear (8.9 %), plum (8.8 %), cherry (8.7 %), wine/beer (8.0 %), peanut (7.0 %), shellfish (6.5 %), carrot (6.4 %), strawberry (6.4 %), and apricot (6.3 %). Concerning the staple and dairy food items, subjects with asthma experienced adverse reactions most commonly against milk (including subjects with suspected lactose intolerance, 11.5 %), shellfish (6.5 %), sour milk/yogurt (6.25 %), cheese (4.5 %), egg (3.3 %), fish (2.9 %), soy (1.4 %), wheat (including subjects with suspected gluten intolerance, 3.23 %) while about 1.4 % to other flours. When excluding subjects with clinically suspected lactose intolerance, we observed that about 2.35 % of the asthmatics reacted to milk. When excluding subjects with suspicious gluten intolerance, as described previously, we observed that only 1.4 % of subjects reported adverse reactions to wheat. In addition 5.9 % of the asthmatics reported reactions to fried/fat food, and 1.6 % to food additives. More detailed data concerning the distribution of the self-reported adverse reactions to all the specific food items in asthmatics compared to non-asthmatics are presented in Table 2.

Association between self-reported food-related gastrointestinal symptoms and asthma

Subjects with asthma also report significantly more gastrointestinal symptom to hazelnut (13.0 % vs 5.2 %, $p < 0.001$), apple (11.4 % vs 6 %, $p < 0.001$), milk (10.4 % including subjects with suspicious lactose intolerance vs 5.7 %,

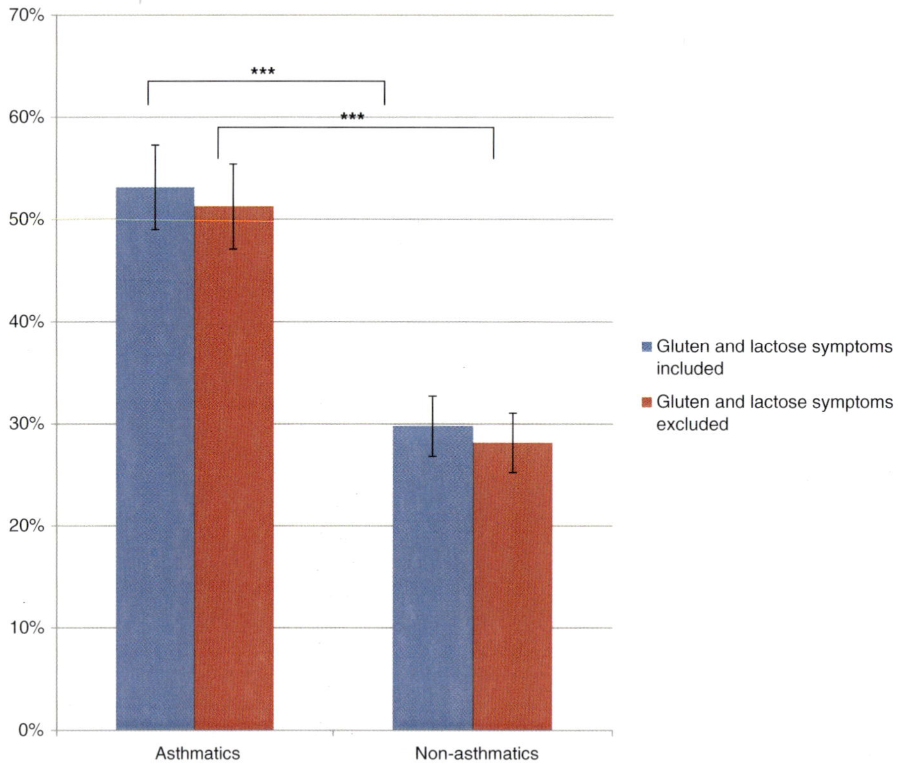

Fig. 2 Prevalence of self-reported adverse reactions to foods among asthmatics and non-asthmatics both including and excluding symptoms typical for suspicious gluten and lactose intolerance. Subjects with asthma reported a much higher prevalence compared to subjects with no asthma (53.1 % vs. 29.8 %, p <0.001 when including all symptoms). ***$p < 0.001$

$p < 0.01$), kiwi (9.7 % vs 5.3 %, $p < 0.01$), peach (8.3 % vs 2 %, $p < 0.001$), plum (6.75 % vs 2.2 %, $p < 0.001$), nectarine (6.7 % vs 1.3 %, $p < 0.001$), pear (6.4 % vs 2.4 %, $p < 0.001$), cherry (6.2 % vs 2.4 %, $p < 0.001$) followed by walnut (5.9 % vs 3.0 %, $p < 0.01$), fried/fat food (5.7 % vs 3.3 %, $p < 0.05$), sour milk/yoghurt (5.6 % vs 2.8 %, $p < 0.01$) and almond (5.45 % vs 2.3 %, $p < 0.01$) compared to non-asthmatics. Details concerning the prevalence of gastrointestinal symptoms between asthmatics and non-asthmatics for all foods are presented in Table 3.

IgE sensitization for the most common foods among asthmatics and non-asthmatics

When assessing the sIgE-sensitization profiles for the most-common foods in panels fx1 and fx5, we observed that subjects with asthma are generally more frequently sensitized to the food items tested compared to non-asthmatics (38.2 % vs 13.9 %, $p < 0.001$). More specifically, when comparing asthmatics with non-asthmatics, it was found that subjects with asthma were significantly more frequently sensitized to hazelnut (31.8 % vs 11.2 %, $p < 0.001$), peanut (9.1 % vs 4.3 %, $p < 0.001$), almond (6.6 % vs 2.4 %, $p < 0.001$), milk (6.0 % vs 1.6 %, $p < 0.001$), wheat (5.5 % vs 1.8 %, $p < 0.001$), egg (5.3 % vs 1.4 %, $p < 0.001$), soy (3,5 % vs 1.1 %, $p = 0.003$), brazil nut (2.2 % vs 0.4 %, $p = 0.003$), fish (1.3 % vs 0.0 %, $p = 0.001$). All data are presented in Fig. 3a and b and in Table 4.

Hazelnut seems to be the most frequent food causing symptoms and is also the food item with the highest frequency of IgE-sensitization in asthmatics. Hazelnut is one of the birch pollen-related foods and IgE to hazelnut correlated strongly with IgE to birch in the asthmatic subjects (r = 0.904, p < 0.001) as well as in non-asthmatic subjects (r = 0.920, $p < 0.001$). A moderate correlation was observed between IgE to birch and IgE to peanut (r = 0.357, $p < 0.001$) in the asthmatic subjects as well as in non-asthmatic subjects (0.395, $p < 0.001$). When looking for possible correlations between IgE-sensitization and self-reported symptoms for the most common foods, we observed the highest correlation between IgE and self-reported symptoms for hazelnut (r = 0.496, $p < 0.001$) in the asthmatic group as well in the non-asthmatic adults (r = 0.499, $p < 0.001$). IgE-sensitization to birch also correlated with self-reported symptoms from hazelnut both in subjects with and without asthma, although slightly weaker (r = 0.455, $p < 0.001$ resp. r = 0.472, $p < 0.001$).

Table 2 Prevalence of adverse reactions (including GI symptoms) to the different foods among asthmatics (asthma), non-asthmatics (no asthma) and in the total sample (all)

Food	% asthma	% no asthma	% all	p	Risk ratio
Hazelnut	20.5	7.2	12.2	<0.001	2.83
Apple	17.5	7.15	11.1	< 0.001	2.45
Kiwi	14.3	6.3	9.3	< 0.001	2.27
Walnut	12.8	4.1	7.3	< 0.001	3.15
Milk	11.5	6.9	8.6	0.003	1.67
Peach	10.7	2.4	5.6	< 0.001	4.39
Brazil nut	9.8	3.5	5.9	< 0.001	2.78
Almond	9.5	2.9	5.4	< 0.001	3.30
Nectarine	9.3	1.8	4.7	< 0.001	5.15
Pear	8.85	2.9	5.1	< 0.001	3.09
Plum	8.8	2.45	4.9	< 0.001	3.61
Cherry	8.65	2.65	4.9	< 0.001	3.26
Wine/beer	8	3.8	5.4	< 0.001	2.08
Peanut	7	2.8	4.3	< 0.001	2.63
Shellfish	6.5	3.1	4.4	0.002	2.09
Carrot	6.4	2.3	3.9	< 0.001	2.73
Strawberry	6.4	1.8	3.5	< 0.001	3.53
Apricot	6.3	1.4	3.3	< 0.001	4.52
Sourmilk/yogurt	6.25	3.5	4.55	0.015	1.78
Fried/fat food	5.9	3.3	4.3	0.018	1.79
Potato	5.5	1.2	2.8	< 0.001	4.70
Cheese	4.5	1.7	2.8	0.001	2.65
Others	4.5	3.1	3.6	0.16	1.46
Sweet pepper	4.4	1.9	2.8	0.006	2.28
Chili/tabasco	4.3	1.8	2.8	0.004	2.40
Tomato	4.15	1.9	2.8	0.011	2.18
Orange	3.8	2.8	3.1	0.26	1.38
Banana	3.8	1.1	2.1	< 0.001	3.56
Bean	3.3	1.6	2.2	0.033	2.06
Egg	3.3	1.1	1.9	0.002	3.09
Flour (wheat)	3.3	1.6	2.2	0.033	2.05
Avocado	3.1	0.5	1.5	< 0.001	5.84
Fish	2.9	0.2	1.25	< 0.001	13.80
Cheese[a]	2.8	0.6	1.5	< 0.001	4.37
Cayenne/red pepper	2.8	1.4	1.9	0.056	2.01
Chocolate	2.8	1.5	2	0.084	1.86
Milk[a]	2.35	1	1.6	0.063	2.15
Pea	2.2	0.4	1.1	0.001	5.27
Additives	1.6	0.4	0.9	0.021	3.66
Curry	1.55	1	1.25	0.41	1.46
Sour milk/yogurt[a]	1.4	0.5	0.9	0.076	2.64
Flour (wheat)[b]	1.4	0.1	0.6	0.002	12.94

Table 2 Prevalence of adverse reactions (including GI symptoms) to the different foods among asthmatics (asthma), non-asthmatics (no asthma) and in the total sample (all) *(Continued)*

Celery	1.4	0.2	0.7	0.006	6.49
Soy	1.4	0.2	0.7	0.006	6.49
Melon	1.4	0.2	0.65	0.006	6.48
Flour (non wheat)	1.4	0.5	0.85	0.083	2.59
Dried fruit	1.2	0.2	0.6	0.014	5.71
Salami	1	0.4	0.7	0.15	2.44
Pork	1	0.5	0.7	0.26	1.94
Sunflower seed	0.9	0	0.3	0.004	-
Chestnut	0.7	0.4	0.5	0.47	1.65
Flour (non wheat)[b]	0.7	0	0.3	0.011	-
Chicken	0.7	0.1	0.3	0.054	6.48
Camomile	0.7	0.5	0.6	0.69	1.30
Sesame seed	0.7	0.1	0.3	0.054	6.49
Anise/caraway	0.5	0.1	0.3	0.13	4.86
Beef	0.35	0.3	0.3	0.93	1.08
Lingonberry	0.3	0.1	0.2	0.31	3.25
Coriander	0.2	0.1	0.1	0.73	1.62
Poppy seed	0.2	0	0.1	0.20	-
Parsley	0.2	0.2	0.2	0.86	0.81

P-value was considered significant when <0.05 comparing the self-reported intolerance for the different foods between asthmatics to non-asthmatics
[a]lactose intolerance symptoms excluded
[b]gluten intolerance symptoms excluded

Seasonal variation of gastrointestinal symptoms in subject with and without asthma

Asthmatics experienced more symptoms from the gastro-intestinal tract during the spring (6.7 % vs 2.2 %, $p < 0.001$), summer (5.1 % vs 1.9 %, $p = 0.001$) and autumn (5.9 % vs 3.2 %, $p = 0.013$), but not during the winter compared to non-asthmatics. In addition, asthmatic subjects with IgE reactivity to birch pollen more frequently report gastrointestinal symptoms compared to birch pollen sensitized subjects without asthma during the spring (5.7 % vs 0.8 %, $p = 0.034$), summer (4.2 % vs 0.0 %, $p = 0.026$) and autumn (3.7 % vs 0.0 %, $p = 0.046$) (Fig. 4 and Additional file 2: Table S1).

Discussion

In the present study, subjects with asthma more frequently reported adverse reactions to foods compared to non-asthmatics (53 % vs 30 %), and patients with asthma more frequently showed IgE reactivity to the most common foods. These results are in line with data from a previous study by Woods et al. in which it was suggested a positive association between IgE sensitization to foods and asthma or allergic disease [22]. The data was supported also by the sensitisation patterns of specific-IgE

Table 3 Prevalence of self-reported gastrointestinal symptoms for the different foods among asthmatics (asthma), non-asthmatics (no asthma) and in the total sample (all)

Food	% asthma	% no asthma	*p*	Ratio
Hazelnut	13	5.2	< 0.001	2.51
Apple	11.4	6	< 0.001	1.91
Milk	10.4	5.7	0.001	1.84
Kiwi	9.7	5.3	0.002	1.82
Peach	8.3	2	< 0.001	4.11
Plum	6.75	2.2	< 0.001	3.02
Nectarine	6.7	1.3	< 0.001	5.27
Pear	6.4	2.4	< 0.001	2.63
Cherry	6.2	2.4	< 0.001	2.55
Walnut	5.9	3	0.006	1.99
Fried/fat food	5.7	3.3	0.026	1.73
Sour milk/yogurt	5.6	2.8	0.007	2.01
Almond	5.45	2.3	0.002	2.33
Brazil nut	5.3	2.6	0.008	2.06
Apricot	3.8	1.3	0.001	2.99
Sweet pepper	3.7	1.7	0.018	2.15
Cheese	3.5	1	0.001	3.27
Tomato	3.5	1.4	0.007	2.51
Strawberry	3.4	0.95	< 0.001	3.61
Peanut	3.3	1.7	0.045	1.95
Carrot	3.3	1.6	0.033	2.06
Others	3.1	1.7	0.074	1.83
Shellfish	3	1.2	0.013	2.53
Chili/tabasco	2.8	1	0.0075	2.90
Egg	2.8	1	0.008	2.89
Banana	2.7	0.95	0.008	2.88
Wine/beer	2.6	1.4	0.090	1.88
Bean	2.6	1.6	0.18	1.62
Potato	2.4	0.5	0.0015	4.52
Flour (wheat)	2.2	1.4	0.21	1.62
Avocado	2.2	0.4	0.001	5.27
Chocolate	1.9	0.85	0.074	2.24
Orange	1.9	1.4	0.43	1.38
Pea	1.9	0.3	0.002	5.95
Cheese[a]	1.6	0	< 0.001	-
Fish	1.55	0.1	< 0.001	14.61
Cayenne/red pepper	1.4	0.7	0.22	1.87
Soy	1.4	0.2	0.006	6.49
Milk[a]	1.3	0.2	0.013	5.78
Melon	1.2	0.2	0.014	5.67
Flour (non wheat)	1.2	0.4	0.083	2.83
Sour milk/yogurt[a]	0.9	0.1	0.021	8.26
Pork	0.9	0.4	0.28	2.02
Salami	0.7	0.2	0.15	3.25
Flour (wheat)[b]	0.7	0	0.011	-
Dried fruit	0.7	0.1	0.053	6.53
Celery	0.7	0.1	0.054	6.49
Curry	0.7	0.4	0.49	1.62
Sunflower seed	0.7	0	0.011	-
Chestnut	0.5	0.3	0.54	1.65
Additives	0.5	0.3	0.55	1.63
Flour (non wheat)[b]	0.5	0	0.027	-
Chicken	0.5	0	0.027	-
Anise/caraway	0.5	0	0.027	-
Beef	0.35	0.3	0.93	1.08
Camomile	0.3	0.1	0.31	3.25
Lingonberry	0.3	0.1	0.31	3.25
Sesame seed	0.3	0.1	0.31	3.24
Coriander	0.2	0.1	0.73	1.62
Parsley	0.2	0	0.20	-
Poppy seed	0.2	0	0.20	-

Table 3 Prevalence of self-reported gastrointestinal symptoms for the different foods among asthmatics (asthma), non-asthmatics (no asthma) and in the total sample (all) ***(Continued)***

P-value was considered significant when <0.05 comparing the self-reported intolerance for the different foods between asthmatics to non-asthmatics
[a]lactose intolerance symptoms excluded
[b]gluten intolerance symptoms excluded

for the most common foods found in the present study. We also show that asthmatics reported symptoms from the GI-tract in a greater frequency compared to non-asthmatics and the most common foods causing self-reported symptoms were nuts, fruits, milk dairy products, alcohol, peanuts and shellfish. The non-asthmatic subjects seem to report adverse reaction to the same food items as asthmatics but at a significantly lower frequency. These data are in the line with previous reports that show a clear relation between food sensitization/allergy and asthma [23, 24]. Here, we demonstrate that the most common foods causing self-reported adverse reactions in subjects with asthma, when excluding those with suspected lactose- and gluten-intolerance, are fruits (as apple, kiwi, peach, nectarine), nuts (hazelnut, walnut, brazil nut), almond, peanut, followed by shellfish, milk dairy products, fried/fat food, potato, tomato, egg, flour and fish. The main allergens found in the reported fruits and nuts, carry allergens with known cross-reactivity with PR-10 allergens which are related to birch pollen. This, may explain the high prevalence of adverse reactions to these foods, since birch pollen sensitization is very common in Sweden [25]. These findings are confirmed in the present study, in which, 32.9 % of the asthmatics and 12.6 % of the non-asthmatics were sensitized to birch pollen. Thus, birch

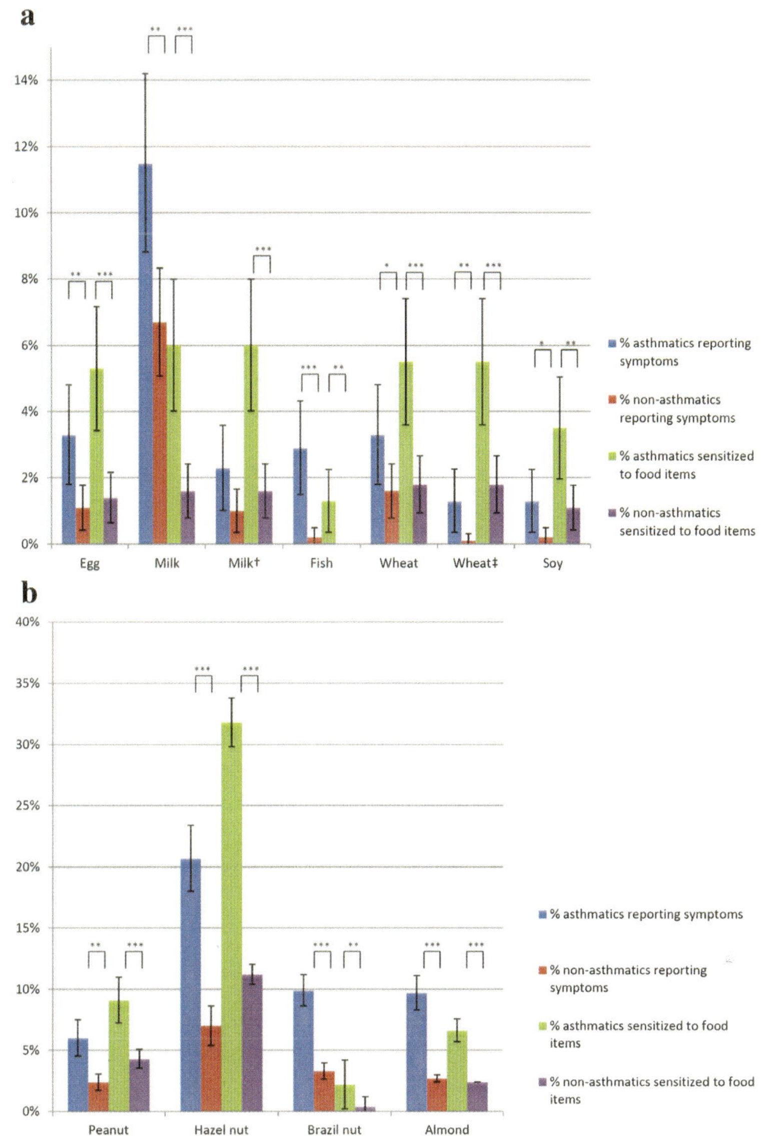

Fig. 3 Prevalence of self-reported symptoms and IgE sensitization for the most common foods among asthmatics and non-asthmatics (95 % CI). **a** staple foods **b** birch-related foods. †: lactose intolerance symptoms excluded. ‡: gluten intolerance symptoms excluded. *$p < 0.05$. **$p < 0.01$. ***$p < 0.001$

sensitization could explain the frequent adverse reactions observed following ingestion of birch related foods [26]. When testing the subjects included, with the allergen panels for the most common staple foods and nuts (fx1 and fx5), we observe interesting differences between asthmatics and non-asthmatics. Generally, adults with asthma are significantly more sensitized to any food, compared to non-asthmatics (38.2 % vs 13.9 %, $p < 0.001$) which may be a result of a general atopic phenotype in asthmatics. Subjects with asthma are more frequently sensitized to hazelnut, peanut, almond and milk compared to non-asthmatics which is mainly in accordance with the results from self-reported symptoms in this study. However, the correlation between IgE sensitization to specific food items and the symptoms they cause are rather low, but significant.

Concerning the staple foods, we show that asthmatic subjects more frequently report symptoms from egg, fish, milk, and wheat as well as soy compared to non-asthmatics and when we exclude subjects with suspected lactose- and gluten-intolerance, we notice an important difference in the results for milk and wheat (Table 2). When excluding subjects with suspicious intolerance to gluten and/or lactose though, the risk of losing some subjects with true allergy is inevitable, however the difference between asthmatics and non-asthmatics still remains. These results are in the line with previous reports

Table 4 Prevalence for self-reported symptoms with 95 % CI and IgE-sensitization profile for the most common foods among asthmatics and non-asthmatics

Food	Self-reported symptoms of the food among asthmatics (95 % CI)	Self-reported symptoms of the food among non-asthmatics (95 % CI)	IgEsensitization to food among asthmatics (95 % CI)	IgEsensitization to food among non-asthmatics (95 % CI)
Egg	3.30 % (1.80 % -4.80 %)	1.10 % (0.42 % -1.78 %)	5.30 % (3.42 % -7.18 %)	1.40 % (0.64 % -2.16 %)
Milk	11.50 % (8.81 % -14.19 %)	6.70 % (5.07 % -8.33 %)	6.00 % (4.01 % -7.99 %)	1.60 % (0.79 % -2.41 %)
Milk[a]	2.30 % (1.01 % -3.59 %)	1.00 % (0.34 % -1.66 %)	6.00 % (4.01 % -7.99 %)	1.60 % (0.79 % -2.41 %)
Fish	2.90 % (1.49 % -4.31 %)	0.20 % (-0.09 % -0.49 %)	1.30 % (0.35 % -2.25 %)	0.00 % (0.00 % -0.00 %)
Wheat	3.30 % (1.80 % -4.80 %)	1.60 % (0.78 % -2.42 %)	5.50 % (3.59 % -7.41 %)	1.80 % (0.94 % -2.66 %)
Wheat[b]	1.30 % (0.35 % -2.25 %)	0.10 % (-0.11 % -0.31 %)	5.50 % (3.59 % -7.41 %)	1.80 % (0.94 % -2.66 %)
Soy	1.30 % (0.35 % -2.25 %)	0.20 % (-0.09 % -0.49 %)	3.50 % (1.96 % -5.04 %)	1.10 % (0.42 % -1.78 %)
Peanut	6.00 % (3.99 % -8.01 %)	2.40 % (1.41 % -3.39 %)	9.10 % (6.69 % -11.51 %)	4.30 % (2.98 % -5.62 %)
Hazel nut	20.70 % (17.26 % -24.14 %)	7.00 % (5.34 % -8.66 %)	31.80 % (27.90 % -35.70 %)	11.20 % (9.15 % -13.25 %)
Brazil nut	9.90 % (7.32 % -12.48 %)	3.30 % (2.14 % -4.46 %)	2.20 % (0.97 % -3.43 %)	0.40 % (-0.01 % -0.81 %)
Almond	9.70 % (7.19 % -12.21 %)	2.70 % (1.65 % -3.75 %)	6.60 % (4.52 % -8.68 %)	2.40 % (1.41 % -3.39 %)
Any of the above	37.00 % (32.90 % -41.10 %)	15.40 % (13.04 % -17.76 %)	38.20 % (34.13 % -42.27 %)	13.90 % (11.66 % -16.14 %)

[a]lactose intolerance symptoms excluded
[b]gluten intolerance symptoms excluded

from a Swedish epidemiological survey by Eriksson et al. concerning self-reported food hypersensitivity in north Europe [27]. Interestingly subjects with asthma report significantly more symptoms in high rates after alcohol ingestion as from wine/beer compared to non-asthmatics (7.97 % vs 5.41 %, $p < 0.001$), which is supported by results from previous reports [28–30].

When the IgE sensitization to birch pollen is taken into consideration, we observe that among both asthmatics and non-asthmatics, birch-related foods are the most common causatives for adverse reactions with hazelnut in the first place (20.5 % and 7.2 % respectively) followed by apple (17.5 % and 7.15 % respectively) and other birch related fruits and nuts (Table 2). IgE reactivity

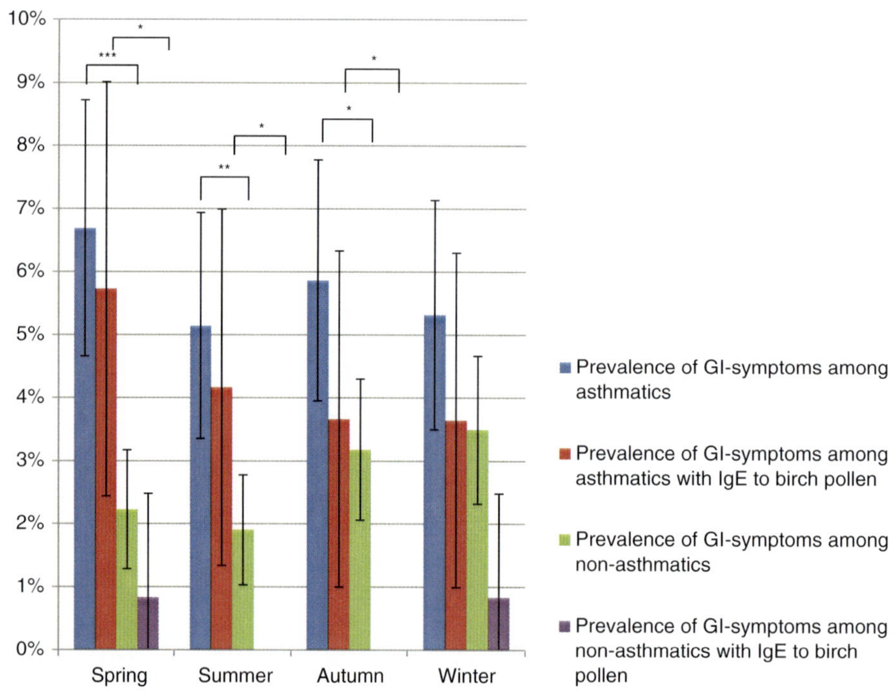

Fig. 4 Prevalence of self-reported gastrointestinal symptoms (GI) among asthmatics and non-asthmatics, and among subjects sensitized to IgE for birch pollen for the different seasons of the year (95 % CI). $^{*}p < 0.05$. $^{**}p < 0.01$. $^{***}p < 0.001$

to hazelnut and birch were also correlated to self-reported symptoms evoked by hazelnut, which is supported by the reported strong correlation between IgE for birch and IgE for hazelnut in both asthmatic and non-asthmatic subjects.

It is worth to comment that the prevalence of allergic asthma is much higher in the paediatric and adolescent population [31] and at about 40 years of age the prevalence of allergic and non-allergic asthma is approximately the same, and thereafter the non-allergic asthma dominates [32–35]. IgE-sensitization to the different foods and even other allergens may be more strongly connected to allergic asthma in the paediatric population [36] and less so in adults, which is supported by several recent studies, that show remission of the allergic disease before adulthood [37], and a decrease in the prevalence of IgE sensitization to foods among adults [38]. However, as shown in the present study adult asthmatics also have a high frequency of adverse reactions to foods that correlate with their IgE sensitization profile.

In this study, asthmatics reported more gastrointestinal symptoms during spring, summer and autumn compared to non-asthmatics. It is still not clear if increased asthma symptoms can be related to the increased frequency of gastrointestinal symptoms observed in the present study. The possible seasonal variation in gastrointestinal symptoms may be related to the pollen season where exposure to pollen may increase the reactivity after the ingestion of pollen related food items [25], which could be aggravated by the increased intestinal permeability seen in asthmatic patients [39] as well as in patients with atopy and IBS [40]. In two other studies, it was demonstrated that asthmatics with allergy to birch pollen experience more symptoms from the gastrointestinal tract, which resemble irritable bowel syndrome (IBS)-like symptoms, during the pollen season [41, 42]. It has also been shown that atopic subjects with IBS and self–reported food hypersensitivity had more severe gastrointestinal symptoms when compared to non-atopic subjects with IBS [40]. Interestingly, besides the reported symptoms from the birch-pollen related foods, asthmatics reported more gastrointestinal symptoms to fried/fat food, rich in carbohydrate, wine/beer, legumes and spices which would signify that these patients may more frequently suffer from IBS [43, 44].

The present study has some limitations that should be taken into consideration. It is well known that self-reported food intolerance yield a much higher prevalence compared to prevalence from performed food challenges and IgE data for food allergies [45]. However, the comparison between asthmatics and non-asthmatics should still be valid, since we have no reason to believe that the self-reporting accuracy differs between these two groups. It would also have been of great value to have asked specifically for lactose and gluten intolerance, and not only get input from the free text fields. Nevertheless, the reported symptoms do affect the subjects, whether it is a true allergy or not. The large number of participants in the study makes the findings reliable and fascinating as there are very few studies to date having examined the relation between food hypersensitivity and IgE sensitization to the most common foods in adults.

Conclusions

The novelty of this study, as one of the largest epidemiological studies in the adult population, is that it examines the relation between self-reported adverse reactions and IgE-sensitization for the most common foods and in adult asthmatic and non-asthmatic subjects as well as the relation between asthma and gastrointestinal symptoms caused by various foods in adults, for which the existing data are still very scarce.

In conclusion, the prevalence of both self-reported symptoms and IgE sensitization to various foods were much higher among asthmatics compared to non-asthmatic Swedish adults, both in total and for most individual food items studied. Hazelnut and other birch pollen related foods most commonly induced gastrointestinal symptoms in asthmatics and we propose that one important factor that may explain these findings is the high frequency of sensitization to birch pollen in asthmatic patients in Northern Europe.

Competing interests

The authors declare that they have no competing interests.

Authors' contributions

All authors were involved in the discussions and contributed to writing the manuscript. All authors read, revised and approved the final version of the manuscript to be published.

Acknowledgements

We would like to thank Ass Prof Ulf Bengtsson for making the questionnaire for the adverse reactions to different foods available to be used in this study. We would also like to thank the research nurses in Krefting Research Centre for their help in collecting all data and interviewing all subjects who participated in this study.

Author details

[1]Section of Allergology, University Hospital of Sahlgrenska, 413 45 Gothenburg, Sweden. [2]Krefting Research Centre, Department of Internal Medicine and Clinical Nutrition, University of Gothenburg, Gothenburg, Sweden. [3]Department for Rheumatology and Inflammation Research, Sahlgrenska Academy, University of Gothenburg, Gothenburg, Sweden. [4]R&D, ImmunoDiagnostics, Thermofischer Scientific, Uppsala, Sweden.

References

1. Chafen JJ, Newberry SJ, Riedl MA, Bravata DM, Maglione M, Suttorp MJ, et al. Diagnosing and managing common food allergies: a systematic review. JAMA. 2010;303(18):1848–56.
2. Nwaru BI, Hickstein L, Panesar SS, Muraro A, Werfel T, Cardona V, et al. The epidemiology of food allergy in Europe: a systematic review and meta-analysis. Allergy. 2014;69(1):62–75.
3. Sicherer SH, Sampson HA. Food allergy: epidemiology, pathogenesis, diagnosis, and treatment. J Allergy Clin Immunol. 2014;133(2):291–307. 2.
4. Berns SH, Halm EA, Sampson HA, Sicherer SH, Busse PJ, Wisnivesky JP. Food allergy as a risk factor for asthma morbidity in adults. J Asthma. 2007;44(5):377–81.
5. Roberts G, Patel N, Levi-Schaffer F, Habibi P, Lack G. Food allergy as a risk factor for life-threatening asthma in childhood: a case-controlled study. J Allergy Clin Immunol. 2003;112(1):168–74.
6. Bock SA, Munoz-Furlong A, Sampson HA. Fatalities due to anaphylactic reactions to foods. J Allergy Clin Immunol. 2001;107(1):191–3.
7. Oehling A, Baena Cagnani CE. Food allergy and child asthma. Allergol Immunopathol (Madr). 1980;8(1):7–14.
8. Roberts G, Lack G. Food allergy and asthma–what is the link? Paediatr Respir Rev. 2003;4(3):205–12.
9. Woods RK, Thien F, Raven J, Walters EH, Abramson M. Prevalence of food allergies in young adults and their relationship to asthma, nasal allergies, and eczema. Ann Allergy Asthma Immunol. 2002;88(2):183–9.
10. Blanco Carmona JG, Juste Picon S, Garces Sotillos M, Rodriguez GP. Occupational asthma in the confectionary industry caused by sensitivity to egg. Allergy. 1992;47(2 Pt 2):190–1.
11. Boulet LP, Laberge F. Occupational asthma to fish. Occup Environ Med. 2014;71(11):804.
12. James JM, Crespo JF. Allergic reactions to foods by inhalation. Curr Allergy Asthma Rep. 2007;7(3):167–74.
13. Caffarelli C, Deriu FM, Terzi V, Perrone F, De Angelis G, Atherton DJ. Gastrointestinal symptoms in patients with asthma. Arch Dis Child. 2000;82(2):131–5.
14. Kivity S, Fireman E, Sade K. Bronchial hyperactivity, sputum analysis and skin prick test to inhalant allergens in patients with symptomatic food hypersensitivity. Isr Med Assoc J. 2005;7(12):781–4.
15. Powell N, Huntley B, Beech T, Knight W, Knight H, Corrigan CJ. Increased prevalence of gastrointestinal symptoms in patients with allergic disease. Postgrad Med J. 2007;83(977):182–6.
16. Tielemans MM, Jaspers Focks J, van Rossum LG, Eikendal T, Jansen JB, Laheij RJ, et al. Gastrointestinal symptoms are still prevalent and negatively impact health-related quality of life: a large cross-sectional population based study in The Netherlands. PLoS One. 2013;8(7):e69876.
17. Louis E, Louis R, Drion V, Bonnet V, Lamproye A, Radermecker M, et al. Increased frequency of bronchial hyperresponsiveness in patients with inflammatory bowel disease. Allergy. 1995;50(9):729–33.
18. White AM, Stevens WH, Upton AR, O'Byrne PM, Collins SM. Airway responsiveness to inhaled methacholine in patients with irritable bowel syndrome. Gastroenterology. 1991;100(1):68–74.
19. Wallaert B, Desreumaux P, Copin MC, Tillie I, Benard A, Colombel JF, et al. Immunoreactivity for interleukin 3 and 5 and granulocyte/macrophage colony-stimulating factor of intestinal mucosa in bronchial asthma. J Exp Med. 1995;182(6):1897–904.
20. Ronmark EP, Ekerljung L, Lotvall J, Toren K, Ronmark E, Lundback B. Large scale questionnaire survey on respiratory health in Sweden: effects of late- and non-response. Respir Med. 2009;103(12):1807–15.
21. Landis JR, Koch GG. The measurement of observer agreement for categorical data. Biometrics. 1977;33(1):159–74.
22. Woods RK, Stoney RM, Raven J, Walters EH, Abramson M, Thien FC. Reported adverse food reactions overestimate true food allergy in the community. Eur J Clin Nutr. 2002;56(1):31–6.
23. Liu AH, Jaramillo R, Sicherer SH, Wood RA, Bock SA, Burks AW, et al. National prevalence and risk factors for food allergy and relationship to asthma: results from the National Health and Nutrition Examination Survey 2005–2006. J Allergy Clin Immunol. 2010;126(4):798–806. 4.
24. Patelis A, Gunnbjornsdottir M, Malinovschi A, Matsson P, Onell A, Hogman M, et al. Population-based study of multiplexed IgE sensitization in relation to asthma, exhaled nitric oxide, and bronchial responsiveness. J Allergy Clin Immunol. 2012;130(2):397–402. 2.
25. Vieths S, Scheurer S, Ballmer-Weber B. Current understanding of cross-reactivity of food allergens and pollen. Ann N Y Acad Sci. 2002;964:47–68.
26. Eriksson NE, Holmen A. Skin prick tests with standardized extracts of inhalant allergens in 7099 adult patients with asthma or rhinitis: cross-sensitizations and relationships to age, sex, month of birth and year of testing. J Investig Allergol Clin Immunol. 1996;6(1):36–46.
27. Eriksson NE, Moller C, Werner S, Magnusson J, Bengtsson U, Zolubas M. Self-reported food hypersensitivity in Sweden, Denmark, Estonia, Lithuania, and Russia. J Investig Allergol Clin Immunol. 2004;14(1):70–9.
28. Lieberoth S, Backer V, Kyvik KO, Skadhauge LR, Tolstrup JS, Gronbaek M, et al. Intake of alcohol and risk of adult-onset asthma. Respir Med. 2012;106(2):184–8.
29. Linneberg A, Berg ND, Gonzalez-Quintela A, Vidal C, Elberling J. Prevalence of self-reported hypersensitivity symptoms following intake of alcoholic drinks. Clin Exp Allergy. 2008;38(1):145–51.
30. Vally H, Thompson PJ. Allergic and asthmatic reactions to alcoholic drinks. Addict Biol. 2003;8(1):3–11.
31. Ronmark E, Bjerg A, Perzanowski M, Platts-Mills T, Lundback B. Major increase in allergic sensitization in schoolchildren from 1996 to 2006 in northern Sweden. J Allergy Clin Immunol. 2009;124(2):357–63. 63.e1-15.
32. Ekerljung L, Bossios A, Lotvall J, Olin AC, Ronmark E, Wennergren G, et al. Multi-symptom asthma as an indication of disease severity in epidemiology. Eur Respir J. 2011;38(4):825–32.
33. Kamdar TA, Peterson S, Lau CH, Saltoun CA, Gupta RS, Bryce PJ. Prevalence and characteristics of adult-onset food allergy. J Allergy Clin Immunol Pract. 2015;3(1):114. 5.e1.
34. Pallasaho P, Juusela M, Lindqvist A, Sovijarvi A, Lundback B, Ronmark E. Allergic rhinoconjunctivitis doubles the risk for incident asthma–results from a population study in Helsinki. Finland Respir Med. 2011;105(10):1449–56.
35. Warm K, Backman H, Lindberg A, Lundback B, Ronmark E. Low incidence and high remission of allergic sensitization among adults. J Allergy Clin Immunol. 2012;129(1):136–42.
36. Strinnholm A, Winberg A, West C, Hedman L, Ronmark E. Food hypersensitivity is common in Swedish schoolchildren, especially oral reactions to fruit and gastrointestinal reactions to milk. Acta Paediatr. 2014;103(12):1290–6.
37. Winberg A, Strinnholm A, Hedman L, West C, Perzanowski M, Ronmark E. High incidence and remission of reported food hypersensitivity in Swedish children followed from 8 to 12years of age - a population based cohort study. Clin Trans Allergy. 2014;4(1):32.
38. Patelis A, Gunnbjornsdottir M, Borres MP, Burney P, Gislason T, Toren K, et al. Natural history of perceived food hypersensitivity and IgE sensitisation to food allergens in a cohort of adults. PLoS One. 2014;9(1):e85333.
39. Benard A, Desreumeaux P, Huglo D, Hoorelbeke A, Tonnel AB, Wallaert B. Increased intestinal permeability in bronchial asthma. J Allergy Clin Immunol. 1996;97(6):1173–8.
40. Lillestol K, Helgeland L, Arslan Lied G, Florvaag E, Valeur J, Lind R, Berstad, A. Indications of 'atopic bowel' in patients with self-reported food hypersensitivity. Aliment Pharmacol Ther. 2010;31(10):1112–22.
41. Magnusson J, Lin XP, Dahlman-Hoglund A, Hanson LL, Telemo E, Magnusson O, et al. Seasonal intestinal inflammation in patients with birch pollen allergy. J Allergy Clin Immunol. 2003;112(1):45–50.
42. Rentzos G, Lundberg V, Stotzer PO, Pullerits T, Telemo E. Intestinal allergic inflammation in birch pollen allergic patients in relation to pollen season, IgE sensitization profile and gastrointestinal symptoms. Clin Trans Allergy. 2014;4:19.
43. Bohn L, Storsrud S, Tornblom H, Bengtsson U, Simren M. Self-reported food-related gastrointestinal symptoms in IBS are common and associated with more severe symptoms and reduced quality of life. Am J Gastroenterol. 2013;108(5):634–41.
44. Simren M, Mansson A, Langkilde AM, Svedlund J, Abrahamsson H, Bengtsson U, et al. Food-related gastrointestinal symptoms in the irritable bowel syndrome. Digestion. 2001;63(2):108–15.
45. O'Keefe AW, De Schryver S, Mill J, Mill C, Dery A, Ben-Shoshan M. Diagnosis and management of food allergies: new and emerging options: a systematic review. J Asthma Allergy. 2014;7:141–64.

The development of a standardised diet history tool to support the diagnosis of food allergy

Isabel J Skypala[1*], Carina Venter[2], Rosan Meyer[3], Nicolette W deJong[4], Adam T Fox[5], Marion Groetch[6], J N Oude Elberink[7], Aline Sprikkelman[8], Louiza Diamandi[9], Berber J Vlieg-Boerstra[10] and the Allergy-focussed Diet History Task Force of the European Academy of Allergy and Clinical Immunology

Abstract

The disparity between reported and diagnosed food allergy makes robust diagnosis imperative. The allergy-focussed history is an important starting point, but published literature on its efficacy is sparse. Using a structured approach to connect symptoms, suspected foods and dietary intake, a multi-disciplinary task force of the European Academy of Allergy and Clinical Immunology developed paediatric and adult diet history tools. Both tools are divided into stages using traffic light labelling (red, amber and green). The red stage requires the practitioner to gather relevant information on symptoms, atopic history, food triggers, foods eaten and nutritional issues. The amber stage facilitates interpretation of the responses to the red-stage questions, thus enabling the practitioner to prepare to move forward. The final green stage provides a summary template and test algorithm to support continuation down the diagnostic pathway. These tools will provide a standardised, practical approach to support food allergy diagnosis, ensuring that all relevant information is captured and interpreted in a robust manner. Future work is required to validate their use in diverse age groups, disease entities and in different countries, in order to account for differences in health care systems, food availability and dietary norms.

Keywords: History, Diet, Tool, Allergy, Food, Diagnosis

Introduction

Adverse reactions to foods are frequently reported, however only those involving immunological mechanisms, including both immunoglobulin E (IgE) and non-IgE mediated, can be defined as food allergy (FA) [1]. The prevalence of FA varies worldwide, but the rate of true FA in children and adults is consistently lower than self-reported rates [2-5]. A European systematic review found the overall point prevalence in Europe of self-reported FA to be 5.9% (95% CI: 5.7-6.1), compared with a food challenge confirmed FA rate of 0.9% (95% CI: 0.8-1.1) [6]. Reported FA persists over time in adults [7], and age-related changes can affect the immune system, increasing the potential for newly diagnosed food allergy in older adults [8].

This disparity between reported and actual levels of FA make a robust diagnosis imperative in order to avoid overt and/or unnecessary dietary restrictions leading to either continuation of symptoms due to the wrong food being eliminated or nutritional deficiencies [9,10]. Guidelines [1,11-13] provide expert evidence-based support for the diagnosis of FA, which includes taking an allergy focussed history, performing appropriate tests and food reintroduction or controlled food challenge. Although international consensus agrees that the allergy-focussed history is a key part of the diagnostic pathway [1,12], the lack of standardisation, and variable expertise of the history taker, may prevent the ascertainment of sufficient information, leading to poor interpretation of the facts.

However, when the right questions are posed and the answers are systematically linked to appropriate actions, an allergy history can be invaluable [11,14], and for some conditions, history has been demonstrated to be wholly diagnostic [15]. Included in the additional supporting information of recent European Academy of Allergy and Clinical Immunology (EAACI) FA guidelines was a useful list of key questions for the clinical history [1] Therefore these guidelines not suggest an allergy-focussed

* Correspondence: i.skypala@rbht.nhs.uk
[1]Royal Brompton & Harefield NHS Foundation Trust, London, UK
Full list of author information is available at the end of the article

history is fundamental to the establishment of a diagnosis, they also provide a starting point for a structured approach to history-taking. Recognition of the importance of the diet and clinical history by EAACI led to the formation of an EAACI Task Force to develop paediatric and adult diet history tools for use by health care professionals.

Methods

The Allergy-focussed Diet History Task Force, an international multi-professional group of food allergy experts, agreed that evidence-based tools would need to be developed. In order to gather evidence of links between reported symptoms, trigger foods and dietary intake, and the existence of any published diagnostic questionnaires, a search on Pub Med and Medline was undertaken. The search terms shown in Table 1 were used, and papers from 1990 to January 2012 were selected in the order given below:

1) Randomized controlled trials
2) Non-randomized controlled clinical trials
3) Before and after clinical trials
4) Prevalence studies employing oral food challenge
5) Systematic reviews and other meta analyses
6) Observational studies – cohort or case reports
7) Other subject reviews

The search resulted in 36 publications, but only one study measured the diagnostic efficacy of history against validated test methods [15]. Access to more rigorous methodology employed by the EAACI Food Allergy Guidelines Task Force [6], yielded no additional appropriate papers. In the absence of a lack of suitable published evidence, the Task Force undertook to develop age-specific diet history tools based on expert opinion, with the factors considered being supported by guidelines or underpinned by evidence from individual studies. A structure for the tools was established to enable rapid assimilation and interpretation of answers to standard questions on symptoms, atopic history, family history of atopy, co-factors, suspected or known food triggers, quantity of food involved, foods currently consumed and avoided, cross-reacting foods, growth and development and likelihood of nutritional risk. The pooled knowledge and expertise of the panel greatly contributed to the construction of the questions, especially where evidence was lacking.

Table 1 Search terms for review

Tree	food hypersensitivities
Tree	food hypersensitivity
Tree	hypersensitivity food
allergies food	questionnaire
allergy food	questionnaires
assessing	recognition
assessment	recognise
detect	recognising
detecting	screen
detection	screening
diagnose	signs
diagnoses	symptoms
diagnosing	work up
diagnosis	workup
diagnostic intent	
evaluating	
evaluation	
food allergies	
food allergy	

Results

Two allergy-focussed diet history tools for paediatric and adult patients were developed (see Additional files 1 and 2) based on a traffic light scheme similar to those used to inform consumers about healthy eating or energy efficiency:

Red - gather information through questioning the patient on their allergic history, foods habitually eaten, nutritional status, and relevant co-factors.

Amber – facilitates interpretation of the responses to the red-stage questions by linking the information gained to match potential diagnostic pathways, utilising the algorithms and tables provided to refine and formulate a potential diagnosis thus enabling the practitioner to prepare to move forward.

Green - the way ahead is clear to institute appropriate testing and/or onward referral to a specialist allergy centre, gastroenterologist or a specialist dietitian.

Red stage - questioning and linking

Symptoms and atopic history

Symptoms

The characterization of symptoms is an essential first step when taking a history from someone presenting with adverse reactions to foods.

Presenting symptoms: IgE-mediated FA

A number of guidelines have summarised these symptoms [1,11-13], primarily those seen in children, which can be skin related (pruritus, erythema, acute urticaria, acute angioedema), gastro-intestinal (anal pruritus, colicky abdominal pain, diarrhoea and vomiting) or upper and lower respiratory symptoms. In adults, skin reactions are also associated with IgE-mediated food allergy [16], but gastrointestinal symptoms are predominant especially dysaesthesia of the tongue, oropharyngeal pruritus and vomiting [17-20]. Rhinitis, conjunctivitis and asthma are also presenting features of adult food allergy [5,15] Tachycardia, hypotension, throat tightness, bronchospasm, laryngeal oedema, shortness of breath, syncope and anaphylaxis can affect all ages [21,22].

Presenting symptoms: non-IgE mediated FA

Proctocolitis [23] is characterised by blood and mucous in the stools and occasional diarrhoea, although the infant appears well. The symptoms of food protein-induced enterocolitis syndrome (FPIES) include late onset gastro-intestinal symptoms of profuse vomiting, diarrhoea, pallor and occasionally hypovolemic shock [24]. Children and infants with Eosinophilic Oesophagitis (EoE) often show signs of chronic vomiting, abdominal pain, poor appetite, food refusal, other feeding refusal behaviours as well as dysphagia [25]. Up to one third of young children with Atopic Dermatitis (AD) may present with a FA, particularly those with moderate to severe eczema unresponsive to topical treatment [26,27]. Adults have less well documented non-IgE-mediated food allergies, but dysphagia and oesophageal food impaction are particularly associated with adult-onset EoE [28].

Presenting symptoms: other symptoms caused by food

Sometimes symptoms of an allergic disorder can resemble those due to non-immune mediated adverse reactions to foods, thus complicating the diagnostic process. For example, dietary histamine has been reported to provoke rhino-conjunctivitis, flushing, pruritus, urticaria, asthma, hypotension and abdominal cramping [29]. The food additive sodium metabisulphite has been linked to symptoms of rhinitis, nasal blockage, wheeze and abdominal pain [30]. Abdominal symptoms are a notable feature of Irritable Bowel Syndrome (IBS), a diagnosis which is positively associated with pain in the lower abdomen, pain relieved by bowel movements, frequent pain and abdominal bloating [31].

Onset of symptoms

It is important to establish the temporal relationship between eating a food and the onset of symptoms. It is generally agreed that the sooner the symptoms occur after eating, the greater the likelihood that an IgE-mediated mechanism is provoking the reaction [1,12]. Non-IgE-mediated FA symptoms are usually delayed; children with FPIES typically experience severe vomiting 1–4 hours after ingestion of the suspect food [32]. However occasionally symptom speed of onset does not provide such clear signposting; co-factors such as exercise can mislead if the symptoms only occur during exercise, but the food involved could have been eaten up to 2 hours earlier [33]. Another example is delayed anaphylaxis to red meat occurs in relation to IgE antibodies to the oligosaccharide galactose-alpha-1,3-galactose (alpha-gal) generated by tick bites [34]. Conversely, some non-immune-mediated adverse food reactions may manifest soon after eating, i.e. gastrointestinal symptoms triggered by lactose intolerance [35], or wheeze provoked by the food additive sodium metabisulphite [30].

Other important factors relating to symptoms include ascertainment of the quantity of food required to trigger symptoms, frequency and reproducibility of the reactions and the interval since the last reaction [1,11-13]. The age of onset of symptoms, feeding/diet history, history of any food elimination and any previous therapeutic interventions are also significant.

Atopic history

For children, in addition to a physical examination focusing on growth and development, any allergy related co-morbidities and family history of atopy should be ascertained [1,11]. The likelihood of food allergy is enhanced in children with moderate to severe eczema [26]. For adults, a physical examination is also helpful, but it is also vital to establish atopic status due to the strong association between atopic disease and the manifestation of food allergy in adults [36]. Allergic rhinitis is increasingly prevalent in food allergic adults, reportedly affecting 41% of UK adults suffering from adverse reactions to foods in 2009, compared to 25% in 1991 [37,38]. Asthmatics with food allergy are also more likely to have severe and uncontrolled asthma [39] and suffer from fatal or near fatal food anaphylaxis [22].

Known aeroallergen sensitisations

There is an increasing level of aeroallergen sensitisation in all age groups, which persists into old age [40,41]. Thus establishing sensitisation to pollens, mites and animal dander is vital when interpreting the history, especially as geographical variation in aeroallergen sensitisation across Europe affects prevalence and foods involved [42]. Positive tests to pollen [15], latex [43] or house dust mite [44], can be linked to homologous reactions to fruits, vegetables, nuts or shellfish. More unusual cross-reactions include sensitisation to bird feathers inducing symptoms to the egg yolk allergen alpha livetin [45], individuals sensitised to galactose-alpha-1,3-galactose (alpha-gal), reacting to beef and pork [34], and reactions to pork associated with sensitisation to cats [46]. The sensitising agent might be a food-related parasite such as cereal mites [47] or the *Anisakis* nematode worm [48].

Extrinsic (co) factors and routes of exposure

In adults, exercise, alcohol, stress, aspirin or non-steroidal anti-inflammatory drugs (NSAIDs) can enhance or precipitate an allergic reaction to food [49]. Food-dependant exercise-induced anaphylaxis (FDEIA) is characterised by a lack of reaction to the trigger food unless it is consumed in close proximity to taking exercise [50]. Wheat, crustaceans, tomatoes, celery, strawberries, cheese have all been implicated [33,49-53]. Alcohol can also act as a co-factor, but symptoms to alcohol could also be due to an allergy to grapes or barley [54,55], sensitivity to vasoactive amines or sodium metabisulphite [29,30], or caused by a congenital deficiency of the enzyme alcohol dehydrogenase [56]. Food additives have also been shown to act as co-factors in cases of anaphylaxis [53]. Co-factors may be less relevant in children [57], but exposure to allergens other than via the oral route require consideration in both children and adults; these include inhalation of aerosolized allergens, transfer of allergens during cooking or by skin contact [58-60].

Food & symptoms

Food triggers – IgE-mediated FA

Although there are a large range of foods which can be implicated in IgE-mediated FA, only a limited number regularly provoke reactions in most people. Most reactions in children are due to milk, egg and peanut [2], with milk and egg being the most common causes of anaphylaxis [61]. Milk, egg, wheat and soy allergy usually remit in late childhood [62-65], thus a primary allergy to these foods is rare in adults. Wheat allergy in adults is generally associated with FDEIA [52] and adults reporting reactions to soy usually develop symptoms due to homology between soy protein and birch pollen allergens [66]. Peanut and tree nut allergy in adults is usually a persistence of childhood allergy since only 8-10% of cases are newly diagnosed in adolescence or adulthood [67-69]. Up to 30% of adults with a peanut allergy have cross-reactivity to other legumes such as lupine [70]. Lupine allergy also presents in childhood, but is far less prevalent than peanut allergy in the general population, affecting less than 0.3% of patients with reported reactions to foods [71]. Seeds such as sesame and mustard are also a significant cause of IgE-mediated reactions in certain populations [72,73]. Those with a primary allergy to one type of nut, seed or legume can react to other similar foods due to co-sensitisation to homologous allergens [74-79].

Fish and shellfish trigger both paediatric and adult IgE-mediated FA [80,81], often provoking severe reactions [22,82]. Pan allergens in vertebrate fish account for strong interspecies cross-reactivity; thus sensitization to more than one species is common in fish-allergic individuals [80]. The same is true for crustaceans and molluscs, although sensitisation to minor seafood allergens can limit clinical reactivity solely to the seafood which provoked the index reaction [83]. The lack of homology between the pan allergens in vertebrate fish and shellfish usually means fish-allergic individuals can tolerate shellfish and vice versa [80].

Fruits and, to a lesser extent, vegetables, are often the most frequently reported foods to provoke new onset reactions in adults [5,17,18,37]. These reactions are usually due to oral allergy syndrome or pollen-food syndrome (PFS), a common manifestation of cross-reactive plant FA in adults, which can affect 50% or more pollen-sensitized individuals [15,17]. Such reactions are also reported in older children and teenagers, although only limited epidemiological data supports this [84]. Reactions, usually to more than one food, typically occur to tree nuts, apples, peaches and cherries, although peanuts and soy may also be involved [15,17,85-87]. If PFS is suspected then any history of seasonal hay fever should be linked to symptoms to fruits and vegetables, and symptoms may be worse or only occur during the pollen season [61]. Homologous allergens in natural rubber latex (*Hevea brasiliensis*) can also cross-react with foods, in particular kiwi fruit, avocado, chestnuts and bananas [44]. Lipid Transfer Protein (LTP) allergy should also be considered if plant foods provoke severe reactions [88]. LTP allergy, usually associated with sensitisation to the peach LTP allergen Pru p 3 [88,89], is highly prevalent in southern Europe [90], and associated with presence of co-factors such as alcohol and exercise [19,49].

Whilst children might have a reaction to a food soon after the first exposure, older children and adults may suddenly develop symptoms to foods consumed for many years. However, foods habitually eaten are mostly considered as safe and should not be tested. If the reactions are to multiple foods and PFS is not suspected, then a 'hidden' allergen used as an ingredient in composite dishes may be implicated, such as legumes, seeds, celery and natural food colourings.

Food triggers – non-IgE-mediated FA

FPIES typically occurs in response to milk or soy proteins in infant formula, and more rarely to food proteins in breast milk [91,92]. The common provoking allergens in FPIES are milk, rice and soy, but reactions have also been reported to oats, fish, egg and some fruit and vegetables [93]. Although eosinophilic gastrointestinal disorders are seen in both adults and paediatrics, offending foods may differ [94]. In children, milk, egg, wheat and soy have been found to be most relevant, although in some cases fish, nuts and peanuts also play a role, although meat proteins (including, beef, lamb, chicken and pork), carrots, potato, maize and peanuts may also be causative foods [95]. Wheat and milk appear to be major allergens in adults although other triggers could include corn, rice and legumes [96].

Food triggers – non-immune mediated adverse food reactions

Milk is most frequently linked to non-immune mediated conditions in adults including lactose intolerance [35],

IBS [97], and some respiratory conditions [98]. In the absence of IgE-sensitisation to wheat, coeliac disease [99] should be excluded prior to considering differential diagnoses such as non-coeliac gluten sensitivity [100] and IBS [101]. There is some evidence that foods containing high levels of oligo-, di-, mono-saccharides and polyols carbohydrates (FODMAPS™) could provoke some or all of the gut symptoms experienced by IBS sufferers [102]. Oligosaccharides (wheat, rye, onions, garlic, artichokes and legumes) probably affect the majority of IBS sufferers, 45% of whom will also be intolerant to foods high in fructose (honey, apples, pears, watermelon and mango) [103]. Reported reactions to multiple foods in the absence of IgE-sensitisation can indicate a non-immune mediated reaction. Potential mediators may include food additives (azo dyes, benzoates, sulphites and mono-sodium glutamate) [30,104], or naturally-occurring substances such as vasoactive or biogenic amines (fish, pork and fermented or aged meat products, strong cheeses, red wine, spinach, aubergine and yeast extract) [29], or salicylates (coffee, dried herbs and spices, cherries, strawberries and certain apple varieties) [105] although robust evidence on the prevalence of these types of reactions is lacking.

Foods eaten and avoided

All foods and food products which can be consumed without any symptoms should be noted, especially common allergenic foods, or 'hidden' food allergens such as mustard, celery, soy and lupine. Emerging evidence indicates that some children can tolerate foods containing well-cooked milk and egg, but will still react to raw/less well cooked forms [106,107]. Similarly those with PFS may be able to tolerate cooked fruits but not raw [15,17]. Reported avoidance of the trigger food may not be complete exclusion [108] due to lack of awareness of foods that contain small amounts of allergen. A dietetic consultation will establish true abstinence and information from food labels, recipes or food diaries may also be useful [109].

Nutritional issues

Nutritional impairment is a tangible risk in those with suspected FA; the elimination of food allergens often entails the exclusion of foods that contribute essential nutrients for growth and development (Table 2) [9,10]. Poor growth and stunting has been shown to occur in children with IgE-mediated FA who are on exclusion diets [10,110], with the number of foods excluded linked to a low weight for age and height for age in such children [10]. Feeding difficulties may also occur as clinical features of non-IgE mediated FA. Adults generally are not in danger of developing major nutritional deficiencies although individuals avoiding multiple foods can be at risk [111]. Therefore both tools contain a nutritional assessment section which, on completion, should indicate whether onward referral for specialist nutritional intervention is required. A dietitian can ascertain and interpret the diet history to ensure normal growth and development, employing a variety of measures to determine dietary intake [112,113]. The nutritional analysis can signpost the requirement for nutritional supplements

Table 2 Main food allergens and their nutrient content [118]

Allergen	Nutrients involved
Milk	Protein, Carbohydrate, Fats, Vitamin A and vitamin D, riboflavin, pantothenic acid, vitamin B12, calcium, magnesium, phosphate
Egg	Protein, Riboflavin, biotin, vitamin A, vitamin B12, vitamin D, vitamin E, pantothenic acid, selenium, iodine, folate
Fish	All fish: Protein, iodine.
	Fish bones: calcium, phosphorus, fluoride.
	Fatty fish: Protein, fat, vitamins A and D, omega-3 fatty acids
Shellfish	Similar nutrients to white fish.
	Crab and mussels: Protein and good sources of omega 3
	Selenium, zinc, iodine and copper
Molluscs	Varying amounts of protein (scallop), calcium (clam), zinc (oysters) and iron (clam)
Wheat	Carbohydrate, Protein Fibre, thiamine, riboflavin, niacin, calcium, iron, folate if fortified
Peanut	Protein, fats, Vitamin E, niacin, magnesium
Soya	Protein, Thiamine, riboflavin, pyridoxine, folate, calcium, phosphorus, magnesium, iron, zinc, fibre
Lupin	Negligible nutritional value when consumed as a condiment or taken in very small amounts
Tree nuts	Depends on type of nut, but similar to peanuts + omega 3 and 6 fatty acids
Sesame seed	Protein, fats, Vitamin E, calcium, potassium, phosphorus, vitamin B and iron and omega 6 fatty acids
Mustard	Negligible nutritional value when consumed as a condiment or taken in very small amounts
Celery/celeriac	Fibre

and give expert advice to ensure a healthy, regular and varied diet is taken as this has been shown to be of importance in the development of allergy [114,115] It is important that the user take into account the important role of under-nutrition in paediatric and adult food allergy since poor nutritional status may aggravate symptoms and a healthy diet could be important in the prevention of allergic disease [10,116,117].

Amber stage - interpretation of history

This stage involves linking the answers to the questions from the 'red' section and includes interpretation of symptoms, medical history, trigger foods and nutritional issues. Typical symptoms and foods associated with IgE mediated FA are listed in the left hand column of this section, and adapted to differences in age-related onset. The right-hand column lists foods and symptoms most associated with adverse food reactions that are not immune-mediated. In general, paediatric patients are far more likely to suffer from non-IgE mediated conditions than non-immune mediated conditions [24]. Thus the paediatric tool also contains a middle column listing foods and symptoms most associated with paediatric non-IgE mediated FA. However, this middle column is not present on the adult tool since these conditions are often most prevalent in childhood [24], the exception being EoE, which does exist in adults, with the adult form usually being diagnosed between the ages of 30–50 years [119].

This section also contains a guide to the foods most likely to be causative of FA at different ages and to support the interpretation of reported food triggers. There is information on cross-reactivity, a PFS diagnostic algorithm [15] and lists of potential allergens in composite meals. Collectively, the information in the amber section enables the user to decide whether the patient has an IgE- or a non IgE-mediated FA, a non-immune mediated adverse food reaction or a differential diagnosis not related to allergy, or combined symptoms.

Green stage - tests and diagnosis

This section contains a test algorithm and care plan to summarise the outcome. Once the green stage is completed, the user should have sufficient information to undertake further tests, or make an onward referral to specialist services as indicated.

Conclusion

The EAACI Food Allergy and Anaphylaxis Guidelines [1] emphasise the importance of taking a careful allergy-focussed history, and asking structured questions. These age-appropriate diet history tools, developed by a multi-professional international group of experts, bring together relevant factors, important in the aetiology of FA. The authors acknowledge that all of the evidence submitted in support of the tools has not been systematically graded, however, this is the first time that all of the relevant questions in an allergy focussed diet history have been agreed, documented, referenced and linked in a systematic way to provide standardised practical tools. The paediatric and adult diet history tools can be adapted to country specific dietary norms, whilst ensuring a standardised approach and screening for nutritional status. The information gained is vital in the formulation of a provisional diagnosis.

These tools can be used by anyone who needs guidance in taking a diet and clinical history, being particularly useful for those who not working in a specialist allergy setting. An accurate history determines the need for allergy testing. Once a diagnosis is made, patients can be managed appropriately or be referred onwards to an allergy specialist physician and/or dietitian as required. Newly diagnosed food allergy is a growing burden for all ages, against a backdrop of complex dietary intake patterns, multiple co-factors, social complications and diverse presenting features. These tools provide a scaffold of questions on which the diagnosis of FA can be built.

Competing interests

The authors declare that they have no competing interests.

Authors' contributions

IS chaired the Task Force, wrote the initial tools and drafted the manuscript. CV participated in the Task Force, provided input into the tools, and helped to draft the manuscript. RM participated in Task Force and contributed to the final version of the paediatric tool. NdJ participated in Task Force and contributed to the final version of the adult tool. AF participated in the Task Force and contributed to the paediatric tool. MG participated in the Task Force and contributed to the paediatric tool. JOE participated in Task Force. AS participated in the Task Force. LD participated in the Task Force. BVB conceived the idea for the Task Force and greatly participated in the development of the tools. All authors read and approved the final manuscript.

Authors' information

Isabel J Skypala and Carina Venter are Joint first authors.

Acknowledgements

The authors are very grateful for the funding and support from EAACI which enabled them to produce the tools that this paper relates to.

Author details

[1]Royal Brompton & Harefield NHS Foundation Trust, London, UK. [2]The David Hide 6. Asthma and Allergy Research Centre, Isle of Wight, UK. [3]Great Ormond Street NHS Foundation Trust, London, UK. [4]Erasmus MC, Rotterdam, NL, Netherlands. [5]Guy's and St Thomas' Hospitals NHS Foundation Trust and Kings College, London, UK. [6]Jaffe Food Allergy Institute, Icahn School of Medicine at Mount Sinai, New York, USA. [7]Department of Allergology, University Medical Centre of Groningen, University of Groningen, Groningen,

NL, Netherlands. [8]Emma Children's Hospital Academic Medical Centre, Amsterdam, NL, Netherlands. [9]University of Athens, Athens, GR, Greece. [10]Emma Children's Hospital, Paediatric Respiratory Medicine and Allergy, Academic Medical Centre, University of Amsterdam, Amsterdam, NL, Netherlands.

References

1. Muraro A, Werfel T, Hoffmann-Sommergruber K, Roberts G, Beyer K, Bindslev-Jensen C, et al. EAACI food allergy and anaphylaxis guidelines: diagnosis and management of food allergy. Allergy. 2014;69:1008–25.
2. Venter C, Pereira B, Voigt K, Grundy J, Clayton CB, Higgins B, et al. Prevalence and cumulative incidence of food hypersensitivity in the first 3 years of life. Allergy. 2008;63:354–9.
3. Eller E, Kjaer HF, Host A, Andersen KE, Bindslev-Jensen C. Food allergy and food sensitization in early childhood: results from the DARC cohort. Allergy. 2009;64:1023–9.
4. Vierk KA, Koehler KM, Fein SB, Street DA. Prevalence of self-reported food allergy in American adults and use of food labels. J Allergy Clin Immunol. 2007;119:1504–10.
5. Zuberbier T, Edenharter G, Worm M, Ehlers I, Reimann S, Hantke T, et al. Prevalence of adverse reactions to food in Germany – a population study. Allergy. 2004;59:338–45.
6. Nwaru BI, Hickstein L, Panesar SS, Muraro A, Werfel T, Cardona V, et al. The epidemiology of food allergy in Europe: a systematic review and meta-analysis. Allergy. 2014;69:62–75.
7. Patelis A, Gunnbjörnsdottir M, Borres MP, Burney P, Gislason T, Torén K, et al. Natural history of perceived food hypersensitivity and IgE sensitisation to food allergens in a cohort of adults. PLoS One. 2014;10(9):e85333.
8. Diesner SC, Untersmayr E, Pietschmann P, Jensen-Jarolim E. Food allergy: only a pediatric disease? Gerontology. 2011;57:28–32.
9. Christie L, Hine RJ, Parker JG, Burks W. Food allergies in children affect nutrient intake and growth. J Am Diet Assoc. 2002;102:1648–51.
10. Meyer R, De Koker C, Dziubak R, Venter C, Dominguez-Ortega G, Cutts R, et al. Malnutrition in children with food allergies in the UK. J Hum Nutr Diet. 2014;27:227–35.
11. NICE clinical guideline 116 – Food allergy in children and young people. National Institute for Health and Clinical Excellence. Diagnosis and Assessment of Food Allergy in Children and Young People in Primary Care and Community Settings. London: National Institute for Health and Clinical Excellence; 2011. www.nice.org.uk/guidance/CG116 guidelines.
12. Boyce JA, Assa'ad A, Burks AW, Jones SM, Sampson HA, Wood RA, et al. NIAID-sponsored expert panel. Guidelines for the Diagnosis and Management of Food Allergy in the United States: Summary of the NIAID-Sponsored Expert Panel Report. J Allergy Clin Immunol. 2010;126:1105–18.
13. Burks AW, Tang M, Sicherer S, Muraro A, Eigenmann PA, Ebisawa M, et al. ICON: food allergy. J Allergy Clin Immunol. 2012;129:906–20.
14. Venter C, Arshad SH. Guideline fever: an overview of DRACMA, US NIAID and UK NICE guidelines. Curr Opin Allergy Clin Immunol. 2012;12:302–15.
15. Skypala IJ, Calderon MA, Leeds AR, Emery P, Till SJ, Durham SR. Development and validation of a structured questionnaire for the diagnosis of Oral Allergy Syndrome in subjects with seasonal allergic rhinitis during the UK birch pollen season. Clin Exp Allergy. 2011;41:1001–11.
16. Soares-Weiser K, Takwoingi Y, Panesar SS, Muraro A, Werfel T, Hoffmann-Sommergruber K, et al. The diagnosis of food allergy: a systematic review and meta-analysis. Allergy. 2014;69:76–86.
17. Eriksson NE, Formaren H, Svenonius E. Food hypersensitivity in patients with pollen allergy. Allergy. 1982;37:437–43.
18. Osterballe M, Hansen TK, Mortz CG, Høst A, Bindeslev-Jensen C. The prevalence of food hypersensitivity in an unselected population of children and adults. Pediatr Allergy Immunol. 2005;16:567–73.
19. Pascal M, Muñoz-Cano R, Reina Z, Palacín A, Vilella R, Picado C, et al. Lipid transfer protein syndrome: clinical pattern, cofactor effect and profile of molecular sensitization to plant-foods and pollens. Clin Exp Allergy. 2012;42:1529–39.
20. Hebling A, McCants ML, Musmand JJ, Schwartz HJ, Lehrer SB. Immunopathogenisis of fish allergy: identification of fish-allergic adults by skin test and radioallergosorbent test. Ann Allergy Asthma Immunol. 1996;77:48–54.
21. Ross MP, Ferguson M, Street D, Klontz K, Schroeder T, Luccioli S. Analysis of food-allergic and anaphylactic events in the National electronic injury surveillance system. J Allergy Clin Immunol. 2008;121:166–71.
22. Pumphrey RS, Gowland MH. Further fatal allergic reactions to food in the United Kingdom, 1999–2006. J Allergy Clin Immunol. 2007;119:1018–9.
23. Meyer R, Schwarz C, Shah N. A review on the diagnosis and management of food-induced gastrointestinal allergies. Curr Allergy Clin Immunol. 2012;25:1–8.
24. Katz Y, Goldberg MR, Rajuan N, Cohen A, Leshno M. The prevalence and natural course of food protein-induced enterocolitis syndrome to cow's milk: a large-scale, prospective population-based study. J Allergy Clin Immunol. 2011;127:647–53.
25. Spergel JM, Brown-Whitehorn TF, Beausoleil JL, Franciosi J, Shuker M, Verma R, et al. 14 years of eosinophilic esophagitis: clinical features and prognosis. J Pediatr Gastroenterol Nutr. 2009;48:30–6.
26. National Institute for Health and Clinical Excellence. Atopic Eczema in Children (CG57). www.nice.org.uk/guidance/CG57. 2007.
27. Werfel T, Ballmer-Weber B, Eigenmann PA, Niggemann B, Rancé F, Turjanmaa K, et al. Eczematous reactions to food in atopic eczema: position paper of the EAACI and GA2LEN. Allergy. 2007;62:723–8.
28. Straumann A, Aceves SS, Blanchard C, Collins MH, Furuta GT, Hirano I, et al. Pediatric and adult eosinophilic esophagitis: similarities and differences. Allergy. 2012;67:477–90.
29. Maintz L, Novak N. Histamine and histamine intolerance. Am J Clin Nutr. 2007;85:1185–96.
30. Vally H, Misso NL. Adverse reactions to the sulphite additives. Gastroenterol Hepatol Bed Bench. 2012;5:16–23.
31. Neri M, Laterza F, Howell S, Di Gioacchino M, Festi D, Ballone E, et al. Symptoms discriminate irritable bowel syndrome from organic gastrointestinal diseases and food allergy. Eur J Gastroenterol Hepatol. 2000;12:981–8.
32. Feuille E, Nowak-Węgrzyn A. Definition, etiology, and diagnosis of food protein-induced enterocolitis syndrome. Curr Opin Allergy Clin Immunol. 2014;14:222–8.
33. Romano A, Scala E, Rumi G, Gaeta F, Caruso C, Alonzi C. Lipid transfer proteins: the most frequent sensitizer in Italian subjects with food-dependent exercise-induced anaphylaxis. Clin Exp Allergy. 2012;42:1643–53.
34. Commins SP, James HR, Stevens W, Pochan SL, Land MH, King C, et al. Delayed clinical and ex vivo response to mammalian meat in patients with IgE to galactose-alpha-1,3-galactose. J Allergy Clin Immunol. 2014;134:108–15.
35. Raithel M, Weidenhiller M, Hagel AF, Hetterich U, Neurath MF, Konturek PC. The malabsorption of commonly occurring mono and disaccharides. Dtsch Arztebl Int. 2013;110:775–82.
36. Schäfer T, Böhler E, Ruhdorfer S, Weigl L, Wessner D, Heinrich J, et al. Epidemiology of food allergy/food intolerance in adults: associations with other manifestations of atopy. Allergy. 2001;56:1172–9.
37. Skypala IJ, Bull S, Deegan K, Gruffydd-Jones K, Holmes S, Small I, et al. The prevalence of pollen-food syndrome (PFS) and prevalence and characteristics of reported food allergy; a survey of UK adults aged 18–75 incorporating a validated PFS diagnostic questionnaire. Clin Exp Allergy. 2013;43:928–40.
38. Young E, Stoneham MD, Petuckevitch A, Barton J, Rana R. A population study of food intolerance. Lancet. 1994;343:1127–30.
39. Berns SH, Halm EA, Sampson HA, Sicherer SH, Busse PJ, Wisnivesky JP. Food allergy as a risk factor for asthma morbidity in adults. J Asthma. 2007;44:377–81.
40. Linneberg A, Gislum M, Johansen N, Husemoen LL, Jørgensen. Temporal trends of aeroallergen sensitization over twenty-five years. Clin Exp Allergy. 2007;37:1137–42.
41. Wüthrich B, Schmid-Grendelmeier P, Schindler C, Imboden M, Bircher A, Zemp E, et al. Prevalence of atopy and respiratory allergic diseases in the elderly SAPALDIA population. Int Arch Allergy Immunol. 2013;162:143–8.
42. Newson RB, van Ree R, Forsberg B, Janson C, Lötvall J, Dahlén SE, et al. Geographical variation in the prevalence of sensitization to common aeroallergens in adults: the GA(2) LEN survey. Allergy. 2014;69:643–51.
43. Wagner S, Breiteneder H. The latex-fruit syndrome. Biochem Soc Tans. 2002;30:935–40.
44. Boquete M, Iraola V, Morales M, Pinto H, Francisco C, Carballás C, et al. Seafood hypersensitivity in mite sensitized individuals: is tropomyosin the only responsible allergen? Ann Allergy Asthma Immunol. 2011;106:223–9.

45. Szépfalusi Z, Ebner C, Pandjaitan R, Orlicek F, Scheiner O, Boltz-Nitulescu G, et al. Egg yolk α-livetin (chicken serum albumin) is a cross-reactive allergen in the bird-egg syndrome. J Allergy Clin Immunol. 1994;93:932–42.
46. Hilger C, Kohnen M, Grigioni F, Lehners C, Hentges F. Allergic cross-reactions between cat and pig serum albumin. Study at the protein and DNA levels. Allergy. 1997;52:179–88.
47. Sánchez-Borges M, SuárezChacón R, Capriles-Hulett A, Caballero-Fonseca F, Fernández-Caldas E. Anaphylaxis from ingestion of mites: pancake anaphylaxis. J Allergy Clin Immunol. 2013;131:31–5.
48. Nieuwenhuizen N, Lopata AL, Jeebhay MF, Herbert De'B R, Robins TC, Brombacher F. Exposure to the fish parasite *Anisakis* causes allergic airway hyper reactivity and dermatitis. J Allergy Clin Immunol. 2006;117:1098–105.
49. Cardona V, Luengo O, Garriga T, Labrador-Horrillo M, Sala-Cunill A, Izquierdo A, et al. Co-factor-enhanced food allergy. Allergy. 2012;67:1316–8.
50. Shadick NA, Laing MH, Partridge AJ, Bingham C, Wright E, Fossel AH, et al. The natural history of food-dependant exercise-induced anaphylaxis: survey results from 10-year follow-up study. J Allergy Clin Immunol. 1999;104:123–7.
51. Romano A, Di Fonso M, Guiffreda F, Papa G, Artesani MC, Viola M. Food-dependent exercise-induced anaphylaxis: clinical and laboratory findings in 54 subjects. Int Arch Allergy Immunol. 2001;25:264–72.
52. Matsuo H, Dahlström J, Tanaka A, Kohno K, Takahashi H, Furumura M, et al. Sensitivity and specificity of recombinant x-5 gliadin-specific IgE measurement for the diagnosis of wheat-dependent exercise-induced anaphylaxis. Allergy. 2008;63:233–6.
53. Hompes S, Dölle S, Grünhagen J, Grabenhenrich L, Worm M. Elicitors and co-factors in food-induced anaphylaxis in adults. Clin Trans Allergy. 2013;3:38.
54. Asero R, Mistrello G, Roncarolo D, Amato S, van-Ree R. A case of allergy to beer showing cross-reactivity between lipid transfer proteins. Ann Allergy Asthma Immunol. 2001;87:65–7.
55. Kalogeromitros DC, Makris MP, Gregoriou SG, Mousatou VG, Lyris NG, Tarassi KE, et al. Grape anaphylaxis: a study of 11 adult onset cases. Allergy Asthma Proc. 2005;26:53–8.
56. Agarwal DP, Harada S, Goedde HW. Racial differences in biological sensitivity to ethanol: the role of alcohol dehydrogenase and aldehyde dehydrogenase isozymes. Alcohol Clin Exp Res. 1981;5:12–6.
57. du Toit G. Food-dependent exercise-induced anaphylaxis in childhood. Pediatr Allergy Immunol. 2007;18:455–63.
58. James JM, Crespo JF. Allergic reactions to foods by inhalation. Curr Allergy Asthma Rep. 2007;7:167–74.
59. Lehrer SB, Kim L, Rice T, Saidu J, Bell J, Martin R. Transfer of shrimp allergens to other foods through cooking oil. J Allergy Clin Immunol. 2007;119:S112.
60. Eriksson NE, Moller C, Werner S, Magnusson J, Bengtsson U. The hazards of kissing when you are food allergic. J Invest Allergol Clin mmunol. 2003;13:149–54.
61. Vetander M, Helander D, Flodström C, Ostblom E, Alfvén T, Ly DH, et al. Anaphylaxis and reactions to foods in children–a population-based case study of emergency department visits. Clin Exp Allergy. 2012;42:568–77.
62. Wood RA, Sicherer SH, Vickery BP, Jones SM, Liu AH, Fleischer DM, et al. The natural history of milk allergy in an observational cohort. J Allergy Clin Immunol. 2013;131:805–12.
63. Sicherer SH, Wood RA, Vickery BP, Jones SM, Liu AH, Fleischer DM, et al. The natural history of egg allergy in an observational cohort. J Allergy Clin Immunol. 2014;133:492–9.
64. Kotaniemi-Syrjanen A, Palosuo K, Jartti T, Kuitunen M, Pelkonen AS, Makela MJ. The prognosis of wheat hypersensitivity in children. Pediatr Allergy Immunol. 2010;21:e421–6.
65. Savage JH, Kaeding AJ, Matsui EC, Wood RA. The natural history of soy allergy. J Allergy Clin Immunol. 2010;125:683–6.
66. Mittag D, Veiths S, Vogel L, Becker W-M, Rhis H-P, Hebling A, et al. Soybean allergy in patients allergic to birch pollen: clinical investigation and molecular characterisation of allergens. J Allergy Clin Immunol. 2004;113:148–54.
67. Skolnick HS, Conover-Walker MK, Koerner CB, Sampson HA, Wesley Burks W, Wood RA. The natural history of peanut allergy. J Allergy Clin Immunol. 2001;107:367–74.
68. Fleischer D, Conover-Walker M, Matsui E, Wood R. The natural history of tree nut allergy. J Allergy Clin Immunol. 2005;116:1087–93.
69. Mullins RJ, Dear KB, Tang ML. Characteristics of childhood peanut allergy in the Australian capital territory, 1995 to 2007. J Allergy Clin Immunol. 2009;123:689–93.
70. Peeters KA, Koppelman SJ, Penninks AH, Lebens A, Bruijnzeel-Koomen CA, Hefle SL, et al. Clinical relevance of sensitization to lupine in peanut-sensitized adults. Allergy. 2009;64:549–55.
71. de Jong NW, van Maaren MS, Vlieg-Boersta BJ, Dubois AEJ, de Groot H, Gerth van Wijk R. Sensitization to lupine flour: is it clinically relevant? Clin Exp Allergy. 2010;40:1571–7.
72. Dalal I, Goldberg M, Katz Y. Sesame seed food allergy. Curr Allergy Asthma Rep. 2012;12:339–45.
73. Morisset M, Moneret-Vautrin D-A, Maadi F, Fremont S, Gunard L, Croizier A, et al. Prospective study of mustard allergy: first study with double-blind placebo-controlled food challenge trials (24 cases). Allergy. 2003;58:295–9.
74. Glaspole IN, de Leon MP, Prickett SR, O'Hehir RE, Rolland JM. Clinical allergy to hazelnut and peanut: identification of T cell cross-reactive allergens. Int Arch Allergy Immunol. 2011;155:345–54.
75. Maleki SJ, Teuber SS, Cheng H, Chen D, Comstock SS, Ruan S, et al. Computationally predicted IgE epitopes of walnut allergens contribute to cross-reactivity with peanuts. Allergy. 2011;66:1522–9.
76. Stutius LM, Sheehan WJ, Rangsithienchai P, Bharmanee A, Scott JE, Young MC, et al. Characterizing the relationship between sesame, coconut, and nut allergy in children. Pediatr Allergy Immunol. 2010;21:1114–8.
77. Barre A, Sordet C, Culerrier R, Rancé F, Didier A, Rougé P. Vicilin allergens of peanut and tree nuts (walnut, hazelnut and cashew nut) share structurally related IgE-binding epitopes. Mol Immunol. 2008;45:1231–40.
78. de Leon MP, Drew AC, Glaspole IN, Suphioglu C, O'Hehir RE, Rolland JM. IgE cross-reactivity between the major peanut allergen Ara h 2 and tree nut allergens. Mol Immunol. 2007;44:463–71.
79. Wallowitz ML, Chen RJ, Tzen JT, Teuber SS. Ses i 6, the sesame 11S globulin, can activate basophils and shows cross-reactivity with walnut in vitro. Clin Exp Allergy. 2007;37:929–38.
80. Turner P, Ng I, Kemp A, Campbell D. Seafood allergy in children: a descriptive study. Ann Allergy Asthma Immunol. 2011;106:494–501.
81. Sicherer SH, Munoz-Furlong A, Sampson HA. Prevalence of seafood allergy in the United States determined by a random telephone survey. J Allergy Clin Immunol. 2004;114:159–65.
82. Thong BY, Cheng YK, Leong KP, Tang CY, Chng HH. Anaphylaxis in adults referred to a clinical immunology/allergy centre in Singapore. Singapore Med J. 2005;46:529–34.
83. Sahabudin S, Misnan R, Yadzir ZH, Mohamad J, Abdullah N, Bakhtiar F, et al. Identification of major and minor allergens of black tiger prawn (Penaeus monodon) and King Prawn (Penaeus latisulcatus). Malays J Med Sci. 2011;18:27–32.
84. du Toit G, Santos A, Roberts G, Fox AT, Smith P, Lack G. The diagnosis of IgE-mediated food allergy in childhood. Pediatr Allergy Immunol. 2009;20:309–19.
85. Ortolani C, Ispano M, Pastorello E, Bigi A, Ansaloni R. The oral allergy syndrome. Ann Allergy. 1988;61:47–52.
86. Mortz CG, Andersen KE, Bindeslev-Jensen C. Prevalence of peanut sensitization and the association to pollen sensitization in a cohort of unselected adolescents – The Odense Adolescence Cohort Study on Atopic Diseases and Dermatitis (TOACS). Pediatr Allergy Immunol. 2005;16:501–6.
87. De Swert LF, Gadisseur R, Sjölander S, Raes M, Leus J, Van Hoeyveld E. Secondary soy allergy in children with birch pollen allergy may cause both chronic and acute symptoms. Pediatr Allergy Immunol. 2012;23:117–23.
88. Fernández-Rivas M, González-Mancebo E, Rodríguez-Pérez R, Benito C, Sánchez-Monge R, Salcedo G, et al. Clinically relevant peach allergy is related to peach lipid transfer protein, Pru p 3, in the Spanish population. J Allergy Clin Immunol. 2003;112:789–95.
89. Javaloyes G, Goikoetxea MJ, García Nuñez I, Aranda A, Sanz ML, Blanca M, et al. Pru p 3 acts as a strong sensitizer for peanut allergy in Spain. J Allergy Clin Immunol. 2012;130:1432–4.
90. Salcedo G, Sanchez-Monge R, Diaz-Perales A, Garcia-Casado G, Barber D. Plant non-specific lipid transfer proteins as food and pollen allergens. Clin Exp Allergy. 2004;34:1336–41.
91. Meyer R, Fleming C, Dominguez-Ortega G, Lindley K, Michaelis L, Thapar N, et al. Manifestation of gastrointestinal food allergies presenting to a single tertiary paediatric gastroenterology unit. World Allergy Organ J. 2013;6:13.
92. Heine RG. Pathophysiology, diagnosis and treatment of food protein-induced gastrointestinal diseases. Curr Opin Allergy Clin Immunol. 2004;4:221–9.

93. Leonard SA, Nowak-Wegrzyn A. Food protein-induced enterocolitis syndrome: an update on natural history and review of management. Ann Allergy Asthma Immunol. 2011;107:95–101.
94. Bohm M, Richter JE. Treatment of eosinophilic esophagitis: overview, current limitations, and future direction. Am J Gastroenterol. 2008;103:2635–44.
95. Spergel JM, Brown-Whitehorn TF, Cianferoni A, Shuker M, Wang ML, Verma R, et al. Identification of causative foods in children with eosinophilic esophagitis treated with an elimination diet. J Allergy Clin Immunol. 2012;130:461–7.
96. Lucendo AJ, Arias Á, González-Cervera J, Yagüe-Compadre JL, Guagnozzi D, Angueira T, et al. Empiric 6-food elimination diet induced and maintained prolonged remission in patients with adult eosinophilic esophagitis: a prospective study on the food cause of the disease. J Allergy Clin Immunol. 2013;131:797–804.
97. Monsbakken KW, Vandvik PO, Farup PG. Perceived food intolerance in subjects with irritable bowel syndrome – aetiology, prevalence and consequences. Eur J Clin Nutr. 2006;60:667–72.
98. Wuthrich B, Schmid A, Walther B, Seiber R. Milk consumption does not lead to mucus production or occurrence of asthma. J Am Coll Nutr. 2005;24:547S–55.
99. Hin H, Bird G, Fisher P, Mahy N, Jewell D. Coeliac disease in primary care: case finding study. BMJ. 1999;318:164–7.
100. Catassi C, Bai JC, Bonaz B, Bouma G, Calabrò A, Carroccio A, et al. Non-Celiac Gluten sensitivity: the new frontier of gluten related disorders. Nutrients. 2013;5:3839–53.
101. NICE Clinical Guideline. Irritable Bowel Syndrome in Adults: Diagnosis and Management Of Irritable Bowel Syndrome In Primary Care. 2008.
102. Gibson PR, Shepherd SJ. Evidence-based dietary management of functional gastrointestinal symptoms: the FODMAP approach. J Gastroenterol Hepatol. 2010;25:252–8.
103. Barrett JS, Irving PM, Shepherd SJ, Muir JG, Gibson PR. Comparison of the prevalence of fructose and lactose malabsorption across chronic intestinal disorders. Aliment Pharmacol Ther. 2009;30:165–74.
104. Di Lorenzo G, Pacor ML, Mansueto P, Martinelli N, Esposito-Pellitteri M, Lo Bianco C, et al. Food additive-induced urticaria: a survey of 838 patients with recurrent chronic idiopathic urticaria. Int Arch Allergy Immunol. 2005;138:235–42.
105. Mitchell J, Skypala I. Aspirin and salicylate in respiratory disease. Rhinology. 2013;51:195–205.
106. Nowak-Wegrzyn A, Bloom KA, Sicherer SH, Shreffler WG, Noone S, Wanich N, et al. Tolerance to extensively heated milk in children with cow's milk allergy. J Allergy Clin Immunol. 2008;122:342–7.
107. Lemon-Mule H, Sampson HA, Sicherer SH, Shreffler WG, Noone S, Nowak-Wegrzyn A. Immunologic changes in children with egg allergy ingesting extensively heated egg. J Allergy Clin Immunol. 2008;122:977–83.
108. Vlieg-Boerstra BJ, van der Heide S, Bijleveld CM, Kukler J, Duiverman EJ, Wolt-Plompen SA, et al. Dietary assessment in children adhering to a food allergen avoidance diet for allergy prevention. Eur J Clin Nutr. 2006;60:1384–90.
109. Groetch M, Nowak-Wegrzyn A. Practical approach to nutrition and dietary intervention in pediatric food allergy. Pediatr Allergy Immunol. 2013;24:212–21.
110. Flammarion S, Santos C, Guimber D, Jouannic L, Thumerelle C, Gottrand F, et al. Diet and nutritional status of children with food allergies. Pediatr Allergy Immunol. 2011;22:161–5.
111. Skypala I. Adverse food reactions–an emerging issue for adults. J Am Diet Assoc. 2011;111:1877–91.
112. Mofidi S. Nutritional management of pediatric food hypersensitivity. Pediatrics. 2003;111:1645–53.
113. Venter C, Laitinen K, Vlieg-Boerstra B. Nutritional aspects in diagnosis and management of food hypersensitivity-the dietitians role. J Allergy (Cairo). 2012;2012:269376.
114. Grimshaw KE, Maskell J, Oliver EM, Morris RC, Foote KD, Mills EN, et al. Diet and food allergy development during infancy: birth cohort study findings using prospective food diary data. J Allergy Clin Immunol. 2014;133:511–9.
115. Roduit C, Frei R, Depner M, Schaub B, Loss G, Genuneit J, et al. Increased food diversity in the first year of life is inversely associated with allergic diseases. J Allergy Clin Immunol. 2014;133:1056–64.
116. Meyer R, Venter C, Fox AT, Shah N. Practical dietary management of protein energy malnutrition in young children with cow's milk protein allergy. Pediatr Allergy Immunol. 2012;23:307–14.
117. Skypala I, Vlieg-Boerstra B. Food intolerance and allergy: increased incidence or contemporary inadequate diets? Curr Opin Clin Nutr Metab Care. 2014;17:442–7.
118. Venter C, Meyer R. Session 1: allergic disease: the challenges of managing food hypersensitivity. Proc Nutr Soc. 2010;69:11–24.
119. Hruz P. Epidemiology of eosinophilic esophagitis. Dig Dis. 2014;32:40–7.

12

Allergen immunotherapy for IgE-mediated food allergy

Sangeeta Dhami[1*], Ulugbek Nurmatov[2], Giovanni Battista Pajno[3], Montserrat Fernandez-Rivas[4], Antonella Muraro[5], Graham Roberts[6,7], Cezmi Akdis[8], Montserrat Alvaro-Lozano[9], Kirsten Beyer[10,11], Carsten Bindslev-Jensen[12], Wesley Burks[13], George du Toit[14], Motohiro Ebisawa[15], Philippe Eigenmann[16], Edward Knol[17,18], Mika Makela[19], Kari Christine Nadeau[20], Liam O'Mahony[21], Nikolaos Papadopoulos[22], Lars Poulsen[23], Cansin Sackesen[24], Hugh Sampson[25], Alexandra Santos[26], Ronald van Ree[27], Frans Timmermans[28] and Aziz Sheikh[29]

Abstract

Background: The European Academy of Allergy and Clinical Immunology (EAACI) is in the process of developing the EAACI Guidelines for Allergen Immunotherapy (AIT) for IgE-mediated food allergy. We seek to critically assess the effectiveness, cost-effectiveness and safety of AIT in IgE-mediated food allergy.

Methods: We will undertake a systematic review, which will involve searching international biomedical databases for published, in progress and unpublished evidence. Studies will be independently screened against pre-defined eligibility criteria and critically appraised using established instruments. Data will be descriptively and, if possible and appropriate, quantitatively synthesised.

Discussion: The findings from this review will be used to inform the development of recommendations for EAACI's Guidelines on AIT.

Keywords: Allergy, Allergen immunotherapy, Food allergy, Therapy, Sensitisation

Background

Food allergy is responsible for considerable morbidity and, in some cases, mortality [1]. Epidemiological studies have demonstrated that the prevalence and severity of food allergy may be increasing, particularly in children [2–5]. Food allergies can be divided into IgE-mediated acute allergic reactions manifesting as urticaria, vomiting, wheezing and anaphylaxis, and non-IgE-mediated food allergy which refers to delayed, cell-mediated reactions. This review is focused on IgE-mediated reactions.

Food allergies can be associated with significant reduction in quality of life, both of individuals who suffer from food allergy and their family members [6]. At present, avoidance measures are the cornerstone of management [7]. Difficulties in avoiding responsible food allergens can result in accidental exposure and the risk of triggering potentially life-threatening anaphylaxis [8]. Many individuals with food allergy therefore need to carry adrenaline (epinephrine) auto-injectors in order to self-manage anaphylaxis reactions. This approach is however perceived as restrictive and still leaves patients at risk if accidental exposure occurs.

Alternative approaches are therefore being investigated. In particular, there is considerable international interest in the role of immunotherapy, which involves repeated administration of very small, but gradually increasing doses of the antigens to which individuals are allergic in the hope of allowing safe exposure to the foods in question. Allergen immunotherapy (AIT) has,

*Correspondence: sangeetadhami@hotmail.com
[1] Evidence-Based Health Care Ltd, Edinburgh, UK
Full list of author information is available at the end of the article

for example, over the last century become established clinical practice in relation to the treatment of severe pollen, insect venom and drug allergy [9]. However AIT has yet to become established in the routine management of food allergy.

The European Academy of Allergy and Clinical Immunology (EAACI) is in the process of developing the EAACI Guidelines for AIT, and this systematic review is one of five inter-linked evidence syntheses that are being undertaken in order to provide a state-of-the-art synopsis of the current evidence base in relation to evaluating AIT for the treatment of food allergy, allergic rhinoconjunctivitis, venom allergy and allergic asthma, and allergy prevention, which will be used to inform the formulation of key clinical recommendations. The focus of this review, which builds on our previous related reviews [10, 11], is on assessing the effectiveness, safety and cost-effectiveness of AIT in the management of IgE-mediated food allergy.

Methods

Search strategy

A highly sensitive search strategy has been developed, and validated study design filters will be applied to retrieve articles pertaining to the use of AIT for IgE-mediated food allergy from electronic bibliographic databases. We have conceptualized the search to incorporate the four elements shown in Fig. 1.

To retrieve randomized controlled trials (RCTs), we will apply the Cochrane highly sensitive search strategy for identifying RCTs in MEDLINE [12]. To retrieve non-randomised studies, i.e. controlled clinical trials (CCT) and quasi-RCTs, we will use the Cochrane Effective Practice and Organisation of Care (EPOC) filter Version 2.4, available on request from the EPOC Group [13, 14]. To retrieve case series, we will use the filter developed by librarians at Clinical Evidence: http://clinicalevidence.bmj.com/x/set/static/ebm/learn/665076.html.

We will search the following databases:

- Cochrane Library including the:
  - CENTRAL (Trials)
  - Methods Studies
  - Health Technology Assessments (HTA)
  - Economic Evaluations Database (EED)

- MEDLINE (OVID)
- Embase (OVID)
- CINAHL (Ebscohost)
- ISI Web of Science (Thomson Web of Knowledge)
- TRIP Database (www.tripdatabase.com)
- Clinicaltrials.gov (NIH web).
- Current controlled trials (www.controlled-trials.com)
- Australian and New Zealand Clinical Trials Registry (http://www.anzctr.org.au)

The search strategy has been developed on OVID MEDLINE and then adapted for the other databases (see Additional file 1: Appendix). In all cases, the databases will be searched from inception to March 31, 2016. Additional references will be located through searching the references cited by the identified studies, and unpublished work and research in progress will be identified through discussion with experts in the field. We will invite experts who are active in the field from a range of disciplines and regions to add to the list of included

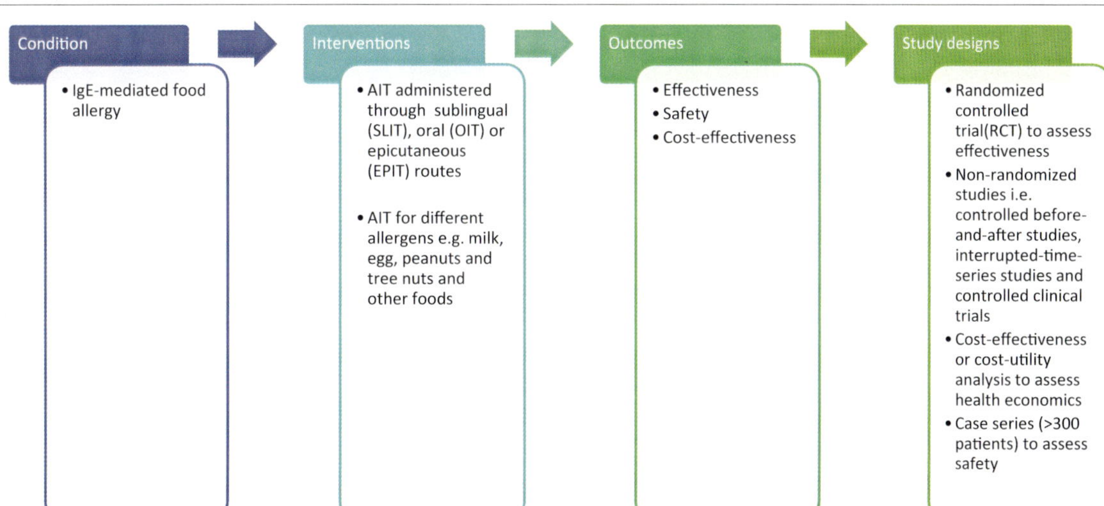

Fig. 1 Conceptualization of systematic review of allergen immunotherapy for IgE mediated food allergy

studies by identifying additional published and unpublished papers and grey literature they are aware of and research in progress. We also, will search Web of Science to find published conference papers and all three major clinical trials repositories [Clinicaltrials.gov (NIH web); Current controlled trials (www.controlled-trials.com); Australian and New Zealand Clinical Trials Registry (http://www.anzctr.org.au) to identify trials in progress]. There will be no language restrictions employed; where possible, relevant literature will be translated into English.

Inclusion criteria

Patient characteristics

We will focus on studies conducted on patients of any age with a physician confirmed diagnosis of IgE-mediated food allergy to milk, eggs, peanuts, tree nuts and other foods in which there is also confirmation of allergic status through positive skin prick tests, specific-IgE or food challenge tests.

Interventions of interest

This review is focused on AIT for different allergens, i.e. milk, eggs, tree nuts, peanuts and other foods, administered through the following routes: oral, sublingual and epicutaneous.

Comparators

We are interested in studies comparing food allergy AIT with placebo or routine care (i.e. adrenaline autoinjector with or without antihistamines) or no treatment.

Study designs

RCTs, will be used to investigate effectiveness (i.e. desensitization and tolerance) and impact on disease specific quality of life; health economic analysis will be used to assess cost-effectiveness; and RCTs and case series with a minimum of 300 patients will be used to assess safety. We will appraise the evidence by looking at higher levels of evidence such as individual RCTs. However, given the likelihood that we will find only a limited number of RCTs, we will also search for and include the following non-randomized studies (NRS): controlled before-and-after studies, interrupted-time-series studies and controlled clinical trials. Given the high inherent risk of bias in making inferences from such NRS, we will be very careful in making inferences from these data [15].

Study outcomes

- Primary Desensitization (i.e. the ability to safely consume foods containing the allergen in question while on AIT) or tolerance (the ability to consume foods containing the allergen in question after discontinuing AIT) at food challenge, as defined in the relevant studies.
- Assessment of changes in disease specific quality of life using a validated instrument; in making this assessment we will focus on the minimal clinically important difference change in quality of life [16].
- Secondary Safety as assessed by local and systemic reactions in accordance with the World Allergy Organization's grading system of side-effects [17, 18].
- Health economic analysis from the perspective of the health system/payer as reported in studies.

Exclusion criteria

The following exclusion criteria will be applied:

- Reviews, systematic reviews, discussion papers, non-research letters and editorials
- Animal studies
- Quantitative studies not employing systematic review or RCT, or employing NRS designs other than those detailed above
- Qualitative studies
- Case series (of <300 patients).

Study selection

All references will be uploaded into the systematic review software Distiller and undergo initial deduplication. Study titles and abstracts will be independently checked by two reviewers according to the above selection criteria and categorized as: included, not included or unsure. Calibration will be undertaken after the first 50 screens to review any discrepancies between reviewers. For those papers in the unsure category, we will retrieve the full-text and re-categorize as above. Any discrepancies will be resolved through discussion and, if necessary, a third reviewer will be consulted. Full text copies of potentially relevant studies will be obtained and their eligibility for inclusion independently assessed. Studies that do not fulfil all of the inclusion criteria will be excluded.

Quality assessment strategy

Quality assessments will independently be carried out on each study by two reviewers using the relevant quality assessment tools. Health economic studies will be assessed using the relevant CASP tool for economic evaluations [19]. RCTs, quasi-RCTs and CCTs will be assessed for generation of allocation sequence, concealment of allocation, baseline outcome measurements, baseline characteristics, incomplete outcome data, blinding of outcome assessor, protection against contamination, selective outcome reporting and other risks of bias. The Cochrane Risk of Bias tool will be used for RCTs and the Cochrane ACROBAT tool will be used for NRS

[12]. Similarly, we will use the quality assessment form produced by the National Institute for Health and Clinical Excellence (NICE) to critically appraise case series [20]. Any discrepancies will be resolved by discussion or, if agreement cannot be reached, a third reviewer will arbitrate

Data extraction, analysis and synthesis

Data will be independently extracted onto a customized data extraction sheet in Distiller by two reviewers, and any discrepancies will be resolved by discussion or, if agreement cannot be reached, by arbitration by a third reviewer.

A descriptive summary with summary data tables will be produced to summarize the literature. If clinically and statistically appropriate, meta-analysis will be undertaken using random-effects modeling given the known clinical heterogeneity between studies. In the event of finding significant statistical heterogeneity between studies (assessed using I^2), this will initially be visually inspected and then, if appropriate, be investigated through the pre-specified subgroup and sensitivity analyses (see below). We will preferentially report on RRs with 95 % CIs A narrative synthesis of the data will also be undertaken.

Sensitivity and subgroup analyses, and assessment for publication bias

Sensitivity analyses will be undertaken by comparing the findings between RCTs and NRS, and by comparing the results from studies that have employed double-blind placebo controlled food challenges versus those using other outcomes to assess for desensitization and/or tolerance.

Subgroup analyses will be undertaken to compare:

- Children (5–11 years) versus adolescents (12–17 years) versus adults (≥18 years)
- Treatment duration: <3 versus ≥3 years
- Years of follow up: end of treatment, 2 versus ≥2 years
- Route of administration: e.g. SCIT versus SLIT
- Allergens used for AIT
- Severity of food allergy: mild/moderate versus severe
- Primary versus secondary IgE-mediated food allergy.

Where possible, publication bias will be assessed through the creation of funnel plots, and tested by Egger's regression test and Begg's rank correlation test [21, 22].

Registration and reporting

This review will be registered with the International Prospective Register of Systematic Reviews (PROSPERO): http://www.crd.york.ac.uk/prospero/. The Preferred Reporting Items for Systematic Reviews and Meta-Analyses (PRISMA) checklist will be used to guide the reporting of the systematic review: http://www.prisma-statement.org/.

Discussion

This review will involve systematically identifying, critiquing and synthesizing the evidence on the effectiveness, cost-effectiveness and safety of AIT for the management of IgE mediated food allergy. It will build on earlier reviews in this area [10, 11]. The findings from this review will be used to inform the development of recommendations for EAACI's Guidelines on AIT. We anticipate that this review will report in 2016.

Authors' contributions

This protocol was drafted by SD and UN and the search strategy was developed by UN. It was revised following critical review by AS and then revised by all co-authors. All authors read and approved the final manuscript.

Author details

[1] Evidence-Based Health Care Ltd, Edinburgh, UK. [2] Division of Population Medicine Neuadd Meirionnydd, School of Medicine, Cardiff University, Heath Park, Cardiff, UK. [3] Allergy Unit, Department of Pediatric, University of Messina, Messina, Italy. [4] Allergy Department, Hospital Clínico San Carlos, IdISSC, Madrid, Spain. [5] Food Allergy Referral Centre Veneto Region, Department of Women and Child Health, Padua General University Hospital, Padua, Italy. [6] The David Hide Asthma and Allergy Research Centre, St Mary's Hospital, Newport Isle of Wight, NIHR Respiratory Biomedical Research Unit, University Hospital Southampton NHS Foundation Trust, Southampton, UK. [7] Faculty of Medicine, University of Southampton, Southampton, UK. [8] Swiss Institute for Allergy and Asthma Research, Davos, Switzerland. [9] Paediatric Allergy and Clinical Immunology Section, Hospital Sant Joan de Déu, Universitat de Barcelona, Barcelona, Spain. [10] Pediatric Pneumology and Immunology, Charité Universitätsmedizin, Berlin, Germany. [11] Icahn School of Medicine at Mount Sinai, New York, NY, USA. [12] Department of Dermatology and Allergy Centre, Odense University Hospital, Odense, Denmark. [13] Department of Pediatrics, School of Medicine, University of North Carolina at Chapel Hill, Chapel Hill, NC, USA. [14] Division of Asthma, Allergy and Lung Biology, Department of Paediatric Allergy, MRC and Asthma Centre in Allergic Mechanisms of Asthma, King's College London and St Thomas NHS Foundation Trust, London, UK. [15] Department of Allergy, Clinical Research Center for Allergy and Rheumatology, Sagamihara National Hospital, Sagamihara, Kanagawa, Japan. [16] University Hospitals of Geneva and Medical School, University of Geneva, Geneva, Switzerland. [17] Department of Dermatology and Allergology, University Medical Center Utrecht, Utrecht, The Netherlands. [18] Department of Immunology, University Medical Center Utrecht, Utrecht, The Netherlands. [19] Skin and Allergy Hospital, Helsinki University Hospital, Helsinki, Finland. [20] Division of Immunology, Allergy and Rheumatology, Department of Pediatrics, Stanford University, Stanford, CA, USA. [21] Swiss Institute of Allergy and Asthma Research (SIAF), University of Zurich, Davos, Switzerland. [22] Department of Allergy, 2nd Pediatric Clinic, University of Athens, Athens, Greece. [23] Allergy Clinic, Copenhagen University Hospital, Gentofte, Denmark. [24] Koç University Hospital, Istanbul, Turkey. [25] World Allergy Organization (WAO), Milwaukee, WI, USA. [26] Division of Asthma Allergy and Lung Biology, Department of Paediatric Allergy, King's College London/Guy's, and St Thomas' Hospital NHS Foundation Trust, London, UK. [27] Department of Otorhinolaryngology, Academic Medical Center, Amsterdam, The Netherlands. [28] Nederlands Anafylaxis Netwerk - European Anaphylaxis Taskforce, Dordrecht, The Netherlands. [29] Allergy and Respiratory Research Group, The University of Edinburgh, Edinburgh, UK.

Competing interests
S. Dhami: support to undertake the systematic review; U. Nurmatov: support to undertake the review; Giovanni Pajno: none; Montserrat Fernandez-Rivas: Participation in immunotherapy clinical trials sponsored by ALK-Abello; A. Muraro: Acting in consulting capacity for ALK, Meda Pharma, Nestle, Nutricia, Novartis. Grants from: Nestlé: Co-investigator for research protocol, Nutricia: Co-investigator for research protocols; G. Roberts: Materials for research programme (ALK-Abello), research grant (ALK-Abello), advisory board (ALK-Abello), speaker (Allergy Therapeutics, ALK-Abelo); C. Akdis: consulting fee Novartis, Boehringer-Ingelheim; stocks Davos Diagnostics, Allimentary Health Pharma Davos; research grant Novartis, Allergopharma; M. Alvaro-Lozano: none; K. Beyer: European Union, German Research Foundation,Berliner Sparkasse, Danone, ThermoFisher Diagnostics, Foundation for the Treatment of Peanut Allergy, author of A European perspective on immunotherapy for food allergies; C. Bindslev-Jensen: Grant from Hal Allergy. Consultancy for Hal Allergy; W Burks: none; G. du Toit: Equity in the FoodMaestro Application. Grants supporting the LEAP Study paid to Kings College, London. Author of the 2015 NEJM LEAP Study manuscripts that do not primarily deal with immunotherapy; M. Ebisawa: none; P. Eigenmann: Grants from LETI, Nestlé, ThermoFisher2, Consulting fee or honorarium from Danone, Novartis, ALK,DBV technologies, Stallergenes, Allergopharma; Edward Knol: Research grant for analysis modified peanut and cows milk allergens from HAL Allergy, Numico research. Consultancy fee from HAL Allergy, advice on peanut allergens; M. Makela: not known; K. Christine Nadeau: none; L. O'Mahony: Consultancy to Alimentary Health Ltd, a probiotic company; N. Papadopoulos: Grant from GSK, NESTLE, MERCK. Consulting fee from GSK, ABBVIE, Novartis, Menarini, Meda, AlK-ABELLO, Allergopharma, Uriach, Stallergenes. Payment for development of educational presentations for Abbvie, Sanofi, Menarini & Meda; L. Poulsen: Grants for Clinical trials in collaboration with ALK, Stallergenes, BioMay, and Anergis; C. Sackesen: Funding from MSD to support laboratory tests for the study 'Effects of the montelukast therapy on asthma and allergic inflammation in children with food allergy'; H. Sampson: received grants or other research support from NIAID; National Institutes of Health, published an editorial accompanying LEAP study publication; A. Santos: none; R. van Ree: Consultancy for HAL Allergy; F. Timmermans: none with respect to this study; A. Sheikh: support to co-ordinate the undertaking of the systematic review and development of the guidelines.

Funding
EAACI.

References

1. Bock SA, Munoz-Furlong A, Sampson HA. Further fatalities caused by anaphylactic reactions to food, 2001–2006. J Allergy Clin Immunol. 2007;119:1016–8.
2. Sicherer SH, Sampson HA. Peanut allergy: emerging concepts and approaches for an apparent epidemic. J Allergy Clin Immunol. 2007;120:491–503.
3. Nwaru BI, Hickstein L, Panesar SS, Muraro A, Werfel T, Cardona V, et al. The epidemiology of food allergy in Europe: a systematic review and meta-analysis. Allergy. 2014;69:62–75.
4. Kotz D, Simpson CR, Sheikh A. Incidence, prevalence, and trends of general practitioner-recorded diagnosis of peanut allergy in England, 2001 to 2005. J Allergy Clin Immunol. 2011;127(623–30):e1.
5. Nwaru BI, Hickstein L, Panesar SS, Roberts G, Muraro A, Sheikh A, on behalf of The EAACI Food Allergy & Anaphylaxis Guidelines Group. Prevalence of common food allergies in Europe: a systematic review and meta-analysis. Allergy. 2014;69:992–1007.
6. DunnGalvin A, Dubois AE, Flokstra-de Blok BM, Hourihane JO. The effects of food allergy on quality of life. Chem Immunol Allergy. 2015;101:235–52.
7. Muraro A, Werfel T, Hoffmann-Sommergruber K, Roberts G, Beyer K, Bindslev-Jensen C, et al. EAACI food allergy and anaphylaxis guidelines: diagnosis and management of food allergy. Allergy. 2014;69:1008–25.
8. Primeau MN, Kagan R, Joseph L, Lim H, Dufreshne C, Duffy C, et al. The psychological burden of peanut allergy as perceived by adults with peanut allergy and the parents of peanut allergic children. Clin Exp Allergy. 2000;30:1135–43.
9. Calderón MA, Boyle RJ, Penagos M, Sheikh A. Immunotherapy: the meta-analyses. What have we Learned? Immunol Allergy Clin N Am. 2011;31(2):159–73.
10. Nurmatov U, Devereux G, Worth A, Healy L, Sheikh A. Effectiveness and safety of orally administered immunotherapy for food allergies: a systematic review and meta-analysis. Br J Nutr. 2014;111:12–22.
11. Nurmatov U, Venderbosch I, Devereux G, Simons FE, Sheikh A. Allergen-specific oral immunotherapy for peanut allergy. Cochrane Database Syst Rev. 2012;9:CD009014.
12. Higgins JPT, Green S, editors. Cochrane handbook for systematic reviews of interventions. Version 5.1.0 [updated March 2011]. The Cochrane Collaboration, 2011. www.cochrane-handbook.org. Accessed on 3 Sept 2015.
13. EPOC Group. http://epoc.cochrane.org/literature-searching-systematic-reviews.
14. Cochrane Effective Practice & Organisation of Care (EPOC) Group: Personal communication Michelle Fiander, Information Specialist & Trial Search Co-ordinator. Ottawa, Canada: EPOC; 2012.
15. Effective Practice and Organisation of Care Group. What study designs should be included in an EPOC review and what should they be called. http://epoc.cochrane.org/sites/epoc.cochrane.org/files/uploads/EPOC%20Study%20Designs%20About.pdf. Accessed on 9 Dec 2015.
16. Salvilla SA, Dubois AE, Flokstra-de Blok BM, Panesar SS, Worth A, Patel S, et al. Disease-specific health-related quality of life instruments for IgE-mediated food allergy. Allergy. 2014;69(7):834–44.
17. Passalacqua G,Baena-Cagnani C, Bousquet J, Walter Canonica G, Casalet T, Cox L, Durham S, Larenas-Linnemann D, Ledford D, Pawankar R, Potter P, Rosario N, Wallace D, Lockey R. Grading local side effects of sublingual immunotherapy for respiratory allergy: Speaking the same language J Allergy Clin Immunol; 2013. http://www.jacionline.org/article/S0091-6749(13)00528-9/pdf.
18. World Allergy Organization Subcutaneous Immunotherapy Systemic Reaction Grading System. https://www.aaaai.org/Aaaai/media/MediaLibrary/PDF%20Documents/Immunotherapy%20Forms/7b-World-Allergy-Organization-Systemic-Reaction-Grading-systemx.pdf.
19. CASP checklist for Economic evaluations. http://media.wix.com/ugd/dded87_3b2bd5743feb4b1aaac6ebdd68771d3f.pdf. Last Accessed on 3 Sept 2015.
20. Higgins JPT, Green S. Cochrane handbook for systematic reviews of interventions. Version 5.0.2 (Chapter 11, Section 11).
21. Egger M, Davey Smith G, Schneider M, et al. Bias in meta-analysis detected by a simple, graphical test. BMJ. 1997;315:629–34.
22. Begg CB, Mazumdar M. Operating characteristics of a rank correlation test for publication bias. Biometrics. 1994;50:1088–101.

13

Sensitivity to food additives, vaso-active amines and salicylates: a review of the evidence

Isabel J. Skypala[1*], M. Williams[2], L. Reeves[3], R. Meyer[4] and C. Venter[5]

Abstract

Although there is considerable literature pertaining to IgE and non IgE-mediated food allergy, there is a paucity of information on non-immune mediated reactions to foods, other than metabolic disorders such as lactose intolerance. Food additives and naturally occurring 'food chemicals' have long been reported as having the potential to provoke symptoms in those who are more sensitive to their effects. Diets low in 'food chemicals' gained prominence in the 1970s and 1980s, and their popularity remains, although the evidence of their efficacy is very limited. This review focuses on the available evidence for the role and likely adverse effects of both added and natural 'food chemicals' including benzoate, sulphite, monosodium glutamate, vaso-active or biogenic amines and salicylate. Studies assessing the efficacy of the restriction of these substances in the diet have mainly been undertaken in adults, but the paper will also touch on the use of such diets in children. The difficulty of reviewing the available evidence is that few of the studies have been controlled and, for many, considerable time has elapsed since their publication. Meanwhile dietary patterns and habits have changed hugely in the interim, so the conclusions may not be relevant for our current dietary norms. The conclusion of the review is that there may be some benefit in the removal of an additive or a group of foods high in natural food chemicals from the diet for a limited period for certain individuals, providing the diagnostic pathway is followed and the foods are reintroduced back into the diet to assess for the efficacy of removal. However diets involving the removal of multiple additives and food chemicals have the very great potential to lead to nutritional deficiency especially in the paediatric population. Any dietary intervention, whether for the purposes of diagnosis or management of food allergy or food intolerance, should be adapted to the individual's dietary habits and a suitably trained dietitian should ensure nutritional needs are met. Ultimately a healthy diet should be the aim for all patients presenting in the allergy clinic.

Keywords: Food, Additives, Allergy, Histamine, Salicylate

Background

The recent food allergy guidelines from the European Academy of Allergy and Clinical Immunology give clear advice on how to diagnose an immune-mediated food allergy [1]. However, non-immune mediated reactions to foods are not addressed. Food additives and naturally occurring 'food chemicals' are attributed by many patients as the cause of their symptoms. Studies have assessed the potential for food additives and food chemicals to cause adverse symptoms, but robust research is difficult to conduct due to a number of factors: performing double blind placebo controlled challenges using foods or varying dosages of individual additives, setting inclusion criteria, standardizing the outcome and ruling out potential co- factors. Also the mechanisms involved have been poorly studied; although some preliminary data indicates the possible role of IgE involvement, many other mechanisms have also been proposed [2].

A vast range of adverse reactions have been attributed to the consumption of these added or natural 'food chemicals'. The most frequent clinical features are chronic urticaria or angioedema [3], but symptoms can also include atopic eczema, [4] flushing, hypotension, abdominal pain, diarrhoea and asthmatic reactions, and occasionally severe or anaphylactoid or severe (anaphylactic) reactions

*Correspondence: i.skypala@rbht.nhs.uk
[1] Royal Brompton and Harefield NHS Foundation Trust, Sydney Street, London SW3 6NP, UK
Full list of author information is available at the end of the article

[5, 6]. Due to the difficulty in diagnosing these conditions, the true prevalence of adverse reactions caused by food chemicals is unknown. A recent cross-sectional study from Japan estimated that the prevalence of chemical intolerances was 7.5 %, with fatigue, depressed mood and somatic symptoms positively correlated with a diagnosis of the condition [7]. Some groups appear to be at higher risk for example steroid-dependent asthmatics, those with marked airway hyper-responsiveness, and those with chronic asthma appear to be at greater risk of sulphite sensitivity [6]. Such prevalence data is even harder to come by in the paediatric population, where adverse reactions to food chemicals are poorly studied.

The range of the additives and natural substances potentially involved in non-immune mediated reactions in both children and adults makes it very difficult to undertake a systematic review of the literature. The following review provides an overview of the prevalence and foods thought to be involved in sensitivity to food additives, vaso-active amines and salicylates adults. It also considers separately the evidence for the dietary exclusion of these substances in the paediatric population.

Food additives

Sulphites

Sulphur dioxide has long been regarded as an air pollutant, but sensitivity to sulphites in foods was first described in 1973 (Kochen). Sulphites, readily metabolised to sulphate (SO_4) by sulphite oxidase [8] mainly occur in the human diet due to the addition of sodium/potassium sulphite/metabisulphite to foods to prevent enzymatic and non-enzymatic browning, control oxidation and prevent bacterial growth. Sulphites added to foods will be present either as a free form mix of sulphur dioxide, bisulphite and sulphite, or bound to carbohydrates or proteins [9]. A plethora of reports in the 1980s demonstrated that sulphites in foods were provoking adverse reactions; by 1984 the US Food and Drug Administration had received more than 250 reports of suspected sulphite reactions including six deaths [10]. Thus both the European Union and the US Food and Drug Administration have regulated the use of sulphites, requiring foods containing more than 10 ppm (10 mg/kg) to be labelled, but there is significant variation between levels for the same foods [11–15]. Foods containing a high level of free form sulphite are more likely to provoke a reaction and this dictates how much sulphite can be added [16]. Foods usually containing significant levels of added sulphite include cider, white wine, and dried fruits—see Table 1 [5, 17, 118].

Sensitivity to sulphites mainly affects patients with asthma, especially those with severe steroid-dependant asthma. Bush and colleagues undertook single-blind challenges with encapsulated sodium metabisulphite in 203 asthmatic subjects and reported a prevalence of 3.9 % in asthmatic patients, with those who were steroid dependant being most at risk [18]. Buckley et al., using similar methodology, found a similar prevalence of 4.6 % in a large cohort of asthmatic patients [19]. A recent review by Vally and Misso suggested that 3–10 % of asthmatics experience symptoms on exposure to ingested sulphites [5]. An analysis of sulphite-sensitive cases in Korea found that two phenotypes of sulphite sensitivity existed, those with sulphite sensitive asthma was the most common, affecting two-thirds of their cohort, with the remainder having sulphite-sensitive urticaria [20]. Sulphites can cause urticaria and angio-oedema both through topical application of sulphite containing cosmetics or skin reactions following oral ingestion of sulphite [5]. Other reactions are less common but include anaphylaxis [6] and rhinitis [21].

It is postulated that the inhalation of sulphur dioxide, generated from ingested sulphites may cause respiratory symptoms [6, 22]. Other mechanisms suggested include IgE-mediated reactions [6, 23, 24], a deficiency of sulphite oxidase [25], and a role for leukotrienes [26]. Due to the unpredictability of the level of available sulphite in different foods, and because sulphite sensitive individuals will not all respond in the same way to sulphite-containing foods, few trials have used foods when evaluating sulphite sensitivity [27]. Taylor and colleagues undertook double-blind, placebo-controlled food challenges (DBPCFC) with foods known to be high in sulphites (lettuce, dehydrated potato, shrimp, dried apricots, white grape juice) in eight subjects whose sulphite sensitivity was established through the use of DBPCFC with encapsulated potassium metabisulphite [28]. Four patients failed to respond to any of the challenges, four responded to sulphited lettuce and there was a varying degree of response to the other foods. Using DBPCFC Vally and Thompson found only 16 % of wine sensitive asthmatics responded to sulphite additives in wine [29].

Benzoates

Benzoic acid is produced by many plants and has also been detected in animals, so is present in many foods, including berries and milk products, usually in relatively low concentrations of up to 40 mg/kg [30–32]. Benzoate can also be a product of digestion, e.g. cinnamic acid from cinnamon is oxidised to a benzoate salt in the liver [33]. Benzoates are also added in much higher concentrations to soft drinks, jams, sweets, chocolates, ice creams, pickles, baked goods due to their antimicrobial properties—see Table 1 [34, 35].

Benzoates have been linked to chronic urticaria, asthma, atopic dermatitis, rhinitis and anaphylaxis

Table 1 Foods more likely to contain high levels of natural or added sulphites, benzoates and monosodium glutamate

	Sulphites (E220–E227) [11, 17, 118, 119]	Benzoates (E210–E219) [30, 31, 33, 119, 120]	Monosodium glutamate (E621–E623, E627, E635) [49, 121]
Meat, poultry and seafood	Prawns, lobster, dried salt cod, crab sticks, squid, meat burger, sausages	Dishes with a spicy sauce, ready to eat meals containing benzoates	Fish sauce
Milk and eggs		Yoghurt, cheese	Parmesan cheese
Fruits	Dried apricots, sultanas, figs, prunes, dates, dried banana, candied or glace fruit desiccated coconut, currants	Cranberries, bilberries, prunes, papaya, dried fruit, avocado	
Vegetables, nuts, seeds and savoury snacks	Dried mushrooms and other fungi, frozen, tinned or vacuum packed potatoes, French fries, instant mash, gnocchi, potato cakes, potato croquettes, vegetarian burgers and sausages, tinned asparagus, broad beans, French beans, chestnuts, walnuts	Pumpkin, kidney beans, soy beans, soy flour, broccoli, spinach, baked beans in tomato/spicy sauce, dry roasted and spicy nuts, Bombay mix, crisps (except ready salted), potato or corn snacks,	Mushrooms, spinach, savoury snacks, crisps
Condiments and miscellaneous	Horseradish sauce, caramel colouring (E150)	Curry powder, allspice, mixed spice, nutmeg, clove, cinnamon, chocolate, cocoa, ketchup, soy sauce, Worcestershire sauce, salad dressing, salad cream, mayonnaise, jam, pickles	Soups, stock, gravy, rubs, coatings, ready-meals, soy sauce, black bean sauce, oyster sauce, tomato sauce, miso, marmite, instant rice and noodle dishes
Drinks	Cider, wine, beer, fruit squash and cordials, soft drinks, grape juice, fruit juice drinks, cola drinks	Tea, squash, cordial, carbonated drinks, milkshake syrup, beer, ready-to-drink alcohol and mixers, spirits with added spices	

Foods with added sulphite, benzoates and MSG will vary from country to country although there is limited good quality evidence to support these findings. Wuthrich et al. proposed that benzoates may be involved via a type IV sensitisation causing allergic contact dermatitis [36] and Van Bever et al. used DBPCFC to show that benzoates may cause atopic dermatitis [37]. Worm et al. also undertook DBPCFC to show a late phase response in atopic dermatitis, but the capsules used contained a mixture of additives including benzoates rather than benzoates alone [38]. In a more recent study using a DBPCFC to a mixture of food additives including benzoates, Park et al. showed they had no effect on atopic dermatitis [39].

In another study, Weber et al. hypothesised that benzoates could exacerbate asthma, however in the DBPCFC study, only 1/43 subjects had a positive result, with individual testing negative on re-challenge 2 years later [40]. In 1981 Tarlo et al. found only 1/28 subjects with chronic asthma reacted to benzoates, but did not respond symptomatically to a benzoate-free diet [41]. Persistent rhinitis has also been linked to consumption of benzoates; Pacor et al. showed that 8.8 % (20 subjects) reacted to a DBPCFC challenge to monosodium benzoate. The subjects with a positive challenge had previously reported an improvement in symptoms within in 1 month of using an additive free diet and a return in rhinitis symptoms with the adoption of a food additive rich diet [42].

Only two robust studies have assessed the link between chronic urticaria and benzoates using blinded placebo controlled trials. Ortolani et al. reported that 3/72 (4 %) patients reacted to benzoates [43], but Simon et al. found no positive reactions in their study [44]. Several studies using dietary elimination in chronic urticaria showed positive outcomes to benzoates, but they had either no clear outcome measures, lack of blinding and/or no placebo [45–47]. Rajan and colleagues showed that although 2/100 patients had a positive response to single-blinded challenges with the individual additives including sodium benzoate, neither responded to DBPCFC [48]. They concluded that food and drug additives were a rare cause of chronic urticaria and that avoidance should not be recommended. It is unclear why these studies offer contradictory evidence and also whether natural benzoate is also likely to provoke adverse reactions in the same way that added benzoate might.

Monosodium glutamate

Monosodium glutamate (MSG—E621) is a common added ingredient to savoury foods. Glutamate also occurs naturally in other foods, with ripening of fruits such as tomatoes and the curing of meat such as ham, being associated with an increase in the free amino acids such as glutamate [49]—see Table 1. The L-glutamate derived from dried kelp or seaweed, was originally used to make MSG prior to synthetic derivatives being developed [50]. Originally described as 'Chinese Restaurant Syndrome' in 1968 [51], results from studies utilising DBPCFC have suggested some individuals could experience symptoms from the ingestion of MSG, although only in quantities greater than the normal dietary intake [50, 52]. Other studies have found MSG does not provoke any symptoms [53]. Geha et al. conducted a DBPC crossover study on 130 subjects with reported MSG sensitivity; 2/130 responded to a large dose given without food, with no responses noted when MSG was given with food [54]. Although the glutamate in MSG is chemically indistinguishable from glutamate present in food proteins and is metabolized in the same way [55], it is currently unknown whether foods high in natural bound or free form glutamate can cause the same symptoms as MSG.

This additive has been linked to asthma, headache, urticaria and angioedema, rhinitis, psychiatric disorders and convulsions [56, 57]. A link with asthma was first noted by Allen and Baker [58] although subsequent studies have shown mixed outcomes. Schwartzstein et al. reported that DBPC with MSG were negative in 12 subjects with asthma [59]. Similarly, Woods et al. reported no changes in forced expired volume in one second (FEV1) values and no immediate or late asthmatic reactions in their cohort of 12 subjects [60]. Germano et al. found 1/30 participants experienced a significant reduction in FEV1 during single blind provocation, but this was not reproducible during DBPC challenges [61].

Persistent rhinitis linked to MSG has been demonstrated in DBPC challenges by Asero, but only in a handful of subjects [62]. Pacor et al. found 8/226 non-atopic subjects exhibiting subjective symptoms of rhinitis after a DBPC MSG challenge, and concluded that reactions to additives could precipitate rhinitis in some patients [42]. Case reports have linked MSG to urticaria [21], but Simon et al. showed only 2/65 subjects had a positive response in single blinded challenge, neither of whom were positive to a DBPC challenge [44].

Headache has been the most commonly reported symptom in relation to MSG [63] Yang et al. undertook DBPCFC in 61 subjects with self-reported sensitivity to MSG; 18/61 had no response, 21/61 had a placebo response and 22/61 a positive response to the active challenge only. On re-challenge a threshold dose of 2.5 g MSG was established [64]. Baad-Hansen et al. conducted a DBPCFC in 14 healthy individuals and reported a significant increase in reported headache and pericranial muscle tenderness after taking an individually tailored dose of MSG (150 mg/kg) [65]. However, despite these studies, an authoritative view is that the weight of the literature does not presently support the use of an MSG free diet for patients with chronic headaches [50].

Naturally occurring 'food chemicals'

Biogenic/vasoactive amines

Biogenic or vasoactive amines are produced by bacteria during fermentation, storage or decay [6, 66–68]. They include beta-phenylethylamine, tyramine, tryptamine, putrescine, cadaverine, spermine and spermidine, but histamine is the one most frequently linked to food-related symptoms. When plasma histamine levels are raised above the normal range (0.3–1.0 ng/mL) this produces certain effects. For example a level of 1–2 ng/mL causes increased gastric acid secretion and heart rate, with, flushing, headache, urticaria, pruritus and tachycardia occurring at a level of 3–5 ng/mL), bronchospasm at a level of 7–12 ng/mL and cardiac arrest occurring at levels of 100 ng/mL [6]. Thus large amounts of ingested histamine can cause significant symptoms in otherwise well individuals. For example symptoms of flushing, sweating, urticaria, GI symptoms, palpitations and in severe cases bronchospasm may occur following the consumption of spoiled fish [69]. This condition, known as scombroid poisoning, occurs due to the high level of histidine in certain fish species being converted into histamine by marine bacteria [70]. Due to the nature of the symptoms caused, reactions involving vasoactive amines may therefore be incorrectly diagnosed as a food allergy.

Although 75 mg of liquid histamine can provoke symptoms in healthy volunteers [71], defining a safe threshold level for sensitive individuals is difficult [72]. Foods generally considered to contain high levels of vaso-active amines are shown in Table 2, however the amounts of histamine found in different foods varies according to the type of bacteria, food composition and conditions for fermentation [73]. Bodmer et al. found that mean levels of histamine were 3.63 mg/L for French wines, 2.19 mg/L for Italian wines and 5.02 mg/L for Spanish wines [68]. Symptoms to wine may not always be a reliable indicator of sensitivity to histamine. In a placebo-controlled study, Kanny et al. found no correlation between wine histamine content and wine intolerance, and concluded that other vaso-active amines or sulphites may be more relevant in intolerance to wine [74]. It has been proposed that other foods may be able to cause histamine release directly from tissue mast cells [6] although evidence for this is lacking [75].

Wantke et al. found a diet low in vasoactive amines alleviated chronic headache in 73 % of patients [76]. Another study reported that 27/44 (61 %) of subjects had a significant improvement in idiopathic urticaria, angiooedema and pruritus on a diet low in dietary amines, although foods containing additives or high in natural salicylate were also restricted [72]. King and colleagues reported subjects with chronic urticaria/angioedema had a marginally significant reduction in their use of antihistamines on a histamine-reducing diet compared to a control group who eliminated artificial sweeteners from their diet. However response to the diet varied and the numbers in each group were very low [77]. Another study found that 58 % of adult patients with irritable bowel syndrome (IBS) considered foods rich in vasoactive amines, such as wine, beer, salami and cheese, to be a cause of their symptoms [78].

The diagnosis of sensitivity to vasoactive amines is usually made through history and dietary exclusion; however some studies have suggested that the measurement of diamine oxidase (DAO) levels may be helpful. One study found a DAO level <3 kU/mL was associated with reported symptoms to high histamine foods, whereas a level of >10 kU/mL indicated histamine intolerance was unlikely [6]. Patients with chronic idiopathic urticaria and GI symptoms have been shown to have reduced DAO activity [79, 80]. Another study reported that the size of the skin prick test wheal to histamine after 50 min, the 'histamine 50-skin-prick test', was a useful diagnostic indicator; 82 % of subjects with histamine intolerance maintained a wheal size greater than 3 mm compared with 18 % of controls [81].

Salicylates

Salicylate intolerance has been defined as 'a nonspecific antigen-induced pseudo-allergic hypersensitivity reaction to salicylic acid, its derivatives or other related organic or inorganic acids of similar chemical structure' [82]. Salicylic acid is widely distributed in plant foods and, like its synthetic counterpart acetyl salicylate (Aspirin™) has anti-inflammatory activity. Acetyl salicylate is a potent inhibitor of COX-1, an isoform of the enzyme cyclooxygenase (COX), which prevents the conversion of arachidonic acid to cyclic prostanoids, whereas salicylic acid inhibits COX-2 gene expression [83, 84]. A diet rich in spices, which contain high levels of in salicylic acid, has been linked to lower levels of colorectal cancer in rural inhabitants of Southern India [85], although caution has been advised with regard to an over-emphasis on the importance of dietary salicylates compared with other bioactive plant phenolics in the diet [86].

The reported level of salicylates in different foods is highly variable between studies. Swain et al. published the salicylate content of 333 foods [87] and these data continue to underpin dietary salicylate avoidance advice. Subsequent studies have reported different results for the same foods [88–90], possibly due to diverse analytical methods and the origin, processing and storage of the foods tested [91–93]. Table 2 gives a list of high salicylate foods based on all of the published data. There is also uncertainty regarding the bioavailability of dietary salicylate; Jansen et al. reported that urinary salicylate

Table 2 Foods more likely to contain high levels of vaso-active amines and salicylate

	Vaso-active amines [6, 75, 122–126]	Salicylate [85, 87–90, 97]
Meat, poultry and seafood	All cured meat especially pork products e.g. ham, salami, pepperoni, game, bacon, sausages, fresh pork, fresh or canned tuna, canned sardines, anchovies, mackerel, salmon, herring, processed fish products (fish pastes, smoked, dried or pickled fish), fish sauce	
Milk and eggs	Blue cheese, parmesan, brie, camembert, emmenthal, old gouda, cheddar cheese and other hard cheeses	
Fruits	Oranges, bananas, tangerines, pineapple, grapes, strawberries	Granny smith apples, cherries, strawberries, currants, raisins, kiwi, Gala melon, peaches and nectarines, raspberries
Vegetables, nuts, seeds and savoury snacks	Tomatoes, pickled cabbage, aubergine, spinach, broad beans, peanuts, tree nuts	Asparagus, sweet corn, raw tomatoes, tomato puree
Condiments and miscellaneous	Fermented soy products including miso and tempeh	Ginger, mixed herbs, mustard, oregano, curry powder, black pepper, cardamom pods, cinnamon, cumin, fenugreek, mint, nutmeg, paprika, rosemary, thyme, turmeric, liquorice, peppermint, Worcestershire sauce, honey, tomato ketchup
Drinks	Green tea, champagne, coffee, cocoa, chocolate, wine, beer, fresh fruit juices, smoothies	Coffee, pineapple juice, cider, Benedictine liqueur, lemon tea, black tea, apple juice, cranberry juice, orange juice, tomato juice, fizzy drinks, Drambui liqueur, wine, rum

excretion showed that the bioavailability of dietary salicylate in most people is low [94], whereas Lawrence and colleagues showed bioavailability to be high [95]. Curry spices, universally agreed as being high in natural salicylate, not only have a high bioavailability, they also inhibit both COX-1 and COX-2, which may indicate they could be a more important dietary factor than other high salicylate foods [85].

Baenkler has proposed that 2.5 % of Europeans may have salicylate sensitivity [96], but the evidence on which this assertion is based is sparse. Aspirin exacerbated respiratory disease (AERD), an inflammatory disease exacerbated by aspirin or other non-steroidal anti-inflammatory drugs (NSAIDS), usually presents in adult life, and affects up to 20 % of asthmatic subjects and 40 % of those with nasal polyps [97]. It has been shown that AERD subjects have down regulation of COX-2 expression in nasal polyps [98]' so it could be hypothesised that such individuals might be more likely to be affected by dietary salicylate but there is conflicting evidence. Corder and Buckley reported that a challenge with salicylic acid had a significant effect on the lung function, whereas Dahlen et al. found no such reactions [99, 100].

Salicylate intolerance has also been proposed as a cause of other conditions; Raithel et al. proposed that 2–7 % of all patients with inflammatory bowel syndrome and food allergies could be affected by salicylate intolerance [82]. Gibson and Barrett suggest that since there are no published studies demonstrating efficacy of salicylate avoidance in gut disease, they recommend the dietary restriction of fermentable oligosaccharides, disaccharides, monosaccharides and polyols (FODMAPs™) as first line therapy for the majority of patients with functional bowel symptoms [101, 102].

Chemical diets in children

Evidence for the efficacy of diets free from individual additives or high levels of natural food chemicals in children is sparse. There is a lack of convincing published data on the effect of the avoidance of food additives, although Supramaniam et al. demonstrated that 3/36 (10 %) children exhibited urticaria or angioedema in response to MSG [103], and avoidance of MSG was helpful in the management of 86 % of children aged 2–16 years with cyclical vomiting syndrome (a variant of migraine in children) [104]. A study on benzoates reported that 3/25 children reacted to sodium benzoate, but the reaction criteria were unclear and no reactions occurred during placebo challenges [37]. More rigorous studies concluded sodium benzoate or artificial colours (or both) in the diet may result in increased hyperactivity in young children [105], although genetic variants associated with the breakdown and clearance of histamine were found to moderate the impact of additives on behaviour [106].

Studies on sulphite intolerance in asthmatic children also appear to demonstrate some degree of effect. Sanz et al. [107] found that 4/20 children with asthma (7–14 years of age) had a positive reaction on double-blind challenge to sodium metabisulphite solution. However, in a subsequent study performed on 5 children with challenge confirmed sulphite intolerance; with a dose of 1.5 mg of oral cyanocobalamin followed by a repeated sodium metabisulphite challenge only resulted in bronchospasm in 1/5 of the children. [108]. There is also limited evidence for the efficacy of diets low in natural food chemicals. In 2013, Hoffmann et al. [109] reported that 14/394 children who presented with gastrointestinal discomfort, had both low levels of DAO and subsequently improved on a diet excluding foods high in histamine. However, the improvement was subjective, being based on a non-validated questionnaire and the dietary exclusion was not blinded. Another study has also shown that a low histamine or histamine-free diet improves symptoms in children with DAO levels <10 kU/mL, but only subjective symptoms were noted [110]. An extensive literature review yielded no prospective randomised controlled studies establishing the link between hypersensitivity reactions in children and salicylates.

Despite this lack of evidence, there has been a rise in the use of low chemical diets for children for a variety of conditions, in particular for atopic dermatitis, gastrointestinal symptoms and hyperactivity [111]. These diets typically remove foods high in salicylates, histamine, sulphites and MSG from the diet and may be used in conjunction with the dietary elimination of milk, soy, egg and wheat. A retrospective case review by Gray et al. found that almost half of a group of 74 children placed on a diet that eliminated foods naturally high in salicylates suffered adverse outcomes, including nutritional deficiencies, food aversion and eating disorders [112]. Growth velocity is highest within the first years of life and a failure to achieve this potential has a far reaching impact on development and later health [113, 114]. Many of the foods that contain both additives and naturally occurring food chemicals which are listed in Tables 1 and 2, contribute essential nutrients for growth and development. In addition, a lack of taste exposure during early infancy has been shown to lead to feeding difficulties in later life [115]. Therefore unwarranted dietary eliminations of these chemicals should be avoided in young children unless there is exceptional evidence as to their efficacy.

Conclusion

The lack of well-designed placebo-controlled studies investigating the role of many of these substances makes it impossible to provide evidence-based advice for the efficacy of the removal of food additives, histamine and salicylates from the diet. No convincing data exists on the impact of food chemicals on atopic disorders in children, and in light of the importance of growth and development, these diets should be approached with caution in the paediatric population. For adults, the nutritional aspects might appear to be less of an issue, but significant dietary restrictions can affect nutritional status at any age [116]. Thus, the risk–benefit ratio should be considered when contemplating the dietary exclusion of multiple foods, particularly those foods which may confer some health benefit such as foods high in natural salicylates. The literature suggests that the removal of high histamine foods or those containing high levels of sulphites may provide some symptom relief. There is far less evidence on the beneficial effect of restricting other additives in the diet and no published evidence at all for the efficacy of low salicylate diets.

Studies which utilise DBPCFC have rarely shown food additives to be the cause of pseudoallergic symptoms. However, although DBPCFC with the individual additives or pure forms of histamine are ideal, they do not provide a 'real-life' scenario, where the additive or natural food chemical will be consumed as part of the food or food matrix. Ideally the potential cause and effect of foods should be reviewed on an individual basis and any diagnostic diet tailored to the individual, taking account of their symptoms and particular foods suspected, rather than adopting a blanket approach of a few foods diet. There are some foods which are a rich source of additives and/or natural food chemicals (Table 3) and so a limited removal of a few 'high' risk foods in adults might be a good first step to determine whether diet plays a role in symptoms.

Table 3 Foods likely to be high in added and/or natural 'food chemicals'

Food	Amine	Glutamate	Salicylate	Sulphite	Benzoate
Cheese	✓	✓			✓
Wine	✓		✓	✓	
Soy	✓	✓			✓
Tea		✓	✓		
Tomatoes	✓	✓	✓		✓
Herbs and spices			✓		✓
Strawberries and pineapple	✓		✓		
Spinach	✓	✓			✓
Worcestershire sauce		✓	✓		✓
Dried fruit			✓	✓	✓

The elimination of an additive or food chemical often requires a major change to the whole diet, so any benefits arising from the intervention, may be due to lifestyle changes incurred as a result of an improvement in diet, rather than to the removal of the offending additive. In addition, the placebo effects of dietary interventions are as yet an unknown quantity, and require further study. The importance of healthy diets and diversity of foodstuffs has recently been demonstrated in infants and young children, but the lifelong effects may also be important in adults [117]. A healthy diet will usually contain lower levels of additives and therefore a pragmatic approach should focus on improving the nutritional quality of the diet alongside any specific dietary exclusion is an important goal in all dietary interventions for non-immune mediated reactions to foods.

Authors' contributions
IS wrote the abstract, the sections on salicylates and sulphites, the conclusion, collated all of the other sections to produce a cohesive paper and submitted the manuscript. MW wrote the sections on benzoates and monosodium glutamate, LR wrote the section on benzoates and RW wrote the section on chemical diets in children. CV generated the idea for the review and wrote the introduction. All authors read and approved the final manuscript.

Author details
[1] Royal Brompton and Harefield NHS Foundation Trust, Sydney Street, London SW3 6NP, UK. [2] Somerset Partnership NHS Foundation Trust, Somerset, UK. [3] Oxford Health NHS Foundation Trust, Oxford, UK. [4] Great Ormond Street NHS Foundation Trust, London, UK. [5] The David Hide Asthma and Allergy Research Centre, Isle of Wight, UK.

Compliance with ethical guidelines

Competing interests
The authors declare that they have no competing interests.

References

1. Muraro A, Werfel T, Hoffmann-Sommergruber K, Roberts G, Beyer K, Bindslev-Jensen C, Cardona V, Dubois A, duToit G, Eigenmann P, Fernandez Rivas M, Halken S, Hickstein L, Høst A, Knol E, Lack G, Marchisotto MJ, Niggemann B, Nwaru BI, Papadopoulos NG, Poulsen LK, Santos AF, Skypala I, Schoepfer A, Van Ree R, Venter C, Worm M, Vlieg-Boerstra B, Panesar S, de Silva D, Soares-Weiser K, Sheikh A, Ballmer-Weber BK, Nilsson C, de Jong NW, Akdis CA, EAACI Food Allergy and Anaphylaxis Guidelines Group. EAACI food allergy and anaphylaxis guidelines: diagnosis and management of food allergy. Allergy. 2014, 69:1008–25.
2. Kang MG, Song WJ, Park HK, Lim KH, Kim SJ, Lee SY, et al. Basophil activation test with food additives in chronic urticaria patients. Clin Nutr Res. 2014;3:9–16.
3. Werfel T. Skin manifestations in food allergy. Allergy. 2001;56(Suppl 67):98–101.
4. Cardinale F, Mangini F, Berardi M, Sterpeta LM, Chinellato I, Dellino A Cristofori F, Di Domenico F, Mastrototaro MF, Cappiello A, Centoducati T, Carella F, Armenio L. Intolerance to food additives: an update. Minerva Pediatr. 2008;60:1401–09.
5. Vally H, Misso NL. Adverse reactions to the sulphite additives. Gastroenterol Hepatol Bed Bench. 2012;5:16–23.
6. Maintz L, Novak N. Histamine and histamine intolerance. Am J Clin Nutr. 2007;85:1185–96.

7. Azuma K, Uchiyama I, Katoh T, Ogata H, Arashidani K, Kunugita N. Prevalence and characteristics of chemical intolerance: a Japanese population-based study. Arch Environ Occup Health. 2014. doi:10.1080/19338244.2014.926855.
8. Schroeter LC. Sulfur dioxide: applications in foods, beverages and pharmaceuticals. New York: Pergamon Press; 1966.
9. Karovicova J, Simko P. Preservatives in food. In: Nollet LML, editor. Handbook of food analysis. New York; 1996. p. 1745–47.
10. Yang WH, Purchase EC. Adverse reactions to sulfites. CMAJ. 1985;133:865–7.
11. Verger P, Chambolle M, Babayou P, Le Breton S, Volatier JL. Estimation of the distribution of the maximum theoretical intake for ten additives in France. Food Addit Contam. 1998;15:756–9.
12. Zhang JB, Zhang H, Wang HL, Zhang JY, Luo PJ, Zhu L, Wang ZT. Risk analysis of sulfites used as food additives in China. Biomed Environ Sci. 2014;27:147–54.
13. Directive 2003/89/EC of the European Parliament and of the Council of 10 November 2003. Amending directive 2000/13/EC as regards indication of the ingredients present in foodstuffs. OJ L 2003;308:15–8.
14. Food and Drug Administration. New sulfite regulations. FDA Drug Bull. 1986;16:17–8.
15. Manzi P, Masci V, Quattrucci E. Valutazione dell'ingestione potenziale media de alcuni conservanti basata sulla dieta italana di riferimento. In: Consiglio Nazionale delle Ricerche. Agrobiotecnologie nei processi di valorizzazione dei prodotti e sottoprodotti agricoli. Progetto R.A.I.S.A. (Riecerche Avanzante per Innovazioni nei Sisterna Agricolo), Sottoprogetto 4. (Roma: CNR) 1992;II:1093–96.
16. Martin LB, Nordlee JA, Taylor SL. Sulfite residues in restaurant salads. J Food Prot. 1986;49:126–9.
17. Simon RA. Update on sulfite sensitivity. Allergy. 1998;53:72–4.
18. Bush RK, Taylor SL, Holden K, Nordlee JA, Busse WW. The prevalence of sensitivity to sulfiting agents in asthmatics. Am J Med. 1986;81:816–20.
19. Buckley CE III, Saltzman HA, Seiker HO. The prevalence and degree of sensitivity to ingested sulfites. J Allergy Clin Immunol. 1985;75:144.
20. Ban GY, Kim MA, Yoo HS, Ye YM, Park HS. Letter to the editor. Two major phenotypes of sulfite hypersensitivity: asthma and urticaria. Yonsei Med J. 2014;55:542–4.
21. Asero R. Multiple intolerance to food additives. J Allergy Clin Immunol. 2002;110:531–2.
22. Simon R. Adverse reactions to food and drug additives. Immunol Allergy Clin N Am. 1996;16:137–76.
23. Yang W, Purchase E, Rivington R. Positive skin tests and Prausnitz–Kustner reactions in metabisulfite-sensitive subjects. J Allergy Clin Immunol. 1986;78:443.
24. Boxer M, Bush R, Harris K, Patterson R, Pruzansky J, Yang W. The laboratory evaluation of IgE antibody to metabisulfites in patients skin test positive to metabisulfites. J Allergy Clin Immunol. 1988;82:622–6.
25. Prenner B, Stevens J. Anaphylaxis after ingestion of sodium bisulfite. Ann Allergy. 1976;37:180.
26. Gong H Jr, Linn WS, Terrell SL, Anderson KR, Clark KW. Anti-inflammatory and lung function effects of montelukast in asthmatic volunteers exposed to sulphur dioxide. Chest. 2001;119:402–8.
27. Howland WA, Simon RA. Restaurant-provoked asthma: sulfite sensitivity? J Allergy Clin Immunol. 1985;75:145.
28. Taylor SL, Bush RK, Selner JC, et al. Sensitivity to sulfited foods among sulfite-sensitive subjects with asthma. J Allergy Clin Immunol. 1988;81:1159–67.
29. Vally H, Thompson PJ. Role of sulfite additives in wine induced asthma: single dose and cumulative dose studies. Thorax. 2001;56:763–9.
30. Sieber R, Butikofer U, Bosset JO, Ruegg M. Benzoic acid as a natural component of foods—a review. Mitt Lebensmittelunters Hyg. 1989;80:345–62.
31. Wibbertmann A, Kielhorn J, Koennecker G, Mangelsdorf I, Melber C. Concise International Chemical Assessment Document 26. Benzoic acid and sodium benzoate. Vol. 26. Geneva: World Health Organisation; 2000. p. 1–48.
32. Rangan C, Barceloux DG. Food additives and sensitivities. Dis Mon. 2009;55:292–311.
33. Khasnavis S, Pahan K. Sodium benzoate, a metabolite of cinnamon and a food additive, upregulates neuroprotective Parkinson disease protein DJ-1 in astrocytes and neurons. J Neuroimmune Pharmacol. 2012;7:424–35.
34. European Parliament and Council Directive. European Parliament and Council Directive No 95/2/EC of 20 February 1995 on food additives other than colours and sweeteners. Off J Eur Union 1995;L61/18:1.
35. The European Parliament and the Council of the European Union. Directive 2003/15/EC of the European Parliament and of the Council of 27 February 2003, amending Council Directive 76/768/EEC on the approximation of the laws of the member.
36. Wuthrich B. Food-induced cutaneous adverse reactions. Allergy. 1998;53:131–5.
37. Van Bever HP, Docx M, Stevens WJ. Food and food additives in severe atopic dermatitis. Allergy. 1989;44:588–94.
38. Worm MEI, Sterry W, Zuverbier T. Clinical relevance of food additives in adult patients with atopic dermatitis. Clin Exp Allergy. 2000;30:407–14.
39. Park HW, Park CH, Park SH, Park JY, Park HS, Yang HJ, et al. Dermatologic adverse reactions to 7 common food additives in patients with allergic diseases: a double-blind, placebo-controlled study. J Allergy Clin Immunol. 2008;121:1059–61.
40. Weber RWHM, Raine D. Incidence of bronchoconstriction due to aspirin, azo dyes, non-azo dyes, and preservatives in a population of perennial asthmatics. J Allergy Clin Immunol. 1979;64:32–7.
41. Tarlo SMBI. Tartrazine and benzoate challenge and dietary avoidance in chronic asthma. Clin Allergy. 1982;12:303–12.
42. Pacor MLDLG, Martinelli N, Mansueto P, Rini GB, Corrocher R. Monosodium benzoate hypersensitivity in subjects with persistent rhinitis. Allergy. 2004;59:192–7.
43. Ortolani CPE, Luraghi MT, Della-Torre F, Bellani M, Zanussi C. Diagnosis of food intolerance to food additives. Ann Allergy. 1984;53:587–91.
44. Simon RA. Additive-induced urticaria: experience with monosodium glutamate (MSG). J Nutr. 2000;130:1063S–6S.
45. Ros AJL, Michaelsson G. A follow-up study of patients with recurrent urticaria and hypersensitivity to aspirin, benzoates and azo dyes. Br J Dermatol. 1976;95:19–24.
46. Ehlers INB, Binder C, Zuberbier T. Role of nonallergic hypersensitivity reactions in children with chronic urticaria. Allergy. 1998;53:1074–7.
47. Gibson A, Clancy R. Management of chronic idiopathic urticaria by the identification and exclusion of dietary factors. Clin Allergy. 1980;10:699–704.
48. Rajan JP, Simon RA, Bosso JV. Prevalence of sensitivity to food and drug additives in patients with chronic idiopathic urticaria. J Allergy Clin Immunol Pract. 2014;2:168–71.
49. Yamaguchi S, Ninomiya K. Umami and food palatability. J Nutr. 2000;130:921S–6S.
50. Metcalfe DD Sampson H, Simon RA, Lack G. Food allergy: adverse reaction to foods and food additives. 5th ed. New York: Wiley-Blackwell; 2014.
51. Kwok R. Chinese restaurant syndrome. New Eng J Med. 1968;278:796.
52. Kenney RA. Placebo-controlled studies of human reaction to oral monosodium L-glutamate. Glutamic Acid: Adv Biochem Physiol; 1979. p. 363–73.
53. Morselli PLGS. Monosodium glutamate and the Chinese Restaurant Syndrome. Nature. 1970;227:611–2.
54. Geha RS, Beiser A, Ren C, Patterson R, Greenberger PA, Grammer LC, Ditto AM, Harris KE, Shaughnessy MA, Yarnold PR, Corren J, Saxon A. Multicenter, double-blind, placebo-controlled, multiple-challenge evaluation of reported reactions to monosodium glutamate. J Allergy Clin Immunol. 2000;106:973–80.
55. http://www.fda.gov/. Accessed 1 July 2015.
56. Wilson BGBS. Adverse reactions to food additives. Ann Allergy Asthma Immunol. 2005;95:499–507.
57. Gultekin F, Doguc DK. Allergic and immunologic reactions to food additives. Clin Rev Allergy Immunol. 2013;45:6–29.
58. Allen DHDJ, Baker G. Monosodium L-glutamate-induced asthma. J Allergy Clin Immunol. 1987;80:530–7.
59. Schwartzstein RMKM, Weinberger SE, Weiss JW, Drazen JM. Airway effects of monosodium glutamate in subjects with chronic stable asthma. J Asthma. 1987;24:167–72.
60. Woods RKWJ, Thien F, Abramson M, Walters EH. The effects of monosodium glutamate in adults with asthma who perceive themselves

to be monosodium glutamate-intolerant. J Allergy Clin Immunol. 1998;101:762–71.
61. Germano PCS, Hahn B, Metcalfe DD. An evaluation of clinical reactions to monosodium glutamate (MSG) in asthmatics, using blinded placebo-controlled challenge. J Allergy Clin Immunol. 1991;87:177.
62. Asero RBG. Chronic rhinitis with nasal polyposis associated with sodium glutamate intolerance. Int Arch Allergy Immunol. 2007;144:159–61.
63. Gray D. Food and Drug Administration Memorandum, glutamate in food. Fed Regist. 1996;61:48102–10.
64. Yang WHDM, Herbert M, Mao Y, Karsh J. The monosodium glutamate symptom complex: assessment in a double-blind, placebo-controlled, randomised study. J Allergy Clin Immunol. 1997;99:757–62.
65. Baad-Hansen L, Cairns B, Ernberg M, Svensson P. Effect of systemic monosodium glutamate (MSG) on headache and pericranial muscle sensitivity. Cephalalgia. 2010;30:68–76.
66. Jansen SC, van Dusseldorp M, Bottema KC, Dubois AE. Intolerance to dietary biogenic amines: a review. Ann Allergy Asthma Immunol. 2003;91:233–40.
67. Fogel WA, Lewinski A, Jochem J. Histamine in food: is there anything to worry about? Biochem Soc Trans. 2007;35:349–52.
68. Bodmer S, Imark C, Kneubühl M. Biogenic amines in foods: histamine and food processing. Inflamm Res. 1999;48:296–300.
69. Skypala I. Other causes of food hypersensitivity. In: Skypala I, Venter C, editors. Food hypersensitivity: diagnosing and managing food allergies and intolerance. West Sussex: Wiley-Blackwell; 2009. p. p210–40.
70. Attaran RR, Probst F. Histamine fish poisoning: a common but frequently misdiagnosed condition. Emerg Med J. 2000;19:474–5.
71. Wöhrl S, Hemmer W, Focke M, Rappersberger K, Jarisch R. Histamine intolerance-like symptoms in healthy volunteers after oral provocation with liquid histamine. Allergy Asthma Proc. 2004;25:305–11.
72. Vickerstaff Joneja J, Carmona-Silva C. Outcome of a histamine-restricted diet based on chart audit. J Nutr Environ Med. 2001;11:249–62.
73. Yang J, Ding X, Qin Y, Zeng Y. Safety assessment of the biogenic amines in fermented soya beans and fermented bean curd. J Agric Food Chem. 2014;62:7947–54.
74. Kanny G, Gerbaux V, Olszewski A, Frémont S, Empereur F, Nabet F, Kanny G, Gerbaux V, Olszewski A, Frémont S, Empereur F, Nabet F, Cabanis JC, Moneret-Vautrin DA. No correlation between wine intolerance and histamine content of wine. J Allergy Clin Immunol. 2001;107:375–8.
75. Vlieg-Boerstra BJ, van der Heide S, Oude Elberink JN, Kluin-Nelemans JC, Dubois AE. Mastocytosis and adverse reactions to biogenic amines and histamine-releasing foods: what is the evidence? Neth J Med. 2005;63:244–9.
76. Wantke F, Götz M, Jarisch R. Histamine-free diet: treatment of choice for histamine-induced food intolerance and supporting treatment for chronic headaches. Clin Exp Allergy. 1993;23:982–5.
77. King W, McCargar L, Joneja JM, Barr SI. Benefits of a histamine-reducing diet for some patients with chronic urticaria and angioedema. Can J Diet Pract Res. 2000;61:24–6.
78. Böhn L, Störsrud S, Törnblom H, Bengtsson U, Simrén M. Self-reported food-related gastrointestinal symptoms in IBS are common and associated with more severe symptoms and reduced quality of life. Am J Gastroenterol. 2013;108:634–41.
79. Lessof MH, Gant V, Hinuma K, Murphy GM, Dowling RH. Recurrent urticaria and reduced diamine oxidase activity. Clin Exp Allergy. 1990;20:373–6.
80. Cho HJ, Cho SI, Kim HO, Park CW, Lee CH. Lack of association of plasma histamine with diamine oxidase in chronic idiopathic urticaria. Ann Dermatol. 2013;25:189–95.
81. Kofler L, Ulmer H, Kofler H. Histamine 50-skin-prick test: a tool to diagnose histamine intolerance. ISRN Allergy 2011:353045.
82. Raithel M, Baenkler HW, Naegel A, Buchwald F, Schultis HW, Backhaus B, Kimpel S, Koch H, Mach K, Hahn EG, Konturek PC. Significance of salicylate intolerance in diseases of the lower gastrointestinal tract. J Physiol Pharmacol. 2005;56:89–102.
83. Amann R, Peskar BA. Anti-inflammatory effects of aspirin and sodium salicylate. Eur J Pharmacol. 2002;447:1–9.
84. Hare LG, Woodside JV, Young IS. Dietary salicylates. J Clin Pathol. 2003;56:649–50.
85. Paterson JR, Srivastava R, Baxter GJ, Graham AB, Lawrence JR. Salicylic acid content of spices and its implications. J Agric Food Chem. 2006;54:2891–6.
86. Duthie GG, Wood AD. Natural salicylates: foods, functions and disease prevention. Food Funct. 2011;2:515–20.
87. Swain AR, Dutton SP, Truswell AS. Salicylates in foods. J Am Diet Assoc. 1985;85:950–60.
88. Venema DP, Hollman PCH, Janssen KPLTM, Katan MB. Determination of acetylsalicylic acid and salicylic acid in foods, using HPLC with fluorescence detection. J Agric Food Chem. 1996;44:1762–7.
89. Scotter MJ, Roberts DPT, Wilson LA, Howard FAC, Davis J, Mansell N. Free salicylic acid and acetyl salicylic acid content of foods using gas chromatography-mass spectrometry. Food Chem. 2007;105:273–9.
90. Wood A, Baxter G, Thies F, Kyle J, Duthie G. A systematic review of salicylates in foods: estimated daily intake of a Scottish population. Mol Nutr Food Res. 2011;55:S7–14.
91. Janssen KTLPM, Hollman PCH, Venema DP, van Staveren WA and Katan MB. Salicylates in foods. Nut Rev. 1996;54:357–9.
92. Baxter GJ, Graham AB, Lawrence JR, Wiles D, Paterson JR. Salicylic acid in soups prepared from organically and non-organically grown vegetables. Eur J Nutr. 2001;40:289–92.
93. Heiska S, Rousi M, Turtola S, Meier B, Tirkkonen V, Julkunen-Titto R. The effect of genotype and cultivation method on the total salicylate yield of dark leaved willows. Plant Med. 2005;71:1134–9.
94. Janssen KTLPM, Hollman PCH, Reichmann E, Venema DP, van Staveren WA and Katan MB. Urinary salicylate excretion in subjects eating a variety of diets shows the amounts of bioavailable salicylates in foods are low. Am J Clin Nutr. 1996;64:743–7.
95. Lawrence JR, Peter R, Baxter G, Robson J, Graham AB, Paterson JR. Urinary excretion of salicyluric and salicylic acids by non-vegetarians, vegetarians and patients taking low-dose aspirin. J Clin Pathol. 2003;56:651–3.
96. Baenkler H-W. Salicylate intolerance. Dtsch Arztebl Int. 2008;105:137–42.
97. Mitchell JE, Skypala I. Aspirin and salicylate in respiratory disease. Rhinology. 2013;51:195–205.
98. Picado C, Fernandez-Morata JC, Juan M, Roca-Ferrer J, Fuentes M, Xaubet A, Mullol J. Cyclooxygenase-2 mRNA is down expressed in nasal polyps from aspirin-sensitive asthmatics. Am J Resp Crit Care Med. 1999;160:291–6.
99. Corder EH, Buckley CE. Aspirin, salicylate, sulfite and tartrazine-induced broncho-constriction. Safe doses and case definition in epidemiological studies. J Clin Epidemiol. 1995;48:1269–75.
100. Dahlén B, Boréus LO, Anderson P, Andersson R, Zetterström O. Plasma acetylsalicylic acid and salicylic acid levels during aspirin provocation in aspirin-sensitive subjects. Allergy. 1994;49:43–9.
101. Gibson PR. Food intolerance in functional bowel disorders. J Gastroenterol Hepatol. 2011;26:128–31.
102. Barrett JS, Gibson PR. Fermentable oligosaccharides, disaccharides, monosaccharides and polyols (FODMAPs) and nonallergic food intolerance: FODMAPs or food chemicals? Ther Adv Gastroenterol. 2012;5:261–8.
103. Supramaniam GWJ. Artificial food additive intolerance in patients with angio-oedema and urticaria. Lancet. 1986;2:907–9.
104. Paul SP, Barnard P, Soondrum K, Candy DC. Antimigraine (low-amine) diet may be helpful in children with cyclic vomiting syndrome. J Pediatr Gastroenterol Nutr. 2012;54:698–9.
105. McCann D, Barrett A, Cooper A, Crumpler D, Dalen L, Grimshaw K, Kitchin E, Lok K, Porteous L, Prince E, Sonuga-Barke E, Warner JO, Stevenson J. Food additives and hyperactive behaviour in 3-year-old and 8/9-year-old children in the community: a randomised, double-blinded, placebo-controlled trial. Lancet. 2007;370:1560–7.
106. Food Standards Agency. Final technical report for additives and behaviour study submitted by School of Psychology, University of Southampton, 2007.
107. Sanz J, Martorell A, Torro I, Carlos CJ, Alvarez V. Intolerance to sodium metabisulfite in children with steroid-dependent asthma. J Investig Allergol Clin Immunol. 1992;2:36–8.
108. Anibarro B, Caballero T, Garcia-Ara C, Diaz-Pena JM, Ojeda JA. Asthma with sulfite intolerance in children: a blocking study with cyanocobalamin. J Allergy Clin. Immunol. 1992;90:103–9.

109. Hoffmann KM, Gruber E, Deutschmann A, Jahnel J, Hauer AC. Histamine intolerance in children with chronic abdominal pain. Arch Dis Child. 2013;98:832–3.
110. Rosell-Camps A, Zibetti S, Pérez-Esteban G, Vila-Vidal M, Ferrés-Ramis L, García-Teresa-García E. Histamine intolerance as a cause of chronic digestive complaints in pediatric patients. Rev Esp Enferm Dig. 2013;105:201–6.
111. Loblay RH, Soutter VL, Swain AR. Salicylate elimination diets in children. MJA. 2013;198:603.
112. Gray PE, Mehr S, Katelaris CH, Wainstein BK, Star A, Campbell D, Joshi P, Wong M, Frankum B, Keat K, Dunne G, Dennison B, Kakakios A, Ziegler JB. Salicylate elimination diets in children: is food restriction supported by the evidence? MJA. 2013;198:600–2.
113. Barker DJP. Introduction: the window of opportunity. J Nutr. 2007;137:1058–9.
114. Holland D, Chang L, Ernst TM, Curran M, Buchthal SD, Alicata D, Skranes J, Johansen H, Hernandez A, Yamakawa R, Kuperman JM, Dale AM. Structural growth trajectories and rates of change in the first 3 months of infant brain development. JAMA Neurol. 2014;71:1266–74.
115. Ventura AK, Worobey J. Early influences on the development of food preferences. Curr Biol. 2013;23:R40140–8.
116. Kim J, Kwon J, Noh G, Lee SS. The effects of elimination diet on nutritional status in subjects with atopic dermatitis. Nutr Res Pract. 2013;7:488–94.
117. Skypala I, Vlieg-Boerstra B. Food intolerance and allergy: increased incidence or contemporary inadequate diets? Curr Opin Clin Nutr Metab Care. 2014;17:442–7.
118. Leclercq C, Molinaro MG, Piccinelli R, Baldini M, Arcella D, Stacchini P. Dietary intake exposure to sulphites in Italy—analytical determination of sulphite-containing foods and their combination into standard meals for adults and children. Food Addit Contam. 2000;17:979–89.
119. Heimhuber B, Herrmann K. Benzoe-, Phylessig-, 3-Phenylpropan- und Zimts- aure sowie benzoglucosen in einigen Obst-und Fruchtgemuse-arten. Dtsch Le- bensmitt Rundsch. 1990;86:205–9.
120. Campbell HE, Escudier MP, Patel P, Challacombe SJ, Sanderson JD, Lomer MC. Review article: cinnamon- and benzoate-free diet as a primary treatment for orofacial granulomatosis. Aliment Pharmacol Ther. 2011;34:687–701.
121. Williams AN, Woessner KM. Monosodium glutamate 'allergy': menace or myth? Clin Exp Allergy. 2009;39:640–6.
122. Visciano P, Schirone M, Tofalo R, Suzzi G. Biogenic amines in raw and processed seafood. Front Microbiol. 2012;3:188.
123. Linares DM, del Rio B, Ladero V, Martinez N, Fernandez M, Cruz Martin and Alverez MA. Factors influencing biogenic amines accumulation in dairy products. Front Microbiol. 2012;3:180.
124. Chung BY, Cho SI, Ahn IS, Lee HB, Kim HO, Park CW, Lee CH. Treatment of atopic dermatitis with a low histamine diet. Ann Dermatol. 2011;23(Supp 1):S91–5.
125. Shukla S, Kim J-K, Kim M. Occurrence of biogenic amines in soybean food products, soybean and health, Prof. Hany El-Shemy (Ed.), ISBN: 978-953-307-535-8, InTech; 2011. doi:10.5772/19021.
126. Halász A, Baráth A, Simon-Sarkadi L, Holzapfe W. Biogenic amines and their production by microorganisms in food. Trends Food Sci Technol. 1994;5(2):42–9.

A practical approach to vitamin and mineral supplementation in food allergic children

Rosan Meyer[1*], Claire De Koker[2], Robert Dziubak[1], Ana-Kristina Skrapac[2], Heather Godwin[1], Kate Reeve[1], Adriana Chebar-Lozinsky[1] and Neil Shah[1,3]

Abstract

Background: The management of food allergy in children requires elimination of the offending allergens, which significantly contribute to micronutrient intake. Vitamin and mineral supplementation are commonly suggested as part of dietary management. However a targeted supplementation regime requires a complete nutritional assessment, which includes food diaries. Ideally these should be analysed using a computerised program, but are very time consuming. We therefore set out to evaluate current practice of vitamin and mineral supplementation in a cohort of children with non-Immunoglobulin E (IgE) mediated food allergies.

Methods: This prospective, observational study recruited children aged 4 weeks – 16 years, who required to follow an elimination diet for non-IgE mediated allergies. Only children that improved according to a symptom score and were on a vitamin and/or mineral supplement were included. A 3-day food diary including vitamin and mineral supplementation was recorded and analysed using Dietplan computer program. We assessed dietary adequacy with/without the supplement using the Dietary Reference Values.

Results: One hundred-and-ten children had completed food diaries and of these 29% (32/110) were taking vitamin and/or mineral supplements. Children on hypoallergenic formulas were significantly ($p = 0.007$) less likely to be on supplements than those on alternative over-the-counter milks. Seventy-one percent had prescribable supplements, suggested by a dietitian/physician. Sixty percent of those without a vitamin supplement had a low vitamin D intake, but low zinc, calcium and selenium was also common. Of the supplemented cohort many continued to be either under or over-supplemented.

Conclusion: This study has raised the question for the first time, whether clinicians dealing with paediatric food allergies should consider routine vitamin and/or mineral supplements in the light of deficient intake being so common in addition to being so difficult to predict.

Keywords: Dietary adequacy, Elimination diet, Food diary, Non-IgE mediated allergy, Vitamin and mineral supplementation

Introduction

Fundamental to the management of food allergy in early childhood is the total elimination of offending allergens [1]. These often include cow's milk, soya, hen's egg, wheat, fish and nuts; foods which contribute significantly to dietary vitamin and mineral intake [2,3]. Low micronutrient intakes as a result of a dietary elimination have been reported in food allergic children; increasing both the risk of vitamin and mineral deficiency and associated functional morbidity [4-7]. Vitamin D, calcium and omega-3 fatty acids are well documented to be deficient micronutrients in children with IgE-mediated food allergies [8], whilst intakes of trace elements including zinc, selenium and magnesium have been found to be of concern in some non-IgE mediated conditions including allergic colitis and atopic dermatitis [7,9].

A nutritional assessment by a qualified dietitian of the allergic child is now recognised by several international guidelines as essential to ensure dietary adequacy and to support parents in finding suitable alternatives [10-12].

* Correspondence: Rosan.Meyer@gosh.nhs.uk
[1]Department Gastroenterology, Great Ormond Street Hospital for Children NHS foundation Trust, London, UK
Full list of author information is available at the end of the article

The ideal dietetic assessment within the time constraints of a consultation should include a growth assessment, biochemical (when available) and dietary intake assessment to guide individualised dietary advice [13]. A dietary intake assessment can be very time consuming and is therefore often limited to a 24-hour recall. These dietary recall methods provide only a snap-shot of intake and are often biased [14,15], but are used in practice because they are quick and easy to do, and they provide the baseline for dietetic recommendations including supplementation of vitamin and/or minerals.

Although dietary intake as assessed by a 3-day food diary or nutritional status measured by blood markers, provide more accurate reflections of usual intake and nutritional status, these also have limitations [16,17]. Food diaries are time consuming and complex and therefore require highly motivated parents with a high level of literacy and understanding to cooperate [15,16]. The limitations for blood markers include nutrient plasma or serum concentrations not being a reliable reflection of intake and tissue stores, requiring a large blood sample from a small child and measurements can be affected by the measuring methods, contamination and health of the child at measurement [16,17]. In practice, blood investigations are mostly not available or results not accessible for the majority of cases at the time of the dietetic appointment. Therefore empirical vitamin and or mineral supplementation is currently based on the type of dietary elimination and intake as assessed during the consultation. We therefore set out to evaluate current practice of vitamin and mineral supplementation in a cohort of children with non-Immunoglobulin E (IgE) mediated food allergies, to assess the impact of micronutrient supplementation on vitamin and mineral intake and also whether those with low intakes based on food intake diaries received supplementation.

Methods

Subjects and study design

A prospective, observational study was performed in the gastroenterology department, at Great Ormond Street Hospital for Children NHS Foundation Trust, London, UK. Ethical approval (number 11/LO/1177) was obtained for this study. Parents of children aged 4 weeks – 16 years, who had no concomitant non-atopic co-morbidities (i.e. Cerebral Palsy), and required to follow an elimination diet for the diagnosis of suspected food protein induced gastrointestinal allergies, were approached to take part in the study. These children were only included if symptoms improved following the elimination diet as judged by a Likert Scale gastro-intestinal symptom questionnaire, that has previously been developed by the same research team [18]. This questionnaire was administered at baseline prior to commencing the elimination diet and again at 4 weeks after commencing the dietary elimination. In addition to this criterion, the cohort we report on was also on a vitamin and/or mineral supplement.

Dietary intake

A 3-day estimated food diary (1 weekend day and 2 week days) was recorded, at a minimum of 4 weeks following the initiation of the exclusion diet. Carers were given detailed instructions on how to complete the diary as accurately as possible, including a portion size guide and a sample menu. Hypoallergenic formula (HF) consumption (including type and volume), milk alternatives (i.e. oat, rice or almond milk) for older children and vitamin and mineral supplements (suggested by dietitian/physician or self-initiated) were also documented. Both over-the-counter and prescribed supplements were further categorised as: calcium, calcium and vitamin D, multivitamin, multivitamin and mineral, iron, and a combination of the aforementioned. All infants that were exclusively breastfed or received ≥ 2 breast feeds per day in addition to their HF were excluded from the dietary analysis, due to difficulties in estimating breast milk consumption in the individual patient. We choose this method, due to studies by Lanigan et al. [19] indicating that a weighed record does not give a significant advantage to an estimated record and also following the study by Ocke et al. [20] indicating a 3-day food dairy being a feasible method in European children.

Food diaries were discussed with parents and any unclear entries were clarified by the research dietitian at the time of the study appointment or by telephone communication after the appointment. The UK Food Portion Sizes published by the Food Standard Agency was used to help guide parents and healthcare professionals in estimating the correct portion size whenever portions needed converting from household measures to grams [21].

Nutritional intake data was assessed using Dietplan 6 Software (Forestfield Software Limited, UK). Any foods, in particular specialist foods free from allergens, as well as HF and vitamin and mineral supplements not available on the software database were manually added by the researcher, and product information was obtained from the manufacturer where necessary.

We assessed the impact of the vitamin and mineral supplements on dietary intake by using the UK Dietary Reference Values in the following way: inadequate intake was defined as achieving less than the Lower Reference Nutrient Intake (LRNI – meeting nutrient requirements for 2.5% of population) and adequate intake as achieving the Reference Nutrient Intake (range between LRNI and excessive intake) [22,23]. There is currently no RNI for vitamin D, for children ≥ 4 years of age in the UK; as a result we used the recommendations from the UK Department of Health which recommended 7 – 8.5 mg for children until 5 years of age and for older children we used 10 ug/day as reference value.

As there is paucity of data regarding Safe Upper Limits for many of the micronutrients in children, we arbitrarily defined excessive intake as more than 200% of the RNI [23].

Biochemical markers of micronutrient intake

We also collected biochemical markers of micronutrient intake, where available, that were performed at Great Ormond Street Hospital for Children, taken within 3 months of the 3 day food diary. As this hospital is a tertiary referral centre, many children may have had biochemical markers of micronutrient intake in their local centres, which we did not have access to.

Statistical analysis

Statistical analysis was performed using IBM SPSS Statistics for Windows, version 22 (Armonk, NY). Continuous and categorical data are described respectively as medians and interquartile range, and percentages and rates. In order to establish the impact of vitamin and mineral supplementation on micronutrient intake, food diaries of those children receiving a vitamin and mineral supplement were compared to the Dietary Reference Ranges with and without the supplements. The Pearson Chi-Square test was used to compare the differences in proportions of gender between groups receiving and not receiving VMS; children on vitamin and mineral supplements that were on a HF/over-counter-milk. The Fisher exact test was used to compare rates of dietary eliminations. Mann–Whitney *U* test was used to compare age between groups receiving and not receiving VMS; and to compare RNI intake of vitamin A and vitamin D between children taking different supplements. All tests were two-sided and significance level was set at 0.05.

Results

We recruited 131 children for this study, but 110 children had a complete food diary and of these 29% (32/110) were taking vitamin and/or mineral supplements. The supplemented group included 21 boys (65.6%) and the median age of this group was 5.1 years (IQR: 1.5 to 8.5). Although the proportion of boys was similar in supplemented and un-supplemented group (p 0.916) the age of the supplemented group was significantly higher ($p = 0.005$) than the median age of the group not receiving any supplementation (1.6, IQR: 0.7 to 4.6) [Table 1]. A total of 9/32 children on supplements (28%) were established on a HF, 17/32 (53%) on over-the-counter milk alternatives (i.e. coconut milk, oat milk or rice milk) and 6 (19%) had no cow's milk alternative. We found that children on over-the-counter milk alternatives/no milk replacement were significantly more likely to be on supplements compared to those on a HF in the whole cohort ($n = 110$): 40.4% (23/57) vs. 17.0% (9/53), $p = 0.007$.The majority of children on supplements (68%, $n = 22/32$) had prescribable supplements, consisting of mainly multivitamins, calcium and vitamin D and in two cases an iron supplement. The remaining 12 children (2 overlapped between categories) were taking over-the-counter preparations of multivitamins and also omega-3-fatty acids. Table 2 outlines the type of supplements used. In 23/32 (71%) the suggestion for a vitamin and/or mineral supplement was made by the dietitian/ physician, in 6 cases both the dietitian and the parents were involved in choosing the supplement and in 3 children the parents started a supplement without dietetic input. From the cohort on supplements, 14 children were eliminating ≥ 3 foods (cow's milk, soya and gluten/ egg/ other), 10 eliminated 2 foods (milk and soya) and 8 excluded 1 food only (i.e. cow's milk). Tables 1 and 2 describe this cohort in further detail, including the elimination diets and the availability of biochemical markers of micronutrient intake blood markers in this cohort.

When we assessed dietary adequacy of micronutrients without a supplement ($n = 110$), based on the definitions outlined in the methodology, we found that no child in the whole group had a deficient vitamin C intake and that low intakes of vitamin B12, B6, thiamine and folate

Table 1 Demographic details, including dietary elimination of the population with and without vitamin supplementation

Description	VMS	Without VMS	p value
Age	5,1 years	1.6 years	0.005**
Male	21/32 (66%)	52/78 (67%)	0.916
Dietary Elimination			
Cow's Milk	6 (19%)	5 (6%)	0.077
Cow's milk and soya	9 (28%)	11 (14%)	0.104
Cow's milk, soya and egg	3 (9%)	5 (6%)	0.689
Cow's milk, soya, egg and wheat/gluten	5 (16%)	9 (12%)	0.544
Other*	9 (28%)	48 (62%)	0.002**

*This group consists of children with other combinations of food eliminations, **$p < 0.01$.

Table 2 Dietary supplementation and biochemical markers of micronutrient intake of the group of children receiving supplements

Description	Patient numbers
Type of Supplement (some may have multiple supplements)	
Calcium	5
Calcium and vitamin D	4
Multivitamin (containing vitamin D)	15
Multivitamin and Mineral	8
Therapeutic iron	2
Other	5
Supplement initiated by:	
Dietitian/Physician	23
Dietitian and parent	6
Parent	3
Biochemical markers of micronutrient intake: (some children	
had multiple biochemical markers taken)	
Total available	7
Iron profile	7
Selected vitamins	2
Selected trace elements	3
Deficiencies:	
Iron	2
Zinc	1

were rare (Table 3). The dietary intake also revealed that in the whole group 60% (66/110) had a low vitamin D intake and that low zinc, copper and selenium were also seen in some patients (Table 3).

We then assessed dietary intake in those children with a supplement (n = 32) and whether those who had a low micronutrient intake also received appropriate vitamin and/or mineral supplementation. Our data suggests that although 25 children did receive a supplement with vitamin D, only 18/66 (27%) from the cohort with insufficient intake, were correctly identified as requiring this supplement and 10 of those receiving the supplement continued to not achieve their vitamin D requirements. We also found that 22 children had a low zinc intake however only 2/22 of this cohort was given a supplement containing zinc. Similarly, from the whole cohort 10 were identified as having a low calcium intake according to the food diary, but from this group only 3 children received a calcium supplement. However, 15 (18 in total) other children with an adequate calcium intake, were given a calcium supplement (Table 3), which is a similar trend for other vitamins and minerals.

Many children had an intake with supplementation exceeding 200% of the RNI for vitamin C, vitamin B6, thiamin, folate, selenium and vitamin A. In fact we found that of the 22 patients on a supplement containing vitamin A, 59% (n = 13) had intakes exceeding 200% of the RNI. We compared intake of Vitamin A for children who took a specific supplement known to be higher in vitamin A (Dalivit™, Boston Healthcare Limited) versus any other

Table 3 Overview of the vitamin and mineral supplementation: deficient intake in the whole cohort and those that received supplementation and the impact of the supplementation on dietary adequacy

Nutrient	Total number of children receiving supplements for each micronutrient	Deficient intake without VMS (whole cohort)	Deficient patients who were taking VMS[§]	>200% RNI with VMS	Adequate intake* with VMS	Intakes < LRNI with VMS
Vitamin C	23	0% (0/110)	N/A (0/0)	96% (22/23)	4% (1/23)	0% (0/23)
Vitamin A	22	10% (11/110)	9% (1/11)	59% (13/22)	41% (9/22)	0% (0/22)
Niacin	21	8% (9/110)	22% (2/9)	62% (13/21)	38% (8/21)	0% (0/21)
Vitamin B6	21	2% (2/110)	0% (0/2)	95% (20/21)	5% (1/21)	0% (0/21)
Thiamin	18	2% (2/110)	0% (0/2)	89% (16/18)	11% (2/18)	0% (0/18)
Calcium	18	9% (10/110)	30% (3/10)	44% (8/18)	50% (9/18)	6% (1/18)
Vitamin B12	17	1% (1/110)	100% (1/1)	94% (16/17)	6% (1/17)	0% (0/17)
Riboflavin	16	6% (7/110)	14% (1/7)	63% (10/16)	38% (6/16)	0% (0/16)
Vitamin D	25	60% (66/110)	27% (18/66)	16% (4/25)	44% (11/25)	40% (10/25)
Folate	12	3% (3/110)	0% (0/3)	67% (8/12)	33% (4/12)	0% (0/12)
Iron	10	7% (8/110)	0% (0/8)	40% (4/10)	60% (6/10)	0% (0/10)
Zinc	7	20% (22/110)	9% (2/22)	14% (1/7)	86% (6/7)	0% (0/7)
Copper	5	10% (11/110)	0% (0/11)	20% (1/5)	80% (4/5)	0% (0/5)
Selenium	3	11% (12/110)	0% (0/12)	67% (2/3)	33% (1/3)	0% (0/3)

*Children that had > LRNI and < 200% of RNI were classified as having adequate intake.
§This is the number of children from the whole cohort that had a deficient intake and were on a VMS.

form of Vitamin A supplementation. Children who received this supplement with vitamin A had significantly higher percentage RNI intakes of Vitamin A (505% RNI vs. 218% RNI, $p = 0.014$). Similarly, children who received Dalivit™ had higher RNI intake of vitamin D (205% RNI vs. 78% RNI, $p = 0.036$).

Four children received high doses of iron; however 2 of these had diagnosed iron deficiency anaemia, so were expected to receive therapeutic dosages.

Discussion

This study found that almost 30% of children from the whole cohort of children with non-IgE mediated food allergies received vitamin and/or mineral supplementation. The mean age of our supplemented cohort was over 5 years with more children receiving a vitamin and/or mineral supplementation when they were on alternative over-the-counter milks (i.e. coconut, oat or rice milk) which are nutritionally not complete [24]. The higher age of the supplemented group is to be expected as a significant number of children in our cohort were below 2 years and on a HF that contain significant amounts of vitamins and minerals [22].

The use of complementary and alternative medicine, including vitamin and mineral supplementation in atopic dermatitis is known to be commonplace in this population [25]. Studies by Johnston et al. [25,26] investigating the use of parent directed dietary elimination for atopic dermatitis, found that 40% of children were on vitamin and/or mineral supplements and that this is more common than in non-atopic children (24%). The key difference between our study and those published on atopic dermatitis were that all of our patients had an individualised dietetic review, whereas in the study by Johnston et al. [24], only 51% had consulted a dietitian. The primary role of the allergy dietitian is not only to discuss elimination of food allergens, but most importantly to suggest food alternatives that replace the nutrients eliminated which would include a HF and other nutritious foods [27].

Not surprisingly, 75% of children on supplements avoided ≥ 2 food allergens, with cow's milk and soya and a combination of cow's milk, soya, egg, wheat and others being the most common foods eliminated. It is known that children with multiple food allergies are at a higher risk of poor growth and a deficient vitamin and mineral intake [4,28]. What is of concern is that from our study many children who were identified by a 3-day food diary as having a low intake for certain micronutrients, did not receive a supplement, whereas others received excessive amounts of micronutrients. For example 11 patients from our whole cohort had a deficient vitamin A intake, but only 1 of these received a supplement containing vitamin A; conversely, 21 children with sufficient vitamin A intake, received a supplement containing vitamin A. This has resulted in 59% of our cohort receiving > 200% of the RNI for vitamin A. This occurrence can easily be explained by the UK government prescribable multivitamins which always contain vitamin A. As vitamin D is a commonly reported deficiency in the allergic cohort, all patients that require vitamin D, will therefore automatically receive vitamin A as well [5]. The question is whether the excessive vitamin A intake through supplementation is harmful for the allergic child. In 2003 "tolerable upper limits" for 1–3 year olds of various vitamins and minerals were published by the Scientific Committee on Food in Brussels. In this report the upper limit for vitamin A for this age was set at 800 ug RE/day, which would be 200% of the RNI for this age [29]. Similarly the Upper Safe Limits set by the Institute of Medicine is set at 600 ug/day for 1–3 year olds and 900 ug/day for 4–9 year olds [30]. However, no observed adverse effects have been reported for intakes up to 6000 ug/day and it is thought that only a chronic dose of 10–20 times the normal dose would lead to toxicity [30]. Levels therefore reported in our study would certainly not lead to toxicity. Excessive intakes of water soluble vitamins like vitamin C, B vitamins and folate are common and rarely are of significant concern, unless the child has reduced fluid intake, abnormal metabolism or metabolic defects [15].

From the whole cohort (supplemented and unsupplemented), 60% of children had a low vitamin D intake, which is not a surprising finding as 52% of those were not on a HF and it is thought that on average only 10% of the daily requirements for vitamin D are contributed by food in older children who are not on breast milk/formula [31,32]. What is of concern in this study is that only 27% of our population with a low dietary intake for vitamin D were identified as at risk and provided with a supplement that contained vitamin D. A recent study by Goldacre et al. [33] indicated that rickets in England is now at its highest in five decades and is not limited to specific ethnic groups, a concern that is reflected in many European countries. Current recommendations in the UK suggest the use of a multivitamin with vitamin D if volume of formula is below 500 ml or if a child is breastfed [34,35]. However, there are no recommendations for vitamin D specifically for children with food allergies, in spite of this being a commonly reported deficiency in this population [36,37].

In this study we also identified children with low intakes of copper, zinc and selenium, which are not commonly associated with IgE-mediated allergies. Deficiencies and low intakes of these minerals have been documented in children with atopic dermatitis and non-IgE mediated gastrointestinal allergies [7,9]. Only 19% of our cohort received supplements with zinc and selenium and none with copper. Meyer et al. [38] has highlighted low intakes of these trace minerals, in particular in children who are not on a hypoallergenic formula. These micronutrients have an important immunomodulatory role and need to be taken into account when assessing dietary intake also in allergic children [39].

Although a low dietary intake may assist in identifying children at risk of a deficiency, it is known that certain nutritional blood markers may be more sensitive and specific in identifying true deficiency. From our cohort only 7 children had biochemical markers of micronutrient intake available to guide dietitians in their supplement recommendation. The reality therefore is that the dietitian will have to rely on dietary intake and foods eliminated from the allergic child's diet to guide a vitamin and/or mineral supplementation regime. The validity of dietary intake assessment through food records, 24 hour recalls and food frequency questionnaires has been debated by many studies and have significant limitations on an individual level [16]. A systematic review in 2009 on dietary assessment methods for micronutrient intake in infants and children found that a weighed dietary record was more accurate than a food frequency questionnaire for vitamin and mineral intake [16]. In clinical practice however, these are rarely available to a dietitian at the time of the appointment, are time consuming to complete for parents, and for dietitians to analyse [17]. As clinical time constraints are increasing and the child's nutritional safety is paramount, this study has raised the question for the first time, whether dietitians and clinicians dealing with paediatric food allergies should consider routine vitamin and/or mineral supplements in the light of deficient intake being so common, especially for vitamin D, calcium, zinc and selenium and toxicities (if supplemented within the RNI/RDA) being theoretical rather than of clinical significance.

The limitations of this study are linked to the dietary assessment methods, the analysis program as well as the low number of children on supplements. A 3-day estimated food diary may not be the most accurate dietary assessment method to reflect usual intake. However, in the absence of a validated food frequency questionnaire for allergic children and also the ability to take repeated 24 hour recalls, which would have been affected by the atopic disease process itself, a 3-day food dairy was the best choice. In addition, a 3-day food diary suggest low intake, but certainly would not indicate a vitamin or mineral deficiency. Future studies should aim to assess the association between dietary intake methods and actual deficiencies in the food allergic population. In addition, it may be that parents did not document all the supplements their child was on, due to a concern that the dietitian would request them to discontinue or change the supplements. Due to no RNI being available for vitamin D > 4 years of age we also had to use a cut-off of 10 ug/day for children older than 5 years. This reference value may have elevated the number of children with deficient intake, as it is generally used as an aim value for adults. In addition whilst the dietary analysis program calculates vitamin D intake from the diet, it cannot account for the contribution of sunlight (Zipitis et al. [32]). In this study only 32 children out of 110 that had vitamin/and or mineral supplementation. Although this can be perceived as a low number, we do believe that in spite of this, the study is important in highlighting the difficulties dietitians have in predicting which child requires supplementation of vitamins, minerals or both, and opens the debate to routine supplementation of allergic children irrespective of their food allergy.

Conclusion

This study investigates the current practice in a tertiary gastroenterology centre of vitamin and/or mineral supplementation in children with non-IgE mediated allergies on an elimination diet. It is the first study that highlights the difficulties in making a decision in regard to appropriate dietary supplementation based on the information a dietitian has during their clinic appointment. We have highlighted that there is a significant discrepancy between children identified with a low intake through a 3-day food diary and those receiving a micronutrient supplement. In the light of vitamin and mineral deficiencies being common in the food allergic cohort, future studies should be performed to assess the impact of routine vitamin and mineral supplementation in children with food allergies using both nutritional blood markers and dietary intake methods.

Abbreviations

HF: Hypoallergenic formula; IgE: Immunoglobulin E; NHS: National Health Service; RDA: Recommended dietary allowance; RNI: Recommended nutrient intake.

Competing interests

Funding for this study was obtained through Great Ormond Street Charitable Fund. None of the authors have any competing interests related to this publication.

Authors' contributions

RM – Involved in data collection and some dietary analysis, conceptualising and writing of article; CDK – Performed majority of data collection and dietary analysis, conceptualising and writing of article; AKS – Involved in data collection and correction of the publication; RD – Statistical Analysis and article corrections; KR – Critical appraisal of publication; HG – Involved in data collection for the study and correction of publication; ACL – Critical appraisal of publication; NS – Team lead, conceptualising research project and review of article. All authors read and approved the final manuscript.

Acknowledgements

This study was funded by the Great Ormond Street Children Hospital Charity. We would also like to acknowledge all parents and children that participated in this study and took the time to fill in the 3-day food diary.

Author details

[1]Department Gastroenterology, Great Ormond Street Hospital for Children NHS foundation Trust, London, UK. [2]Department Nutrition and Dietetics, Chelsea and Westminster Hospital NHS Foundation Trust, London, UK. [3]Institute of Child Health, University College London, London, UK.

References

1. Groetch M, Nowak-Wegrzyn A. Practical approach to nutrition and dietary intervention in pediatric food allergy. Pediatr Allergy Immunol. 2013;24:212–21.
2. Venter C, Meyer R. Session 1: allergic disease: the challenges of managing food hypersensitivity. Proc Nutr Soc. 2010;69:11–24.
3. Venter C, Arshad SH. Epidemiology of food allergy. Pediatr Clin North Am. 2011;58:327–49.
4. Christie L, Hine RJ, Parker JG, Burks W. Food allergies in children affect nutrient intake and growth. J Am Diet Assoc. 2002;102:1648–51.
5. Noimark L, Cox HE. Nutritional problems related to food allergy in childhood. Pediatr Allergy Immunol. 2008;19:188–95.
6. Fox AT, Du TG, Lang A, Lack G. Food allergy as a risk factor for nutritional rickets. Pediatr Allergy Immunol. 2004;15:566–9.
7. Ojuawo A, Lindley KJ, Milla PJ. Serum zinc, selenium and copper concentration in children with allergic colitis. East Afr Med J. 1996;73:236–8.
8. Sova C, Feuling MB, Baumler M, Gleason L, Tam JS, Zafra H. Systematic review of nutrient intake and growth in children with multiple IgE-mediated food allergies. Nutr Clin Pract. 2013;28:669–75.
9. Toyran M, Kaymak M, Vezir E, Harmanci K, Kaya A, Ginis T, et al. Trace element levels in children with atopic dermatitis. J Investig Allergol Clin Immunol. 2012;22:341–4.
10. Koletzko S, Niggemann B, Arato A, Dias JA, Heuschkel R, Husby S, et al. Diagnostic Approach and Management of Cow's-Milk Protein Allergy in Infants and Children: ESPGHAN GI Committee Practical Guidelines. J Pediatr Gastroenterol Nutr. 2012;55:221–9.
11. National Institute for Clinical Excellence: Diagnosis and assessment of food allergy in children and young people in primary care and community settings. 2011, CG116 Page 1-88. Accessed 1/03/2015 http://www.nice.org.uk/guidance/cg116/resources/cg116-food-allergy-in-children-and-young-people-full-guideline3.
12. Boyce JA, Assa'ad A, Burks AW, Jones SM, Sampson HA, Wood RA, et al. Guidelines for the diagnosis and management of food allergy in the United States: summary of the NIAID-sponsored expert panel report. Nutr Res. 2011;31:61–75.
13. Giovannini M, D'Auria E, Caffarelli C, Verduci E, Barberi S, Indinnimeo L, et al. Nutritional management and follow up of infants and children with food allergy: Italian Society of Pediatric Nutrition/Italian Society of Pediatric Allergy and Immunology Task Force Position Statement. Ital J Pediatr. 2014;40:1.
14. Block G. A review of validations on dietary assessment methods. Am J Epidemiol. 1982;115:492–505.
15. Lee RW, Nieman DC. Nutritional Assessment. 4th ed. Singapore: McGraw-Hill Eudcation; 2007.
16. Ortiz-Andrellucchi A, Henriquez-Sanchez P, Sanchez-Villegas A, Pena-Quintana L, Mendez M, Serra-Majem L. Dietary assessment methods for micronutrient intake in infants, children and adolescents: a systematic review. Br J Nutr. 2009;102 Suppl 1:S87–117.
17. Tricon S, Willers S, Smit HA, Burney PG, Devereux G, Frew AJ, et al. Nutrition and allergic disease. Clin Exp Allergy Rev. 2006;6:117–88.
18. Dominguez-Ortega G, Meyer R, Dziubak R, De Koker C, Godwin H, Skrapak AK, et al. Gastrointestinal Food Allergy Assessment by a Symptom Questionnaire. EAACI-WOA Conference Proceedings. Abstract 2013, p 152.
19. Lanigan JA, Wells JC, Lawson MS, Lucas A. Validation of food diary method for assessment of dietary energy and macronutrient intake in infants and children aged 6–24 months. Eur J Clin Nutr. 2001;55:124–9.
20. Ocke M, Brants H, Dofkova M, Freisling H, van RC, Ruprich J, et al. Feasibility of dietary assessment methods, other tools and procedures for a pan-European food consumption survey among infants, toddlers and children. Eur J Nutr 2014. [E-Pub ahead of Print].
21. Food Standards Agency. Food Portion Sizes. 3rd ed. Norwich: The Stationary Office; 2011.
22. Scientific Advisory Commitee on Nutrition: The Nutritional Wellbeing of the British Population; Belfast, TSO, 2008, pp 1–162. ISBN 9780112432814.
23. European Food Safety Authority. Scientific Opinion on Dietary Reference Values. EFSA Journal. 2013;11(1):1–110.
24. Meyer R. Alternative Milks. Complete Nutrition. 2014;13:53–5.
25. Johnston GA, Bilbao RM, Graham-Brown RA. The use of complementary medicine in children with atopic dermatitis in secondary care in Leicester. Br J Dermatol. 2003;149:566–71.
26. Johnston GA, Bilbao RM, Graham-Brown RA. The use of dietary manipulation by parents of children with atopic dermatitis. Br J Dermatol. 2004;150:1186–9.
27. Venter C, Laitinen K, Vlieg-Boerstra B. Nutritional aspects in diagnosis and management of food hypersensitivity-the dietitians role. J Allergy. 2012;269376:1–11.
28. Meyer R, De KC, Dziubak R, Venter C, Dominguez-Ortega G, Cutts R, et al. Malnutrition in children with food allergies in the UK. J Hum Nutr Diet. 2014;27:227–2235.
29. Scientific Committee on Food. Report of the Scientific Committee on Food on the Revision of Essential Requirements of Infant Formulae and Follow-on Formulae.*SCF/CS/NUT/IF/65*. Brussels: European Commission; 2003. p. 1–213.
30. Allen LH, Haskell M. Estimating the potential for vitamin A toxicity in women and young children. J Nutr. 2002;132:2907S–19.
31. Greer FR. 25-Hydroxyvitamin D: functional outcomes in infants and young children. Am J Clin Nutr. 2008;88:529S–33.
32. Zipitis CS, Markides GA, Swann IL. Vitamin D deficiency: prevention or treatment? Arch Dis Child. 2006;91:1011–4.
33. Goldacre M, Hall N, Yeates DG. Hospitalisation for children with rickets in England: a historical perspective. Lancet. 2014;383:597–8.
34. Department of Health: Vitamin D an essential nutrient for all… but who is at risk of vitamin D defi ciency? 2009, https://www.gov.uk/government/news/dangers-of-vitamin-d-deficiency-highlighted
35. Department of Health: Dangers of vitamin D deficiency highlighted. Accessed 11/11/2014. http://webarchive.nationalarchives.gov.uk/+/www.dh.gov.uk/en/Healthcare/Children/Maternity/Maternalandinfantnutrition/DH_111304.
36. Akan A, Azkur D, Ginis T, Toyran M, Kaya A, Vezir E, et al. Vitamin D level in children is correlated with severity of atopic dermatitis but only in patients with allergic sensitizations. Pediatr Dermatol. 2013;30:359–63.
37. Ehlayel MS, Bener A, Sabbah A. Is high prevalence of vitamin D deficiency evidence for asthma and allergy risks? Eur Ann Allergy Clin Immunol. 2011;43:81–8.
38. Meyer R, De KC, Dziubak R, Godwin H, Dominguez-Ortega G, Shah N. Dietary elimination of children with food protein induced gastrointestinal allergy - micronutrient adequacy with and without a hypoallergenic formula? Clin Transl Allergy. 2014;4:31–29.
39. Kamer B, Wasowicz W, Pyziak K, Kamer-Bartosinska A, Gromadzinska J, Pasowska R. Role of selenium and zinc in the pathogenesis of food allergy in infants and young children. Arch Med Sci. 2012;8:1083–8.

Heterogeneous responses and cross reactivity between the major peanut allergens Ara h 1, 2, 3 and 6 in a mouse model for peanut allergy

Joost J Smit[1,2*], Maarten T Pennings[2,3,5], Karina Willemsen[1], Manon van Roest[1], Els van Hoffen[3,4] and Raymond H Pieters[1]

Abstract

Background: The relative contribution and the relation between individual peanut allergens in peanut allergic responses is still matter of debate. We determined the individual contribution of peanut proteins to B, T cell and allergic effector responses in a mouse model for peanut allergy.

Methods: Mice were immunized and challenged by oral gavage with peanut protein extract or isolated allergens Ara h 1, 2, 3 and 6 followed by assessment of food allergic manifestations. In addition, T cell responses to the individual proteins were measured by an *in vitro* dendritic cell-T cell assay.

Results: Sensitization with the individual peanut proteins elicited IgE responses with specificity to the allergen used as expected. However, cross reactivity among Ara h 1, 2, 3 and 6 was observed. T cell re-stimulations with peanut extract and individual peanut proteins also showed cross reactivity between Ara h 1, 2, 3 and 6. Despite the cross reactivity at the IgE level, only Ara h 2 and 6 were able to elicit mast cell degranulation after an oral challenge. However, after systemic challenge, Ara h 1, 2 and 6 and to lesser extent Ara h 3 were able to elicit anaphylactic responses.

Conclusions: Ara h 1, 2, 3 and 6 sensitize via the intra-gastric route, but differ in their capacity to cause allergic effector responses. Interestingly, extensive cross reactivity at T cell and antibody level is observed among Ara h 1, 2, 3 and 6, which may have important implications for the diagnosis and therapy of peanut allergy. Awareness about the relative contribution of individual peanut allergens and cross reactivity between these allergens is of importance for current research in diagnostics and therapeutics for and the mechanism of peanut allergy.

Keywords: Cross-reactivity, IgE, Peanut allergy, Peanut proteins, T cell, Mouse model, Sensitization, Anaphylaxis

Background

Sensitization to peanut is characterized by the presence of IgE to a number of peanut allergens. Up till now, thirteen peanut allergens, designated Ara h 1–13, are recognized by the WHO/IUS allergen nomenclature subcommittee [1]. Literature suggests that the major allergens in peanut are Ara h 1, 2, 3, and 6, as defined by frequent and prominent IgE binding from patient sera [2-4]. Ara h 1 is a member of the 7/8 S globulin (vicilin) family of seed storage proteins belonging to the cupin superfamily. Ara h 2 and Ara h 6 are members of the 2S albumins (conglutinins) belonging to the prolamin superfamily and are 59% homologous to each other. Importantly, the C terminus of Ara h 2 has some homology with other peanut proteins, specifically with Ara h 6 [5]. Ara h 3 is a 11S globulin (legumins/glycinins) that belongs to the cupin superfamily [2,6].

Importantly, mono-sensitization to a single peanut allergen is rare. Moreover, as extensively reviewed in [7,8], cross reactivity between peanut proteins and tree nut proteins and other allergens are common, even among different protein families. However, clinical studies on cross-reactivity at IgE level between peanut proteins

* Correspondence: j.j.smit@uu.nl
[1]Immunotoxicology group, Institute for Risk Assessment Sciences, Utrecht University, Utrecht, The Netherlands
[2]Utrecht Centre for Food Allergy, Utrecht, The Netherlands
Full list of author information is available at the end of the article

themselves are limited to one study [9] and data on cross reactivity at T cell level are completely lacking. Therefore, we studied 1) the potency of peanut extract (PE) and individual native (not recombinant) peanut proteins Ara h 1, 2, 3 and 6 to induce food allergic manifestations and 2) possible cross reactivity of IgE antibodies and T-cells between Ara h 1, 2, 3 and 6 proteins. For this purpose, we used a well-established mouse model, which has been widely used for many years and has been shown to mimic the clinical and immunological characteristics of human peanut allergy [10-13]. The advantage of these models is the generation of mono-sensitized individual mice, essential for the study of possible cross reactivity. For this purpose, we used well-defined, highly purified, native peanut proteins, which have been used in several previous mouse and human studies [3,4,14,15]. In this model, we observed extensive cross reactivity among peanut proteins at both T cell and IgE level in our models of peanut allergy. In addition, we confirmed that Ara h 2 and 6 are the main cause of effector responses such as mast cell degranulation and anaphylaxis.

Awareness about the relative contribution of individual peanut allergens and cross reactivity between the major peanut proteins is of importance for current research in the fields of diagnostics and therapeutics (including immunotherapy) and for our complete understanding of the mechanism of peanut allergy.

Materials and methods

Mice

Five-week-old specific pathogen-free female C3H/HeOuJ mice were purchased from Charles River (France) and housed under specific pathogen-free conditions within the animal care facility at the Utrecht University. Experiments were approved by the Animal Experiments Committee of the Utrecht University.

Peanut, Ara h 1, 2, 3 and 6 sensitization and challenge

Raw peanuts were kindly provided by Intersnack BV (the Netherlands) and peanut extract (PE) was prepared as previously described [16]. Importantly, we used the same Ara h 1, 2, 3 and 6 preparations used and described before, with a purity of 95-99% as determined by SDS-PAGE electrophoresis and coomassie brilliant blue staining [3,4,15]. Lipopolysaccharide content, as determined by a limulus amoebocyte lysate assay (Cambrex Bio Science, Walkersville, MD, USA), of the peanut allergens was below 0.001 EU/mg protein. All proteins were dissolved and dosed in PBS. Cholera toxin (CT) was obtained from List Biological Laboratories, Inc. (CA, USA). To elicit oral sensitization to peanut proteins, 8 mice were intragastrically (i.g.) dosed by gavage with 6 mg PE or 250 μg Ara h 1, 2, 3, or 6 plus 15 μg CT per mouse for three consecutive days, and this was repeated every week for four weeks (exposure on days 0, 1, 2, 7, 14, 21 and 28). Control groups received PBS plus 15 μg CT. Mice received an i.g. challenge dose of 12 mg PE or 500 μg Ara h 1, 2, 3, or 6 on day 35, were bled after 30 minutes and sacrificed one day later. In separate experiments, 8 mice were i.g. sensitized with PE as described above, and challenged i.p. with 500 μg Ara h 1, 2, 3, or 6. After this systemic challenge, body temperature was measured by means of rectal thermometry every 10–20 minutes for 90 minutes after challenge. In addition, clinical symptoms were scored using a scoring system, as used before [17].

Measurement of PE, Ara h 1, 2, 3, and 6-specific antibodies, MMCP-I and histamine in blood

PE, Ara h 1, 2, 3, and 6-specific IgE in serum obtained on day 28 was analyzed by ELISA as described previously [14,18]. This protocol was amended: a positive pool serum derived from PE/alum-sensitized mice was used as reference value to calculate arbitrary units (AU). For detection of specific IgE, PE, Ara h 1, 2, 3 and/or 6 was coupled to DIG. This coupling was performed according to the manufacturer's instructions (Roche, The Netherlands) and coupled proteins were separated on a sephadex G-25 column and labeling efficiency was determined spectrophotometrically at 280 nm. In addition, plasma was collected within 45 minutes after oral challenge, and MMCP-I was determined in this plasma using a ELISA kit according to instructions of the manufacturer (eBioscience, Austria). Histamine was measured in plasma using a commercial EIA assay (Immunotech, France).

Cell culture and cytokine measurement

Spleen single cell suspensions (2.5×10^6/ml) were incubated in the presence or absence of PE, Ara h 1, 2, 3 or 6 (100 μg/ml) for 96 h at 37°C in complete RPMI1640 with 10% FCS. Culture supernatants were harvested and stored at –20°C until analysis. Levels of IL-5 and IL-13 in culture supernatants were determined by sandwich ELISA according to the instructions of the manufacturers (eBioscience, Austria). The detection limit is 5 pg/ml for both ELISA's.

Dendritic cell/T cell assay

This assay was used as described before [13]. In short, 2–3 C3H/HeOuJ mice were immunized with 100 μg PE, Ara h 1, 2, 3 or 6 bound to imject-alum (Pierce, USA) on day 0 and 14. After 29 days, the CD4+ T cells were isolated from spleen single cell suspensions using magnetic beads (Stemcell Technologies, France). Bone marrow cells from C3H/HeOuJ mice was cultured for 6 days with GM-CSF, after which the bone marrow-derived dendritic cells (DC) were pulsed overnight with 50 μg/ml PE Ara h 1, 2, 3 or 6. The CD4+ T cells were incubated for 72 h with protein-pulsed dendritic cells.

Hereafter, IL-5 and IL-13 production was analyzed by sandwich ELISA (eBioscience, Austria).

Statistical analysis

Data are presented as means ± standard error of the mean (SEM) and analyzed using GraphPad Prism software. Antibody, MMCP-I and cytokine levels were logarithmic transformed followed by a one-way ANOVA and Bonferroni as a post-hoc test. Temperature curves were statistically analyzed using a repeated measures ANOVA and clinical scores were statistically analyzed by the Kruskall-Wallis test.

Results

PE, Ara h 1, 2, 3, or 6-specific antibody and T cell responses in mice

Peanut allergen-specific IgE responses were compared in mice intragastrically exposed to PE, Ara h 1, 2, 3 or 6 with CT. Sensitization with PE induced Ara h 1, 2, 3 and 6 specific IgE (Figure 1). Sensitization with the individual peanut proteins led to the induction of IgE antibody responses with specificity to the allergen used (Figure 1). In addition, although generally at levels lower than the sensitizing allergen, extensive cross reactivity was observed between peanut proteins, since Ara h 1, 2, 3 and

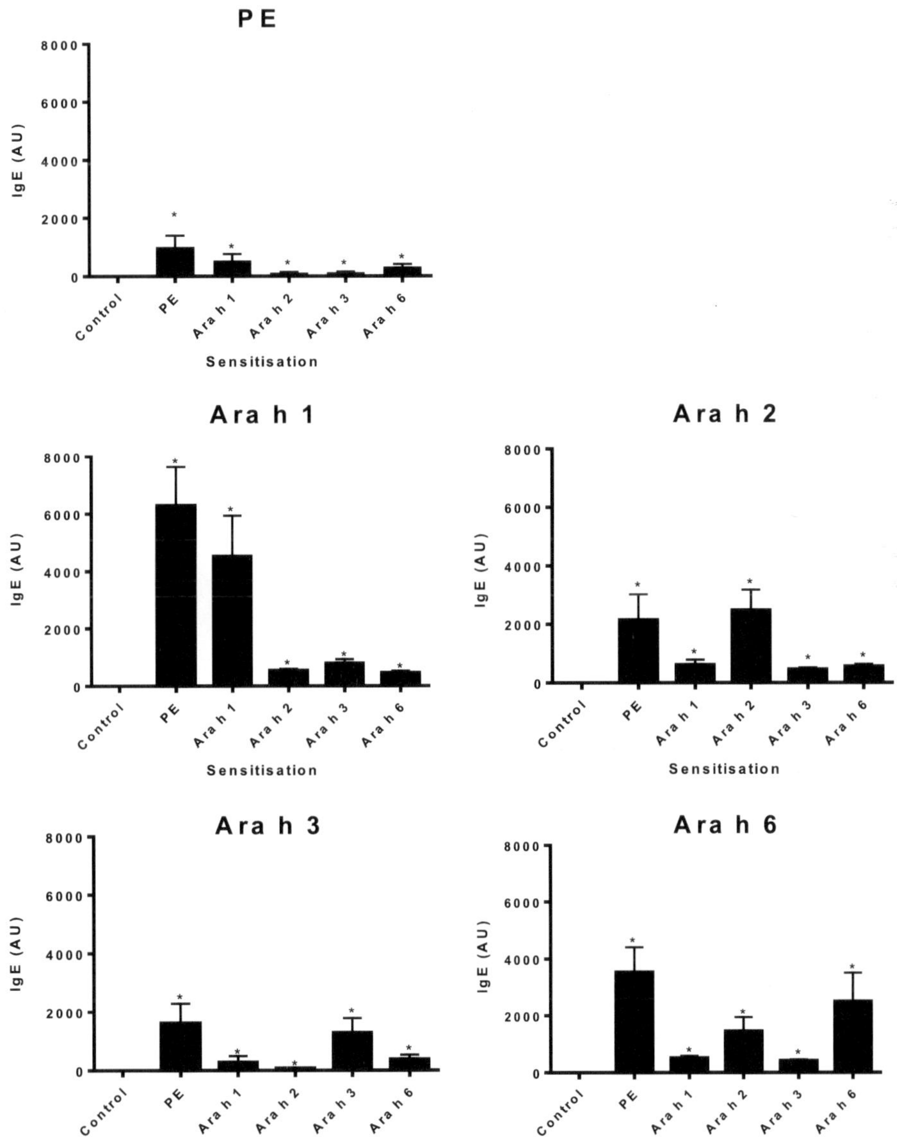

Figure 1 IgE responses after intragastric sensitization. C3H/HeOuJ mice were intragastrically exposed to PBS, (control) PE, or Ara h 1, 2, 3, or 6 and CT during a 4 week period, as described in material and methods. Graphs depict serum levels of PE, Ara h 1, 2, 3, or 6 specific IgE in arbitrary units (AU) at day 36. Data are represented as mean ± SEM of 8 mice. *: $p < 0.01$ compared to control.

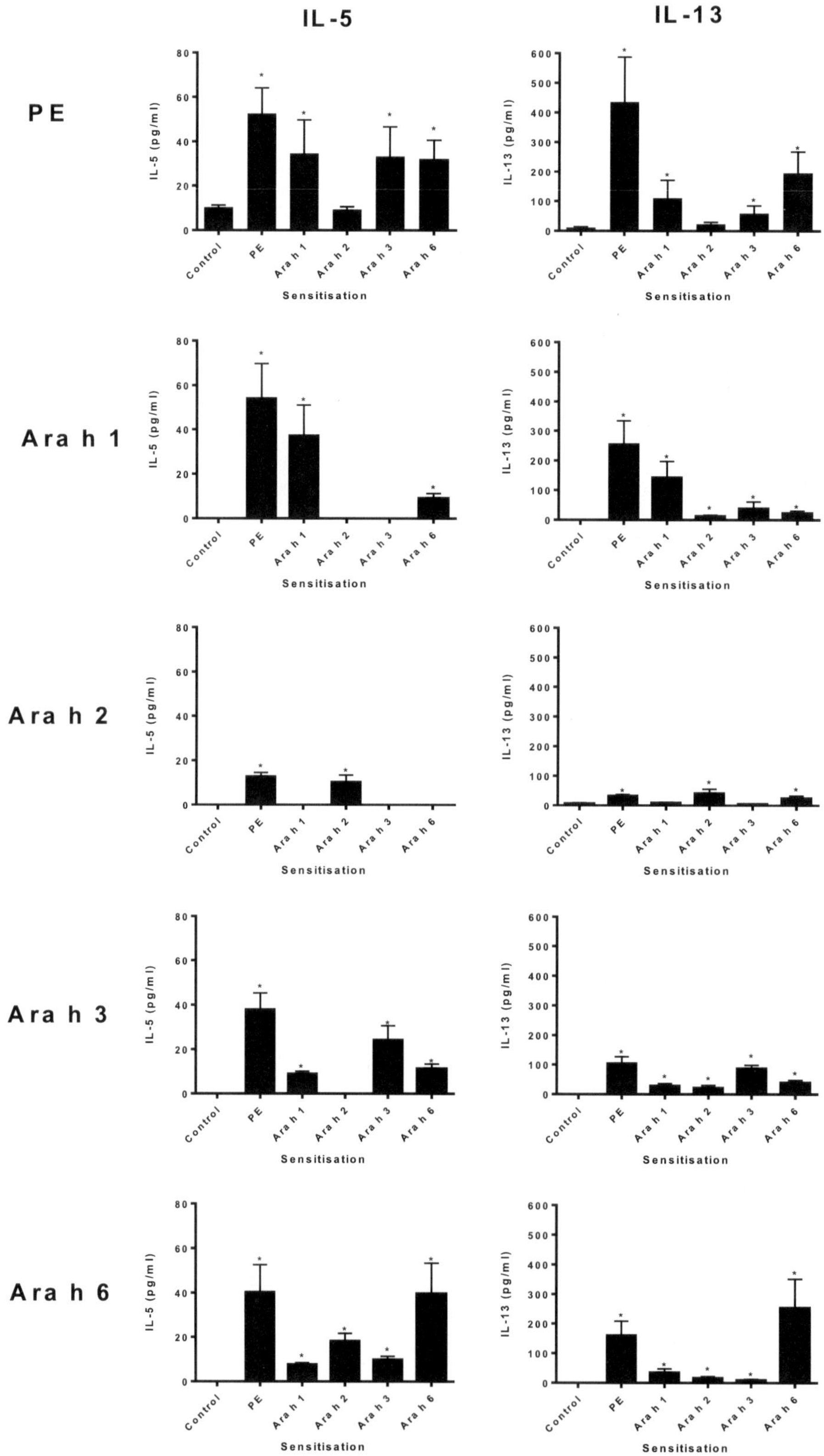

Figure 2 Splenic T cell responses after intragastric sensitization. C3H/HeOuJ mice were intragastrically exposed to PBS (control), PE, or Ara h 1, 2, 3, or 6 and CT during a 4 week period, as described in material and methods. Spleens were isolated and stimulated with medium alone or PE, or Ara h 1, 2, 3, or 6. Graphs depict levels of IL-5 and IL-13 after stimulation. Data are represented as mean ± SEM of 8 mice. *: $p < 0.05$ compared to control.

6 specific IgE antibodies were detected in all sensitized groups (Figure 1).

Next, spleen cells of mice sensitized with PE, Ara h 1, 2, 3, or 6 were restimulated with these respective proteins. Sensitization with PE, followed by restimulation with PE, Ara h 1, 2, 3, or 6 led to induction of the Th2 cytokines IL-5, IL-13 (Figure 2). In addition, PE restimulation of spleens derived from Ara h 1, 3, or 6 sensitized mice induced the same cytokine response. Restimulation with Ara h 2, however, led to lower Th2 cytokine responses in all groups. Furthermore, restimulation with the individual peanut proteins led to the induction of Th2 responses not only in mice of the same sensitizing allergen, but also in mice sensitized with one of the other peanut allergens. This cross reactivity was observed in Ara h 1, 3 and 6 sensitized mice for both IL-5 and IL-13. Despite that responses were generally lower, IL-13 could be measured in Ara h 2-sensitized mice after restimulation with Ara h 1, 3 and 6. IL-5 was measured in small amounts after restimulation with Ara h 2 and 6 in Ara h 2-sensitized mice. Results of both specific IgE and cytokine production *in vivo* are summarized in Table 1.

DC-T cell responses to PE, Ara h 1, 2, 3 and 6

In order to further investigate whether the observed cross reactivity originated at the level of DC-T cell interaction, a sensitive and specific (using purified CD4+ T cells) *in vitro* DC-T cell assay was used. Mice were immunized intraperitoneally by Ara h 1, 2, 3, or 6/alum injection, which led to comparable levels of specific IgG (data not shown) demonstrating that T cell responses to Ara h 1, 2, 3, and 6 did develop. Importantly, no IgG cross-reactivity was observed between mice sensitized for Ara h 1, 2, 3 and 6/alum (data not shown). Restimulation of CD4+ T cells derived from Ara h 1, 2, 3, or 6-immunized mice with PE, Ara h 1, 2, 3, or 6-pulsed DC resulted in production of IL-5 and IL-13 (Figure 3). Both Th2 cytokines were induced most effectively in T cells derived from Ara h 1, 3, or 6 sensitized mice after pulsing of DC with PE or the corresponding allergen. In this assay, pulsing with Ara h 2 did not lead to cytokine production from CD4+ T cells. Importantly, also in this assay, extensive cross reactivity was observed among Ara h 1, 3 and 6, as summarized in Table 2.

Table 1 Summary of PE, Ara h 1, 2, 3 and 6 specific IgE and T cell responses *in vivo* (Figures 1 and 2)

Specific IgE					
→ IgE					
↓ sensitization	PE	Ara h 1	Ara h 2	Ara h 3	Ara h 6
PE	+++	+++	++	++	++
Ara h 1	++	+++	+	+	+
Ara h 2	+	+	++	+	++
Ara h 3	+	+	+	++	+
Ara h 6	++	+	+	+	++
Spleen T cell responses (IL-5 and IL-13)					
→ restim.					
↓ sensitization	PE	Ara h 1	Ara h 2	Ara h 3	Ara h 6
PE	+++	++	+/−	++	++
Ara h 1	++	++	-	+	+
Ara h 2	+	-, +(IL-13)	+/−	+	+
Ara h 3	+	-, +(IL-13)	-	++	+
Ara h 6	++	+	-, +/−(IL-13)	+	++

Mast cell degranulation and systemic anaphylaxis

Subsequently, it was assessed whether the antibody and T cell responses to Ara h 1, 2, 3 and 6 would lead to clinical manifestations of food allergy as well. First, mucosal mast cell degranulation was measured after intra-gastric challenge with PE, Ara h 1, 2, 3 and 6 in correspondingly sensitized mice by measuring mMCP-1 and histamine in plasma. Interestingly, only PE, Ara h 2 and 6 were able to induce mucosal mast cell degranulation and histamine release in sensitized mice (Figure 4).

Intragastric challenge with PE or Ara h 1, 2, 3 or 6 did not lead to anaphylactic symptoms in sensitized mice, as also described before [11]. Therefore, control or PE-sensitized mice were intraperitoneal challenged with PE or Ara h 1, 2, 3, 6 and changes in temperature were measured. An anaphylactic response, reflected by a strong drop in temperature, was observed in PE-sensitized mice after challenge with PE, Ara h 1, 2, 3 and 6 (Figure 5). However, this drop in temperature was significantly less in Ara h 3 challenged mice compared to other sensitized groups. The systemic injection of control, naive mice with peanut or Ara h 1, 2, 3 and 6 did not lead to any anaphylactic responses (Figure 5).

Discussion

In the present study, we demonstrated that Ara h 1, 2, 3 and 6 are individually able to sensitize mice via the intra-gastric route, as measured by induction of IgE and Th2 type cytokines. Despite the sensitizing capacity of Ara h 1, 2, 3 and 6, only Ara h 2 and 6 were able to elicit mast cell degranulation after intra-gastric challenge. These data append earlier studies from our lab and others which showed that sensitization with peanut extract induces Ara h 1, 2, 3, 6 specific responses [14] and that Ara h 2 and 6 are the main cause of effector responses [5,19], including anaphylaxis, in mouse models. In addition, human clinical and *in vitro* data showed that although the large majority of patients show Ara h 1, 2, 3 and 6 specific IgE responses, Ara h 2 and 6 are the main cause of mast cell or basophil effector responses

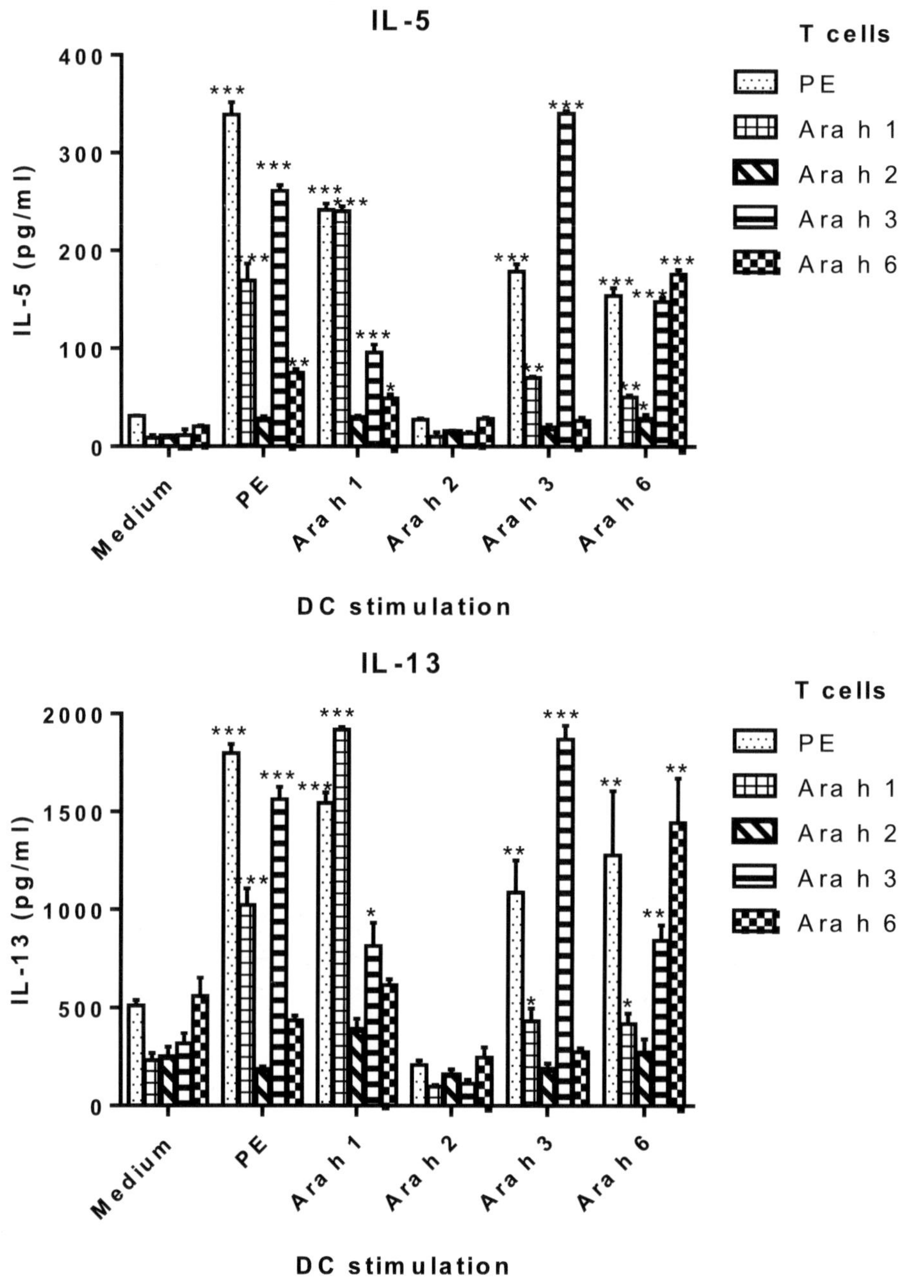

Figure 3 Dendritic cell -T cell responses to peanut proteins ex vivo. Bone marrow derived dendritic cells were pulsed overnight with PE, Ara h 1, 2, 3 or 6. Hereafter, these dendritic cells were incubated for 72 h with splenic CD4+ T cells derived from mice immunized with PE, Ara h 1, 2, 3 or 6. Graphs depict levels of IL-5 and IL-13 after stimulation. Shown is a representative of 3 experiments and data are represented as mean ± SEM of quadruplicates. *: $p < 0.05$, **: $p < 0.01$ or ***: $p < 0.001$ compared to medium control.

[3,4,9]. After systemic challenge however, Ara h 1, 2 and 6 and to lesser extent Ara h 3 were able to elicit anaphylactic responses. Differences in studies may have been caused by the use of native purified proteins in our studies instead of depleted peanut extracts but possibly also by cross reactivity among these proteins, as shown in the present study and discussed above.

Interestingly, restimulation of splenocytes or CD4+ T cells from mono-sensitized mice in our studies showed similar T cell responses compared to the restimulation of short-term Ara h 1, 2, 3 or 6 specific T cell lines from young allergic patients [20]. In both mouse and human assays, Ara h 2 is a poor stimulator of T cell responses, while the other peanut proteins induce significant Th2

Table 2 Summary of PE, Ara h 1, 2, 3 and 6 specific T cell responses after pulsing with dendritic cells (DC) *in vitro* (Figure 3)

→ DC ↓ T cell	PE	Ara h 1	Ara h 2	Ara h 3	Ara h 6
PE	+++	+++	-	++	+++
Ara h 1	++	+++	-	+	+
Ara h 2	-	-	-	-	-
Ara h 3	+++	+	-	+++	++
Ara h 6	-, +(IL-5)	-, +(IL-5)	-	-	+++

type responses. However, others have found T cell responses after stimulation with Ara h 2 [21,22] or Ara h 2/6 [23]. Differences in Ara h 2 preparations (which are made using different denaturing agents for instance), T cell selection, age of the patients and use of short-term versus long-term T cell lines may account for these differences. We cannot explain the lower or even lack of T cell stimulation by Ara h 2 *ex vivo* and *in vitro* in our studies. In contrast, Ara h 6, which is 60% homologous to Ara h 2 [2] was able to stimulate T cells in our and the human studies [20]. Since mice and human do develop T cell-dependent IgE responses to Ara h 2 *in vivo*, we believe that the lack of T cell stimulation by Ara h 2 may be caused by the high stability and lack of degradation of this protein by DC *in vitro* [24].

Importantly, extensive cross reactivity among Ara h 1, 2, 3 and 6 at the level of IgE was observed, although at a level always lower than for the specific sensitizing allergen. Moreover, splenic T cell re-stimulations, *ex vivo* and *in vitro*, also showed cross reactivity between Ara h 1, 3 and 6. This cross reactivity as observed is dependent on purity and possible contamination of Ara h 1, 2, 3 and 6. The purity of the proteins used in this study has been described in several previous publications and varies around 99% [4]. This small percentage of possible contamination is unlikely to have caused the level of cross reactivity observed. In both the animal dosing (<2.5 μg) and detection ELISA (<0.1 μg/ml) the contamination would have been too low to cause contaminative responses almost to the same level as the original protein. Importantly, we did not observe IgG cross-reactivity between mice intraperitoneal sensitized for Ara h 1, 2, 3 in the presence of alum. This indicates that although minute contaminants of other proteins may still be present in individual allergen preparations, these are not responsible for our findings.

The observed cross reactivity is not completely unexpected. Previously, it has been shown that Ara h 1, 2 and 3 display a high extent of cross-reactivity at the IgE level, using peanut allergic patient sera [9]. This may be surprising given the fact that Ara h 1 and 3 belong to the cupin protein family and Ara h 2 and 6 to the 2S albumins, without any clear structural or alignment sequence similarities. Nonetheless, previous studies showed the occurrence of similar epitopes among peanut allergens by IgE binding [9] or biochemical sequence similarities [25]. Functional cross reactivity between proteins of different protein families is rare, but occurs. For instance, it was shown that peanut Ara h 2 was cross-reactive with the walnut allergen Jug r 2 belonging to the different vicilin protein family [26]. However, despite the observed extensive cross reactivity among the peanut allergens in our studies, distinct Ara h 1, 2, 3 and 6-specific epitopes are present which are not shared among the other peanut allergens. This was shown in the already mentioned human IgE inhibition studies [9], but also in our experiments, since the cross reactivity resulted usually in a lower level of IgE or Th2 cytokine production, when compared to the sensitizing allergen. In addition, the observed cross reactivity may even extend to the level of clinical responses, when comparing the occurrence of anaphylaxis between all groups.

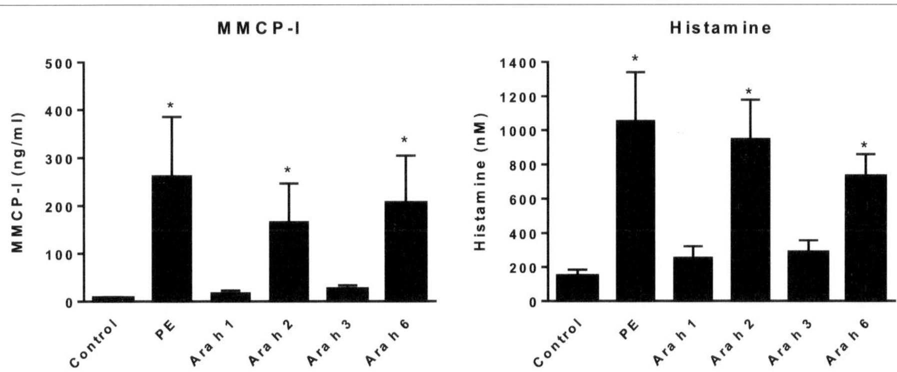

Figure 4 Mucosal mast cell degranulation after intragastric challenge with Ara h 1, 2, 3, or 6. C3H/HeOuJ mice were intragastrically exposed to PBS, (control) PE, or Ara h 1, 2, 3, or 6 and CT during a 4 week period, as described in material and methods. On day 35, mice received an i.g. challenge of PE or Ara h 1, 2, 3, or 6, depending on the protein used during sensitization, followed by blood withdrawal. Graphs depict the level of MMCP-I and histamine in plasma. Data are represented as mean ± SEM of 8 mice. *: $p < 0.05$ compared to control.

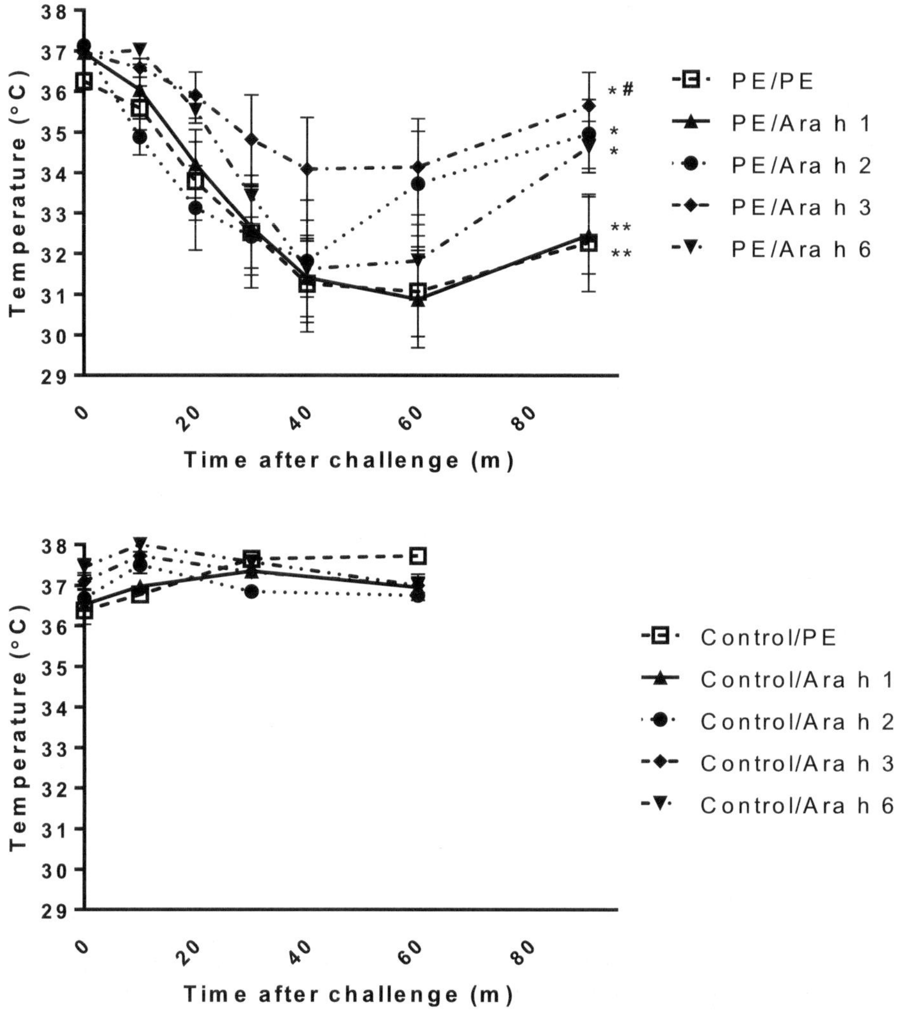

Figure 5 Anaphylaxis after systemic challenge with Ara h 1, 2, 3, or 6. C3H/HeOuJ mice were intragastrically exposed to PBS, (control) or PE and CT during a 4 week period, as described in material and methods. On day 35, mice received a systemic i.p. challenge with PE or Ara h 1, 2, 3, or 6, directly followed by measurement of rectal temperature at indicated time points after challenge. Upper panel shows the PE sensitized mice, lower panel shows the not sensitized control mice. Data are represented as mean ± SEM of 8 mice. *: $p < 0.05$ or **: $p < 0.01$ compared to control. #: $p < 0.05$ compared to PE challenged mice.

Cross reactivity between Ara h 1, 2, 3 and 6 may have several implications. First, cross reactivity may explain the multiple sensitization patterns to peanut. Most peanut allergic patients develop IgE to multiple peanut proteins, mostly to Ara h 1, 2, 3, and 6 [3,27]. In addition, both the increased diversity of epitopes recognized and higher level of IgE binding correlated with the severity of the clinical reaction to peanut [27,28]. Unfortunately, due to the limited amount of mouse serum an extensive mapping of epitope binding could not be performed in our studies. Second, the observed cross reactivity, especially at the level of IgE, may have consequences for the diagnostics of Ara h 1, 2, 3, 6-specific responses. Seemingly specific peanut allergen responses in peanut allergic patients may be caused by cross reactivity in the used assay with other peanut proteins. Third, cross reactivity may be used in (immune-) therapy for peanut allergy. Mouse studies already suggested that immunotherapy with Ara h 2/6 was able to inhibit clinical responses after whole peanut extract challenge in peanut sensitized mice [19]. These clinical responses are dependent only on Ara h 2/6, but we can envision that immunotherapy with Ara h 2/6 could not only be effective in lowering responses to this particular allergen but also to other cross reactive peanut proteins.

Conclusions

In summary, we showed that cross reactivity among the main peanut allergens may exist at the IgE and T cell level, and that DC- T cell interactions underlie this cross reactivity. In addition, we showed that, depending on the route of provocation, Ara h 2 and 6 are the peanut allergens causing clinical responses in our model. These data complement the very limited human clinical studies on peanut allergen cross reactivity, but more research is needed on where and how the immune system recognizes and processes these peanut allergens. This study provides substantial new information on the capacity of peanut allergens to cause sensitization and food allergy, and may have important consequences for diagnostics and immunotherapy of peanut allergy.

Abbreviations

PE: Peanut extract; DC: Dendritic cell; CT: Cholera toxin; AU: Arbitrary units.

Competing interests

All authors of this manuscript declare that they do not have a conflict of interest including relevant financial interests, activities, relationships, and affiliation.

Authors' contributions

JS was responsible for the conception and design, acquisition, analysis, and interpretation of data analyzed and was responsible for writing this manuscript as first author. MP and EH assisted with the acquisition and interpretation of data and critically revising for important intellectual content. KW and MR assisted with the acquisition and analysis of data. RP was responsible for the interpretation of data and critically revising for important intellectual content. All authors have given final approval of the version to be published.

Acknowledgement

The authors would like to acknowledge Stef Koppelman and Aard de Jong at TNO, Zeist, the Netherlands for the initial isolation and purification of Ara h 1, 2, 3 and 6.

Author details

[1]Immunotoxicology group, Institute for Risk Assessment Sciences, Utrecht University, Utrecht, The Netherlands. [2]Utrecht Centre for Food Allergy, Utrecht, The Netherlands. [3]Utrecht University Medical Center, Utrecht, The Netherlands. [4]Current affiliation: NIZO food research BV, Ede, The Netherlands. [5]Current affiliation: HU University of Applied Sciences, Utrecht, The Netherlands.

References

1. Radauer C, Nandy A, Ferreira F, Goodman RE, Larsen JN, Lidholm J, et al. Update of the WHO/IUIS Allergen Nomenclature Database based on analysis of allergen sequences. Allergy. 2014;69:413–9.
2. Zhuang Y, Dreskin SC. Redefining the major peanut allergens. Immunol Res. 2013;55:125–34.
3. Flinterman AE, van Hoffen E, den Hartog Jager CF, Koppelman S, Pasmans SG, Hoekstra MO, et al. Children with peanut allergy recognize predominantly Ara h2 and Ara h6, which remains stable over time. Clin Exp Allergy. 2007;37:1221–8.
4. Koppelman SJ, Wensing M, Ertmann M, Knulst AC, Knol EF. Relevance of Ara h1, Ara h2 and Ara h3 in peanut-allergic patients, as determined by immunoglobulin E Western blotting, basophil-histamine release and intracutaneous testing: Ara h2 is the most important peanut allergen. Clin Exp Allergy. 2004;34:583–90.
5. Porterfield HS, Murray KS, Schlichting DG, Chen X, Hansen KC, Duncan MW, et al. Effector activity of peanut allergens: a critical role for Ara h 2, Ara h 6, and their variants. Clin Exp Allergy. 2009;39:1099–108.
6. Radauer C, Bublin M, Wagner S, Mari A, Breiteneder H. Allergens are distributed into few protein families and possess a restricted number of biochemical functions. J Allergy Clin Immunol. 2008;121:847–52.e7.
7. Bublin M, Breiteneder H. Cross-reactivity of peanut allergens. Curr Allergy Asthma Rep. 2014;14:426.
8. Kulis M, Pons L, Burks AW. In vivo and T cell cross-reactivity between walnut, cashew and peanut. Int Arch Allergy Immunol. 2009;148:109–17.
9. Bublin M, Kostadinova M, Radauer C, Hafner C, Szépfalusi Z, Varga E-M, et al. IgE cross-reactivity between the major peanut allergen Ara h 2 and the nonhomologous allergens Ara h 1 and Ara h 3. J Allergy Clin Immunol. 2013;132:118–24.
10. Li XM, Serebrisky D, Lee SY, Huang CK, Bardina L, Schofield BH, et al. A murine model of peanut anaphylaxis: T- and B-cell responses to a major peanut allergen mimic human responses. J Allergy Clin Immunol. 2000;106(1 Pt 1):150–8.
11. Smit JJ, Willemsen K, Hassing I, Fiechter D, Storm G, van Bloois L, et al. Contribution of classic and alternative effector pathways in peanut-induced anaphylactic responses. PLoS One. 2011;6:e28917.
12. Arias K, Chu DK, Flader K, Botelho F, Walker T, Arias N, et al. Distinct immune effector pathways contribute to the full expression of peanut-induced anaphylactic reactions in mice. J Allergy Clin Immunol. 2011;127:1552–61.e1.
13. Pochard P, Vickery B, Berin MC, Grishin A, Sampson HA, Caplan M, et al. Targeting Toll-like receptors on dendritic cells modifies the T(H)2 response to peanut allergens in vitro. J Allergy Clin Immunol. 2010;126:92–7.e5.
14. Van Wijk F, Hartgring S, Koppelman SJ, Pieters R, Knippels LMJ. Mixed antibody and T cell responses to peanut and the peanut allergens Ara h 1, Ara h 2, Ara h 3 and Ara h 6 in an oral sensitization model. Clin Exp Allergy. 2004;34:1422–8.
15. Koppelman SJ, Knol EF, Vlooswijk RAA, Wensing M, Knulst AC, Hefle SL, et al. Peanut allergen Ara h 3: isolation from peanuts and biochemical characterization. Allergy. 2003;58:1144–51.
16. Mittag D, Akkerdaas J, Ballmer-Weber BK, Vogel L, Wensing M, Becker W-M, et al. Ara h 8, a Bet v 1-homologous allergen from peanut, is a major allergen in patients with combined birch pollen and peanut allergy. J Allergy Clin Immunol. 2004;114:1410–7.
17. Sun J, Arias K, Alvarez D, Fattouh R, Walker T, Goncharova S, et al. Impact of CD40 ligand, B cells, and mast cells in peanut-induced anaphylactic responses. J Immunol. 2007;179:6696–703.
18. Smit JJ, Bol-Schoenmakers M, Hassing I, Fiechter D, Boon L, Bleumink R, et al. The role of intestinal dendritic cells subsets in the establishment of food allergy. Clin Exp Allergy. 2011;41:890–8.
19. Kulis M, Chen X, Lew J, Wang Q, Patel OP, Zhuang Y, et al. The 2S albumin allergens of Arachis hypogaea, Ara h 2 and Ara h 6, are the major elicitors of anaphylaxis and can effectively desensitize peanut-allergic mice. Clin Exp Allergy. 2012;42:326–36.
20. Flinterman AE, Pasmans SGMA, den Hartog Jager CF, Hoekstra MO, Bruijnzeel-Koomen CAFM, Knol EF, et al. T cell responses to major peanut allergens in children with and without peanut allergy. Clin Exp Allergy. 2010;40:590–7.
21. Prickett SR, Voskamp AL, Dacumos-Hill A, Symons K, Rolland JM, O'Hehir RE. Ara h 2 peptides containing dominant CD4+ T-cell epitopes: candidates for a peanut allergy therapeutic. J Allergy Clin Immunol. 2011;127:608–15.e1–5.
22. Starkl P, Felix F, Krishnamurthy D, Stremnitzer C, Roth-Walter F, Prickett SR, et al. An unfolded variant of the major peanut allergen Ara h 2 with decreased anaphylactic potential. Clin Exp Allergy. 2012;42:1801–12.
23. Vissers YM, Blanc F, Skov PS, Johnson PE, Rigby NM, Przybylski-Nicaise L, et al. Effect of heating and glycation on the allergenicity of 2S albumins (Ara h 2/6) from peanut. PLoS One. 2011;6:e23998.
24. Koppelman SJ, Hefle SL, Taylor SL, de Jong GAH. Digestion of peanut allergens Ara h 1, Ara h 2, Ara h 3, and Ara h 6: a comparative in vitro study and partial characterization of digestion-resistant peptides. Mol Nutr Food Res. 2010;54:1711–21.
25. Schein CH, Ivanciuc O, Braun W. Common physical-chemical properties correlate with similar structure of the IgE epitopes of peanut allergens. J Agric Food Chem. 2005;53:8752–9.
26. Maleki SJ, Teuber SS, Cheng H, Chen D, Comstock SS, Ruan S, et al. Computationally predicted IgE epitopes of walnut allergens contribute to cross-reactivity with peanuts. Allergy. 2011;66:1522–9.
27. Shreffler WG, Beyer K, Chu T-HT, Burks AW, Sampson HA. Microarray immunoassay: association of clinical history, in vitro IgE function, and heterogeneity of allergenic peanut epitopes. J Allergy Clin Immunol. 2004;113:776–82.
28. Lewis SA, Grimshaw KEC, Warner JO, Hourihane JO. The promiscuity of immunoglobulin E binding to peanut allergens, as determined by Western blotting, correlates with the severity of clinical symptoms. Clin Exp Allergy. 2005;35:767–73.

16

Atopic dermatitis prevention in children following maternal probiotic supplementation does not appear to be mediated by breast milk TSLP or TGF-β

Melanie Rae Simpson[1,4*], Anne Dorthea Bjerkenes Rø[1,2], Øystein Grimstad[3], Roar Johnsen[1], Ola Storrø[1] and Torbjørn Øien[1]

Abstract

Background: The Probiotics in Prevention of Allergy among Children in Trondheim (ProPACT) study, a randomised, placebo controlled trial, demonstrated that maternal supplementation with probiotic milk reduced the incidence of atopic dermatitis (AD) in infancy. The mechanisms behind this effect are incompletely understood and breast milk cytokines have been postulated as possible mediating factors. In this study we aimed to assess whether breast milk TLSP and TGF-β are affected by a maternal probiotic supplementation regime, and their contribution to the preventive effect of this regime on AD in the offspring.

Methods: TSLP and TGF-β isoforms (TGF-β_1, TGF-β_2 and TGF-β_3) were measured using ELISA and multiplex assays, respectively, in breast milk samples collected at 10 days and 3 months postpartum from women participating in the ProPACT trial ($n = 259$). The natural indirect and direct effects of maternal probiotics on AD, due to changes in breast milk cytokines, were estimated using causal mediation techniques.

Results: Probiotic supplementation tend to lead to high levels of breast milk TSLP at 10 days postpartum ($p = 0.062$), but this change did not contribute to the prevention of AD according to the mediation analysis. Probiotics had no apparent effect on TSLP at 3 months or TGF-βs at either time points. Thus, these are unlikely to be mediators of the effect of maternal probiotics on AD in offspring.

Conclusions: Whilst maternal probiotic supplementation resulted in higher breast milk concentrations of TLSP at 10 days postpartum, this does not appear to be a mechanism for prevention of AD by maternal probiotics.

Trial registration The original trial protocol is registered in ClinicalTrials.gov (identifier NCT00159523)

Background

Perinatal supplementation with probiotics has been shown to reduce the incidence of atopic dermatitis (AD) in infancy [1, 2]. Our own study, the Probiotics in the Prevention of Allergies among Children in Trondheim (ProPACT) trial, demonstrated a 40 % reduction in the development of AD following maternal probiotic supplementation [3]. However, the biological mechanisms behind this effect are incompletely understood. Using samples taken during the ProPACT trial, we have previously reported that the maternal intestinal microbiota is modified by probiotic supplementation, and that children born to mothers who received the probiotics have a higher abundance of *Lactobacillus rhamnosus GG* (LGG) which persists up until 3 months of age [4]. Whilst the transfer of such probiotic bacteria from mother to child may prevent AD, alterations in various components of breast milk have also been postulated as possible mediating factors.

*Correspondence: melanie.simpson@ntnu.no
[4] Det medisinske fakultet, Instiutt for samfunnsmedisin, MTFS, NTNU, Postboks 8905, 7491 Trondheim, Norway
Full list of author information is available at the end of the article

In addition to being a source of nutrition and hydration for newborn infants, breast milk contains a number of immunologically active cells and molecules, such as immunoglobulins, lactoferrins, growth factors and cytokines [5]. Among the cytokines found in breast milk are thymic stromal lymphopoietin (TSLP) and the transforming growth factor-β (TGF-β) cytokines. TSLP has been implicated in the establishment and maintenance of T helper type 2 (Th2) responses, and thus also in defence against helminthic infections and in the pathogenesis of allergy related diseases [6]. Genetic variants of TSLP have been associated with AD and asthma [7] and high levels of epidermal TSLP precede the clinical presentation of childhood AD [8], suggesting that TSLP may be particularly important in the establishment of AD. Other studies have demonstrated that TSLP activates skin dendritic cells promoting a Th2 response and interacts directly with skin-homing Th2 cells to enhance interleukin-4 (IL-4) production which is thought to contribute to the maintenance of inflammation in chronic AD [9, 10]. Consistent with these studies, higher concentrations of TSLP have been reported in both acute and chronic AD lesions [6]. Murine models have shown that over-expression of TSLP in keratinocytes induces an AD-like skin disease and can predispose to allergic airway inflammation after intranasal challenge. Thus, TSLP may also be involved in the progression to other allergy related diseases, a process often referred to as the atopic march [6]. However, the biological effects of breast milk TSLP for the mother and child are unknown [11], and this cytokine is previously unstudied within the context of maternal probiotic supplementation. Neither has the effect of maternal atopy on breast milk TSLP been investigated, nor the association between breast milk TSLP and the development of AD. In contrast to TSLP, the human isoforms of TGF-β (TGF-β_1, TGF-β_2 and TGF-β_3) are primarily implicated in inhibition of allergic inflammation through a wide range of immunoregulatory effects [12]. All three isoforms of TGF-β are found in breast milk. Studies investigating the effect of probiotic supplementation on breast milk TGF-β concentrations and or their association with later allergy related disease in offspring, have produced conflicting results [13–18].

Both TSLP and TGF-βs appear to have important roles in acute and chronic phases of allergy related disease, which makes them interesting as potential mediators of this preventive effect. The aims of the current study were to: (a) determine if perinatal maternal probiotic supplementation alters the concentration of TLSP, TGF-β_1, TGF-β_2 or TGF-β_3 in breast milk at 10 days and 3 months postpartum and (b) investigate if these breast milk cytokines contribute to the preventative effect of maternal probiotic supplementation on the development of AD at 2 years of age through causal mediation analysis.

Methods

Participant recruitment and sample collection

The ProPACT trial enrolled 415 pregnant women who were randomised to receive 250 mL per day of probiotic or placebo milk from 36 weeks gestation until 3 months postpartum [3]. The probiotic milk contained 5×10^{10} colony-forming units (CFUs) of *Lactobacillus rhamnosus GG* (LGG) and *Bifidobacterium animalis* subsp. *lactis* Bb-12 (Bb-12) and 5×10^9 CFU of *L. acidophilus* La-5 (La-5) per serving. The placebo was a fermented skim milk, pasteurised after fermentation and contained no probiotic bacteria. Participants completed lifestyle questionnaires at baseline (~30–36 weeks gestation), 6 weeks, 1 and 2 years postpartum and child health questionnaires at 1 and 2 years of age. The outcome of interest in the current study was the development of AD by 2 years of age as diagnosed by a paediatrician using the United Kingdom (UK) Working Party Diagnostic criteria [19]. Detailed descriptions of the ProPACT study design and clinical outcomes have been published previously [3, 20].

Breast milk samples were collected into a sterile container at 10 days and 3 months postpartum and stored in the participant's home freezer until transported to the laboratory in Styrofoam containers to prevent thawing. Samples were subsequently stored at −80 °C until analysis. All mother-infant pairs that attended the 2 year clinical follow-up and submitted at least one breast milk sample were eligible for inclusion in this study.

Cytokine quantification

Breast milk samples were thawed and centrifuged (16,100*g*, 10 min, 4 °C) to remove the lipids, cells and debris. The aqueous portion was used for subsequent cytokine quantification. TSLP concentrations were measured using a human TLSP ELISA kit (R&D Systems, Minneapolis, USA) according to the manufacturer's instructions. The standards and an internal control were conducted in triplicate. The intra-assay coefficient of variation (CV) was <13.5 % and inter-assay CV was 22 %. A large proportion of the samples had TSLP concentrations outside of the detection limits of the assay, both above and below. We have therefore categorised the TSLP concentrations into the following 4 categories: below detection, low detectable, high detectable and above detection. The internal control sample was chosen as the cut-off between the low and high detectable categories, because it was approximately the median concentration and maximised the inter-assay comparability. For the purpose of mediation analysis TSLP was categorised into a binary variable above and below the internal control.

TGF beta concentrations were measured using a multiplex assay (Bio-Plex Pro TGF-β assay, Bio-Rad Laboratories, Oslo, Norway) following the manufacturer's instructions which included an actvation step. Prior to analysis, 100 μL of the aqueous portion of breast milk was activated using 20 μL 1 N HCl for 10 min at room temperature, followed by neutralisation using 20 μL 1 N NaOH with 0.5 M HEPES. The standard and two internal control samples were conducted in duplicate. Concentrations were calculated using standard curves and scaled by 1.4 due to dilution in the activation-neutralisation process. The intra-assay CVs were <13.6, <13.4 and <14.6 % and the inter-assay CV were <9.9, <5.9 and <14.3 % for TGF-β_1, TGF-β_2 and TGF-β_3, respectively.

Statistical analysis

As described, TSLP concentrations were categorised into a four groups, and the effect of probiotics was assessed using ordinal logistic regression. The distributions of TGF-βs were right-skewed and concentrations are reported as medians and interquartile ranges. Wilcoxon matched-pairs signed-rank test was used to compare the concentration at 10 days and 3 months for the 243 women with TGF-β isoforms measured at both time points. The effect of probiotic supplementation on TGF-β concentrations was assessed using linear regression on log-transformed concentrations. Maternal atopy, maternal smoking during the first year of life and the presence of older siblings were considered to be potential moderators of the effect of probiotics on cytokine concentrations. The effect of probiotics on the breast milk cytokines were therefore also assessed in alternate regression models which included these covariates.

Causal mediation analysis was performed using the user written command, *paramed,* for breast milk cytokines which were found to be altered by probiotic supplementation. This analysis estimated the natural indirect effect (NIE) and natural direct effect (NDE) of maternal probiotic supplementation on the development of AD in offspring, mediated through breast milk cytokine concentrations, using counterfactual definitions of these effects and a log-binomial regression model for AD, given AD is not rare [21–23]. In this study, the NIE represents the effect of the probiotic regime on the development of AD which can be attributed to its effect on the breast milk cytokine. The NDE represents an estimation of what the relative risk (RR) of developing AD after maternal probiotic supplementation would have been, had there been no effect on the concentration of the breast milk cytokine. The *paramed* command does not currently support models with ordinal mediator variables and TSLP concentrations were therefore dichotomised for mediation analysis. Whilst the randomised design ensures that the effect of probiotics on breast milk cytokines and on AD can be estimated without confounding, the relationship between cytokine concentration in breast milk and the development of AD is not randomised. As such, the estimation of NIE and NDE may be confounded by factors which influence both breast milk cytokine concentrations and the risk of developing AD in offspring. The previously mentioned covariates were therefore included in the mediation analysis as potential confounders of the relationship between breast milk composition and AD. All statistical analyses were performed using Stata IC release 13 (StataCorp, College Station, Texas).

Results

Participants

Two hundred and fifty-nine mother-infant pairs were included in this analysis, 129 from the probiotic group and 130 from the placebo group (Fig. 1). This subgroup of participants is representative of the original study population with respect to distribution of baseline characteristics and allergy related disease outcomes [3]. Compliance was high and equivalent in both groups. At baseline, the probiotic group contained more male children and at 2 years of age there were fewer cases of AD (Table 1). In terms of maternal characteristics which have been previously suggested to influence breast milk cytokine concentration, fewer women in the probiotic group had a personal history of atopy (Table 1). There were also fewer women smoking at 6 weeks postpartum in the probiotic group, although the overall prevalence of smoking was very low (8 of 259, 3.2 %).

Thymic stromal lymphopoietin

A greater proportion of breast milk samples taken 10 days postpartum had high concentrations of TLSP compared with the samples taken at 3 months (Fig. 2). The concentration of TSLP was below the lower limit of detection (31.3 pg/mL) in 18.9 % and 26.7 % of samples collected at 10 day and 3 months postpartum, respectively, and above the limit of detection (2000 pg/mL) in 25.6 % and 17.3 %, respectively. Ordered logistic regression revealed a borderline non-significant effect of probiotics on TLSP concentration (OR 1.55 95 % CI 0.98–2.45, $p = 0.062$) at 10 days postpartum which was not sustained at 3 months postpartum (OR 1.35 95 % CI 0.84–2.16, $p = 0.219$). This effect was not significantly altered when adjusting individually or in combination for maternal atopy, maternal smoking or older siblings. The effect of probiotics on breast milk TSLP concentration at 10 days postpartum was marginally enhanced when considering only women compliant with the study protocol ($n = 209$, OR 1.74, 95 % CI 1.06–2.84, $p = 0.028$). We did not find evidence of an association between maternal

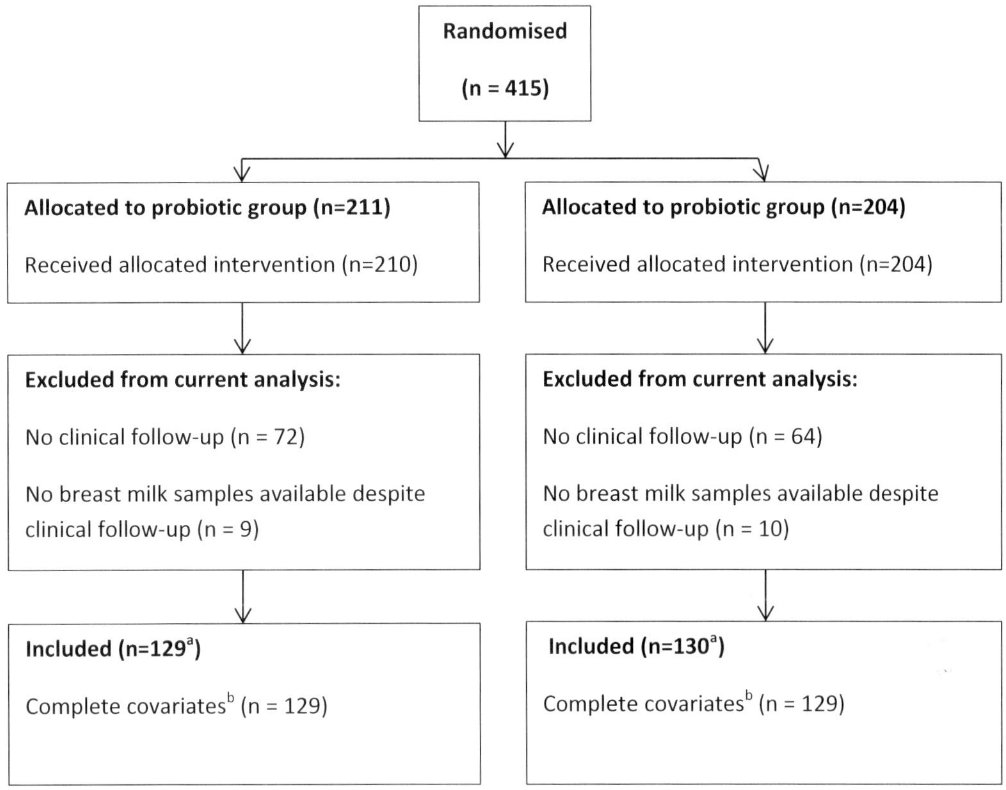

Fig. 1 Flow diagram of participants in the ProPACT study and cytokine analysis of breast milk samples. [a]The provided values represent the number of eligible women who had provided at least one breast milk sample. The precise number of samples analysed for each cytokine at each time point varies and is provided in association with the relevant results. [b]Complete covariates additionally required information on maternal atopy, maternal smoking and the presence of older siblings

Table 1 Baseline characteristics of participating families and allergy related disease in the children at 2 years

Characteristics	Probiotic		Placebo		
	n		n		
Age, mother, yrs mean (SD)	129	30.5 (3.9)	130	30.3 (4.1)	
Sex (male), child, n (%)	129	67 (51.9)	130	53 (40.8)	
Siblings, n (%)	129	60 (46.5)	130	54 (41.5)	
Atopy in family, n (%)	129	91 (70.5)	130	96 (73.9)	
Maternal atopy, n (%)	129	58 (45.0)	129	68 (52.7)	
Maternal smoking[a], n (%)	129	9 (7.0)	130	11 (8.5)	
Compliant[b], n(%)	125	113 (90.4)	128	115 (89.8)	
Allergy related disease at 2 years	**n**	**n (%)**	**n**	**n (%)**	**p-value[c]**
Atopic dermatitis, n (%)	129	29 (22.5)	130	45 (34.6)	0.031
Asthma, n (%)	129	7 (5.4)	130	12 (9.2)	0.240
Allergic rhinoconjunctivits, n (%)	125	1 (0.8)	129	0 (0.0)	0.492
Sensitisation[d], n (%)	122	19 (15.6)	124	15 (12.1)	0.429

[a] Maternal smoking reported during pregnancy, 6 weeks or 12 months postpartum; [b] Compliance with the study protocol was defined by consumption of the study milk on at least 50 % of days from 36 weeks gestation to 12 postpartum, no consumption of other products with probiotics and at least partial breastfeeding until 3 months postpartum; [c] p-value calculated using χ^2-test, except for allergic rhinoconjunctivits where a Fisher's exact *p* value is reported; [d] Allergic sensitisation defined as positive skin prick test (wheal $\geq$ 3 mm) and or positive sIgE ($\geq$ 0.35 kUL^{-1})

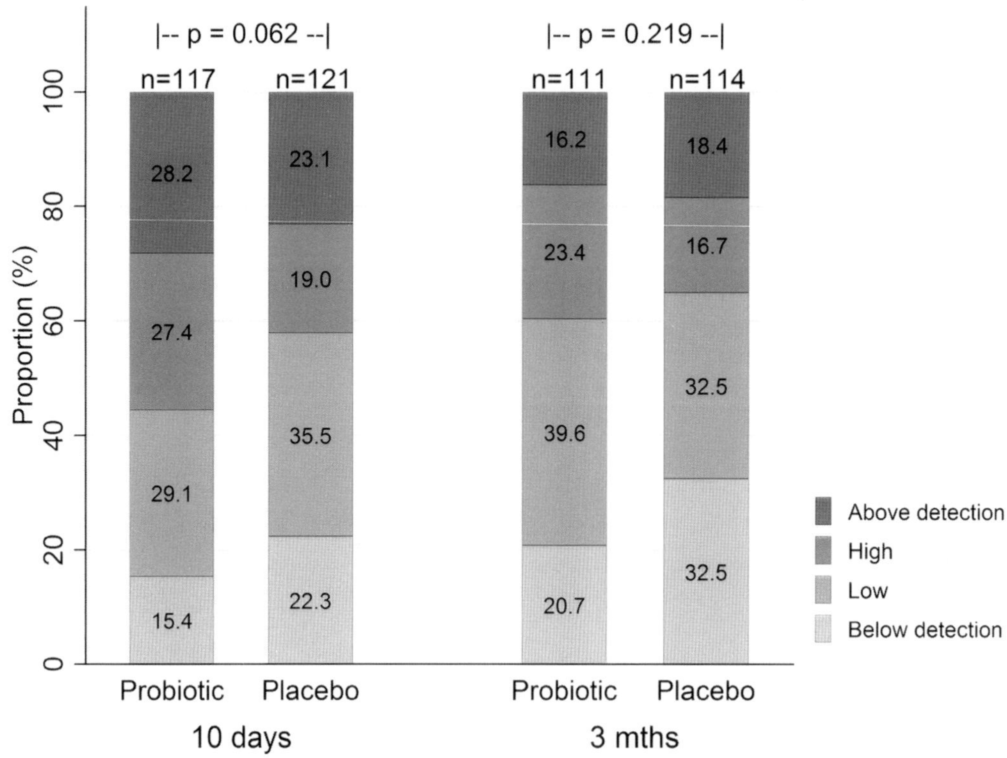

Fig. 2 Breast milk TSLP concentrations at 10 days and 3 months in the probiotic and placebo groups. Proportion of breast milk samples with categorised TSLP concentrations at 10 days and 3 months postpartum in the placebo and probiotic group. Percentages are provided within the *bars*. Overall, higher concentrations of TSLP were measured significantly more often in samples collected at 10 days postpartum ($p < 0.001$ from ordinal logistic regression clustered by individual). Also on subgroup analysis, TSLP concentrations were significantly higher at 10 days in both the probiotic group ($p < 0.001$) and placebo group ($p = 0.005$)

atopy, maternal smoking or the presence of older siblings and TSLP in univariate analysis.

Transforming growth factor β

All three TGF-β isoforms were detectable in all breast milk samples, with the exception of one sample collected at 3 months postpartum which had undetectable TGF-β_3. Similar to TSLP, the concentrations of TGF-β_1, TGF-β_2 and TGF-β_3 were higher at 10 days postpartum compared with 3 months postpartum (Fig. 3). Probiotic supplementation had no observed effect on the concentration of any of the TGF-β subtypes at either time point (Table 2). This lack of effect was not substantially altered when adjusting for potential moderators or when considering the subgroup of women compliant with the study protocol ($n = 219–224$).

Breast milk cytokines as potential mediators of preventative effect on atopic dermatitis

For the purposes of mediation analysis, TSLP concentrations at 10 days were dichotomised. Consistent with the ordinal logistic regression analysis, standard logistic regression on the dichotomised TSLP values also suggested that perinatal probiotic supplementation increased the odds of a high TSLP concentration at 10 days (OR 1.72, 95 % CI 1.03–2.87, $p = 0.039$). However, mediation analysis suggested that the effect of probiotics on TSLP did not result in a significant reduction, or increase, in the risk of developing AD [RR^{NIE} 1.04 (95 % CI 0.94–1.15, $p = 0.45$)], Fig. 4). Breast milk TSLP concentrations at 3 months postpartum and the TGF-β cytokines at both 10 days and 3 months postpartum were not demonstrably affected by probiotic supplementation, indicating that changes in these breast milk cytokines are unlikely to be responsible for the reduced risk of developing AD observed after maternal probiotic supplementation. As such, no estimation of NIE and NDE was conducted for these. Furthermore, none of the cytokines, including TSLP at 10 days, were found to be significantly associated with the development of AD when assessed independently of treatment allocation.

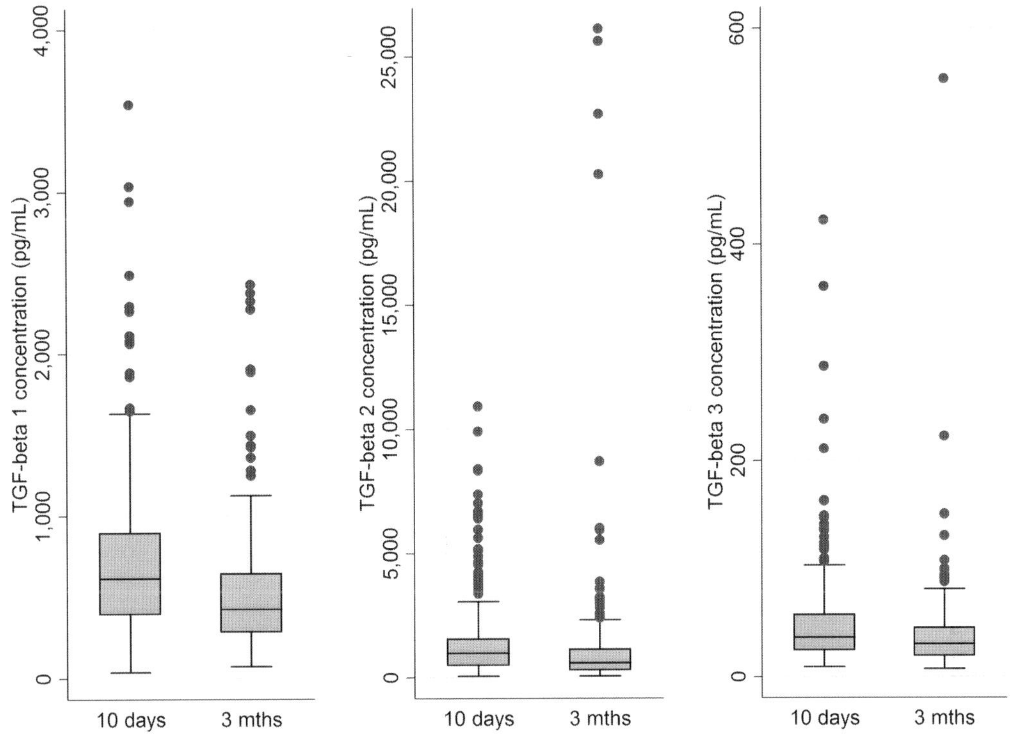

Fig. 3 Concentrations of TGF-β1, 2 and 3 at 10 days and 3 months. All three isoforms of TGF-β are found at statistically significantly lower levels at 3 months postpartum compared to 10 days postpartum ($p < 0.001$ for all isoforms using Mann–Whitney U-test)

Table 2 Breast milk TGF-β concentrations in the probiotic and placebo groups at 10 days and 3 months postpartum

	Days	Treatment				p[a]
		Probiotic		Placebo		
		n	Median (IQR) (pg/mL)	n	Median (IQR) (pg/mL)	
TGF-β_1	10	128	616.9 (407.5–950.4)	127	617.3 (369.7–853.9)	0.34 0.33
	90	123	438.5 (308.0–661.1)	124	417.4 (269.3–641.8)	0.27 0.23
TGF-β_2	10	128	909.8 (451.6–1653.8)	127	999.4 (519.0–1517.1)	0.90 0.83
	90	123	599.6 (311.0–1055.1)	124	532.5 (285.9–1144.2)	0.76 0.69
TGF-β_3	10	128	37.8 (25.3–58.7)	127	35.8 (22.9–57.2)	0.25 0.33
	90	123	29.9 (21.0–42.7)	123	30.8 (18.8–48.7)	0.95 0.86

[a] The upper p-value provided is from the regression analysis of the influence of probiotic ingestion on the log transformed TGF beta concentration by, whilst the lower represents the p-value calculated for the effect of treatment allocation after adjusting for maternal atopy, maternal smoking and presence of siblings

Discussion

Thymic stromal lymphopoietin was the only cytokine with a tendency to be affected by maternal probiotic supplementation, resulting in higher concentrations of TSLP at 10 days postpartum. Causal mediation analysis indicated that the higher concentrations of TSLP at 10 days did not appear to contribute to the beneficial effect of probiotics on the development of AD in offspring. TSLP concentrations at 3 months postpartum and TGF-βs at both time points were not affected by

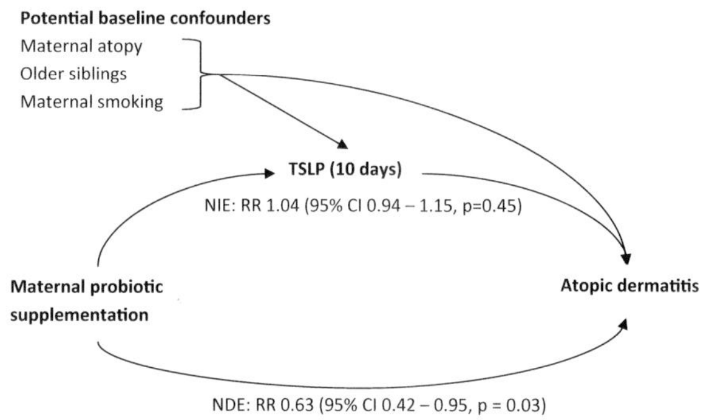

Fig. 4 Hypothetical mediation analysis and estimated natural indirect effect (NIE) and natural direct effect (NDE) of maternal probiotic supplementation. The NIE is an estimate of the effect of maternal probiotic ingestion on the development of AD in offspring mediated by increased TSLP levels in breast milk 10 days postpartum. The NDE is an estimate of the effect of maternal probiotic ingestion on the development of AD not mediated through changes in breast milk TSLP concentration 10 days postpartum. This analysis suggests that TSLP does not significantly contribute to, or oppose, the preventative effect of maternal perinatal probiotic supplementation on the development of atopic dermatitis

probiotic supplementation. As such, these breast milk cytokines are unlikely to be mediators of the beneficial effect of probiotics.

This study provides the first report of the influence of a maternal probiotic supplementation on breast milk TLSP concentrations and investigates its contribution to the prevention of AD. In experimental and observational studies, TSLP has been associated with promotion of a Th2 and allergic type inflammation, particularly in the lung and skin [6, 24]. Therefore, the finding that probiotic supplementation increased the breast milk TSLP concentrations was contrary to what one might have expected. At the same time, high breast milk TSLP may not be as detrimental in the intestinal system where it is described as having a more regulatory function [24, 25]. TSLP released by intestinal epithelial cells in response to commensal bacteria has been shown to promote tolerogenic properties in dendritic cells and macrophages which then produce IL-10 and retinoic acid and promote regulatory T helper (Treg) cell differentiation [25]. Thus the increased TSLP seen in the probiotic group may encourage intestinal immune homeostasis, which in turn is theoretically beneficial for the development of the neonatal immune system and prevention of AD. However, the current data does not suggest that breast milk TSLP contributes to the preventative effect of probiotics on AD, nor does it appear to be associated with the development of AD. It is unclear if the observed lack of mediating effect is due to a loss of information and power due to dichotomisation of TSLP concentration, TLSP degradation prior to reaching the intestines, or a more complex interplay between TSLP, the intestinal microbiota and the immune system. Further studies are required to confirm these findings.

The major strength of this study is that the randomised placebo controlled, double blind design of the ProPACT trial allows an unconfounded assessment of the effect of the probiotic regime on the selected breast milk cytokines. Furthermore, through causal mediation analysis techniques, we are able to estimate if and to what extent the prevention of AD is due to changes in TSLP. The randomised design also means that two of four assumptions required for this mediation analysis [21] are automatically satisfied, namely that there is no residual confounding of the effect of probiotics supplementation on either AD or breast milk TSLP. The other two required assumptions are that there is no unmeasured confounding of the relationship between breast milk TSLP and AD and that there is no confounder of the mediator-outcome relationship that is affected by treatment allocation. Whilst these cannot be excluded, we believe we have measured and included all variables which are likely to affect both breast milk cytokines and AD and that probiotics do not have a strong effect on any other confounders of the relationship between these variables. Another strength of this study is that it is the largest to investigate TSLP concentrations in breast milk and the only one to consider infant outcomes and maternal atopy status. The only other study to report breast milk TSLP concentrations involved 44 women who submitted samples at one of two time points [11]. Whilst they also found that mature milk tended to have lower TSLP concentrations, they reported concentrations which all fell within a relatively narrow range. Our results suggest that there may be a much greater variability between individuals than this small study managed to detect.

One of the limitations of this study is that the breast milk samples were stored between 6 and 8 years before analysis. This has potentially affected the measured concentrations of TSLP and TGF-βs, as has been previously reported for TGF-β_1 [26]. However, there was no difference in the average length of storage between the treatment groups and adjusting for length of storage did not significantly alter the estimated effect of probiotic supplementation on any of the measured cytokines (data not shown). Another limitation is that the time of sample collection was not standardised with respect to time of day and whether fore- or hindmilk was collected. Although diurnal and fore-/hindmilk variation has not been specifically investigated for TSLP and TGF-βs, previous studies suggest that diurnal variation exists in some breast milk cytokines [27] and that the quantity of total protein in the aqueous portion of fore- and hindmilk is reasonably constant [28]. Whilst these factors may have influenced the cytokine concentrations, samples from the probiotic and placebo groups are presumably equally affected and we do not believe they have significantly affected the conclusions of this study. An underlying uncertainty surrounding the measure of breast milk cytokines is another limitation to this study. Previous studies of breast milk TGF-β and other cytokines have produced widely varying concentration measurements. Whilst some of this variability may be explained by factors such as diurnal and fore-/hindmilk variations, ethnicity, maternal atopy status and time point postpartum, it is likely that sample storage, preparation, analysis methods and inter-laboratory differences play a major role in the measured concentrations. As such, it is difficult to compare results between studies, particularly when these variables are inconsistently reported. In studies comparing two exposure groups, be that probiotic versus placebo or maternal atopy versus no atopy, it is reasonable to assume that technical variability between the groups are minimised. Thus, comparing groups within each study is valid and more generally the relative relationship between these groups can be roughly compared across studies.

Five previous studies have reported breast milk TGF-β_1 and or TGF-β_2 concentrations from similar randomised trials of probiotic supplementation. Each of these studies found a statistically significant effect of probiotics on at least one TGF-β isoform in colostrum samples and no effect on concentrations in mature milk. However, they provide conflicting evidence as to whether probiotics increase [14, 15] or decrease [16–18] colostrum TGF-β concentrations. The current study also found no effect of probiotic supplementation on TGF-β concentrations in mature milk, and provides no evidence to suggest either increased or decreased concentrations in breast milk at 10 days postpartum, a time when the milk is sometimes referred as transition milk before colostrum become mature milk. In addition to the previously mentioned sources of variability, the differing results may also reflect a probiotic strain specific effect as none of these studies used the same probiotic species in the same dose or combinations. In terms of methodological differences, it is interesting to note that the two studies reporting reduced TGF-β_2 after probiotic supplementation also reported the manufacturer recommended acid activation of the breast milk samples prior to measurement which means that the reported concentrations represent the entire pool of TGF-β which is naturally found in both a latent and active form. On the other hand, all three studies reporting higher TGF-β_1 or TGF-β_2 do not mention this activation step in their methods. One of these studies, however, used an alternate activation procedure which is thought to additionally release lipid bound TGF-β [17, 29]. All other studies have removed the lipid fraction prior to cytokine analysis. If the conflicting reports of positive or negative associations with probiotics are a reflection of a common effect of probiotics and sample preparation method, rather than strain specific effects, it may imply that probiotics affect the ratio between active and latent TGF-β in breast milk or the proportion of lipid bound TGF-β. Other factors are known to affect the proportion of active versus latent TGF-β, for example, mothers of premature infants having a higher proportion of latent TGF-β [30].

Conclusions

Whilst maternal probiotic supplementation appears to result in higher breast milk concentrations of TLSP at 10 days postpartum, this does not seem contribute to the preventative effect of the probiotic regime on the development of AD. Probiotics did not significantly alter the breast milk concentration of any TGF-β isoforms at 10 days or 3 months postpartum. Further studies are required to both confirm these findings and investigate the other potential mechanism behind the prevention of AD in infancy by perinatal probiotic supplementation.

Abbreviations

AD: atopic dermatitis; Bb12: *Bifidobacterium animalis* subsp. *lactis* Bb-12; ELISA: enzyme-linked immunospot assay; LGG: *Lactobacillus rhamnosus GG*; NDE: natural direct effect; NIE: natural indirect effect; OR: odds ratio; ProPACT: Probiotics in the Prevention of Allergy among Children in Trondheim; RR: risk ratio; TGF-β: transforming growth factor beta; Th2 cells: type 2 T helper cells; TSLP: thymic stromal lymphopoietin.

Authors' contributions

TØ, OS and RJ designed and directed the implementation of the ProPACT trial during which these breast milk samples were collected. TØ and ØG conceived and designed the breast milk analysis experiments. MS and ADBR analysed the data and wrote the initial manuscript draft. All authors have contributed to and approved the final draft of the manuscript.

Author details

[1] Department of Public Health and General Practice, Norwegian University of Science and Technology, Trondheim, Norway. [2] Department of Immunology and Transfusion Medicine, St Olavs Hospital, Trondheim University Hospital, Trondheim, Norway. [3] Department of Dermatology, University Hospital of North Norway, Tromsö, Norway. [4] Det medisinske fakultet, Instiutt for samfunnsmedisin, MTFS, NTNU, Postboks 8905, 7491 Trondheim, Norway.

Acknowledgements

We thank the families for their participation in this study along with the midwives of the Trondheim region for their help in recruitment and distribution of questionnaires and paediatrician Dr. Rakel Berg who examined the children at 2 years. We also thank the project assistants, Guri Helmersen, Else Bartnes and Liv Ryan, who assisted with the logistics of the ProPACT trial and performed the laboratory analysis of the breast milk samples.

Competing interests

The authors declare they have no competing interests.

Funding

This study was funded by the Norwegian University of Science and Technology and the Norwegian Research Council. Tine BA sponsored the study through the supply of study milk and logistics of its distribution. MRS, OS and TØ have attended research seminars sponsored by Tine BA. Siemens Medical Solutions Diagnostics AS provided reagents for the analysis of serum IgE. Employees from the funding sources played no role in the study design, data collection and analysis, decision to publish, or preparation of the manuscript.

References

1. Pelucchi C, Chatenoud L, Turati F, Galeone C, Moja L, Bach JF, La Vecchia C. Probiotics supplementation during pregnancy or infancy for the prevention of atopic dermatitis: a meta-analysis. Epidemiology. 2012;23(3):402–14.
2. Panduru M, Panduru NM, Salavastru CM, Tiplica GS. Probiotics and primary prevention of atopic dermatitis: a meta-analysis of randomized controlled studies. J Eur Acad Dermatol Venereol JEADV. 2015;29(2):232–42.
3. Dotterud CK, Storro O, Johnsen R, Oien T. Probiotics in pregnant women to prevent allergic disease: a randomized, double-blind trial. Br J Dermatol. 2010;163(3):616–23.
4. Dotterud CK, Avershina E, Sekelja M, Simpson MR, Rudi K, Storrø O, Johnsen R, Øien T. Does maternal perinatal probiotic supplementation alter the intestinal microbiota of mother and child. J Pediat Gastroent Nutr. 2015;61(2):200–2007.
5. Hosea Blewett HJ, Cicalo MC, Holland CD, Field CJ. Chapter 2—The immunological components of human milk. In: Steve LT, editor. Advances in food and nutrition research, vol. 54. Cambridge: Academic Press; 2008. p. 45–80.
6. Ziegler SF. Thymic stromal lymphopoietin and allergic disease. J Allergy Clin Immunol. 2012;130(4):845–52.
7. Gao P-S, Rafaels NM, Mu D, Hand T, Murray T, Boguniewicz M, Hata T, Schneider L, Hanifin JM, Gallo RL, et al. Genetic variants in thymic stromal lymphopoietin are associated with atopic dermatitis and eczema herpeticum. J Allergy Clin Immunol. 2010;125(6):1403.e1404–1407.e1404.
8. Kim J, Kim BE, Lee J, Han Y, Jun H-Y, Kim H, Choi J, Leung DYM, Ahn K. Epidermal thymic stromal lymphopoietin predicts the development of atopic dermatitis during infancy. J Allergy Clin Immunol. 2016;137(4):1282.e1284–1285.e1284.
9. Tatsuno K, Fujiyama T, Yamaguchi H, Waki M, Tokura Y. TSLP directly interacts with skin-homing Th2 cells highly expressing its receptor to enhance IL-4 production in atopic dermatitis. J Invest Dermatol. 2015;135(12):3017–24.
10. Schwartz C, Eberle JU, Hoyler T, Diefenbach A, Lechmann M, Voehringer D. Opposing functions of TSLP-responsive basophils and dendritic cells in a mouse model of atopic dermatitis. J Allergy Clin Immunol. 2016. doi:10.1016/j.jaci.2016.04.031.
11. Macfarlane TV, Seager AL, Moller M, Morgan G, Thornton CA. Thymic stromal lymphopoietin is present in human breast milk. Pediatr Allergy Immunol. 2010;21(2 Pt 2):e454–6.
12. Nakao A. The role and potential use of oral transforming growth factor-beta in the prevention of infant allergy. Clin Exp Allergy. 2010;40(5):725–30.
13. Oddy WH, Rosales F. A systematic review of the importance of milk TGF-beta on immunological outcomes in the infant and young child. Pediatr Allergy Immunol. 2010;21(1 Pt 1):47–59.
14. Bottcher MF, Abrahamsson TR, Fredriksson M, Jakobsson T, Bjorksten B. Low breast milk TGF-beta2 is induced by *Lactobacillus reuteri* supplementation and associates with reduced risk of sensitization during infancy. Pediatr Allergy Immunol. 2008;19(6):497–504.
15. Kuitunen M, Kukkonen AK, Savilahti E. Impact of maternal allergy and use of probiotics during pregnancy on breast milk cytokines and food antibodies and development of allergy in children until 5 years. Int Arch Allergy Immunol. 2012;159(2):162–70.
16. Rautava S, Kalliomaki M, Isolauri E. Probiotics during pregnancy and breast-feeding might confer immunomodulatory protection against atopic disease in the infant. J Allergy Clin Immunol. 2002;109(1):119–21.
17. Huurre A, Laitinen K, Rautava S, Korkeamaki M, Isolauri E. Impact of maternal atopy and probiotic supplementation during pregnancy on infant sensitization: a double-blind placebo-controlled study. Clin Exp Allergy. 2008;38(8):1342–8.
18. Prescott SL, Wickens K, Westcott L, Jung W, Currie H, Black PN, Stanley TV, Mitchell EA, Fitzharris P, Siebers R, et al. Supplementation with *Lactobacillus rhamnosus* or *Bifidobacterium lactis* probiotics in pregnancy increases cord blood interferon-gamma and breast milk transforming growth factor-beta and immunoglobin A detection. Clin Exp Allergy. 2008;38(10):1606–14.
19. Williams HC, Burney PG, Hay RJ, Archer CB, Shipley MJ, Hunter JJ, Bingham EA, Finlay AY, Pembroke AC, Graham-Brown RA, et al. The U.K. working party's diagnostic criteria for atopic dermatitis. I. Derivation of a minimum set of discriminators for atopic dermatitis. Br J Dermatol. 1994;131(3):383–96.
20. Simpson MR, Dotterud CK, Storrø O, Johnsen R, Øien T. Perinatal probiotic supplementaion in the prevention of allergy related disease: 6 year follow up of a randomised controlled trial. BMC Dermatol. 2015;15:13.
21. Valeri L, Vanderweele TJ. Mediation analysis allowing for exposure-mediator interactions and causal interpretation: theoretical assumptions and implementation with SAS and SPSS macros. Psychol Methods. 2013;18(2):137–50.
22. VanderWeele T. Explanation in causal inference: methods for mediation and interaction. Oxford: Oxford University Press; 2015.
23. Liu H, Emsley R, Dunn G, VanderWeele T, Valeri L: PARAMED: Stata module to perform causal mediation analysis using parametric regression models. The Stata Journal 2014, Technical paper in preparation:Installation instructions for program code and help file available from: https://ideas.repec.org/c/boc/bocode/s457581.html.
24. Vickery BP, Scurlock AM, Jones SM, Burks AW. Mechanisms of immune tolerance relevant to food allergy. J Allergy Clin Immunol. 2011;127(3):576–84.
25. Peterson LW, Artis D. Intestinal epithelial cells: regulators of barrier function and immune homeostatis. Nat Rev Immunol. 2014;24(3):141–53.
26. Ramirez-Santana C, Perez-Cano FJ, Audi C, Castell M, Moretones MG, Lopez-Sabater MC, Castellote C, Franch A. Effects of cooling and freezing storage on the stability of bioactive factors in human colostrum. J Dairy Sci. 2012;95(5):2319–25.
27. Pontes GN, Cardoso EC, Carneiro-Sampaio MMS, Markus RP. Pineal melatonin and the innate immune response: the TNF-alpha increase after cesarean section suppresses nocturnal melatonin production. J Pineal Res. 2007;43(4):365–71.
28. Saarela T, Kokkonen J, Koivisto M. Macronutrient and energy contents of human milk fractions during the first six months of lactation. Acta Paediatrica (Oslo, Norway: 1992). 2005;94(9):1176–81.
29. Filteau SM, Lietz G, Mulokozi G, Bilotta S, Henry CJK, Tomkins AM. Milk cytokines and subclinical breast inflammation in Tanzanian women: effects of dietary red palm oil or sunflower oil supplementation. Immunology. 1999;97(4):595–600.
30. Namachivayam K, Blanco CL, Frost BL, Reeves AA, Jagadeeswaran R, Mohankumar K, Safarulla A, Mandal P, Garzon SA, Raj JU, et al. Preterm human milk contains a large pool of latent TGF-beta, which can be activated by exogenous neuraminidase. Am J Physiol Gastrointest Liver Physiol. 2013;304(12):G1055–65.

17

Sensitization to PR-10 proteins is indicative of distinctive sensitization patterns in adults with a suspected food allergy

Mark A. Blankestijn[1*], André C. Knulst[1], Edward F. Knol[1,2], Thuy-My Le[1], Heike Rockmann[1], Henny G. Otten[2] and Rob J. B. Klemans[1]

Abstract

Background: The extent of co-sensitization within and between food protein families in an adult population is largely unknown. This study aimed to identify the most frequently recognized components in the PR-10 and storage protein family, as well as patterns in (co-)sensitization, in a birch-endemic area.

Methods: Results of ImmunoCAP ISAC, performed during routine care in Dutch adult outpatients suspected of food allergy, were collected.

Results: A total of 305 patients were selected, aged 16–79 years (median 32 years). Sensitization to one or more PR-10 proteins was most frequent (74% of all subjects), followed by 35% to storage protein and 15% to nsLTPs. Within the PR-10 family, subjects were most often sensitized to Bet v 1 (73% of 305), Cor a 1.04 (72%) and Mal d 1 (68%). Sensitization to PR-10s from soy, celery and kiwi occurred distinctively less often (< 55% of Bet v 1 sensitized subjects) compared to other food PR-10s (all > 70%). Subjects sensitized to these 'less common PR-10 proteins' were sensitized to more food and inhalant components on the ISAC, compared to subjects sensitized to 'common PR-10 proteins' (median 22 vs 13 out of 112, $p < 0.0001$). Seven subjects demonstrated sensitization to food PR-10 proteins, without concomitant sensitization to pollen PR-10s. Within the storage proteins, sensitization to multiple peanut allergens was most common (on average 3 out of 4).

Conclusions: Sensitization to PR-10 food proteins could occur without concomitant sensitization to common PR-10 from pollen in a subset of subjects. Less commonly recognized PR-10 proteins appear to be an indication of polysensitization.

Keywords: ImmunoCAP ISAC, Food allergy, PR-10, Specific IgE, Storage proteins

Background

In food allergy diagnostics, component-resolved diagnostics (CRD) allows the clinician to assess the presence of specific IgE (sIgE) to allergenic proteins (components), instead of crude extracts. A consensus document by the WAO-ARIA-GA2LEN Task Force elaborates the role of CRD in three major aspects of allergy diagnostics: distinguishing between genuine versus cross-reactive sensitization, assessing the possible risk of a severe allergic reaction upon exposure in selected patients and identifying allergens for specific immunotherapy [1]. The ImmunoCAP Immuno-Solid phase Allergen Chip (ISAC; Thermo Fisher Scientific, Uppsala, Sweden) is a multiplex technology to assess the presence of specific IgE to a large number of components at the same time [2]. Studies have demonstrated a good concordance between the ImmunoCAP and ImmunoCAP ISAC in assessing sensitization to components [3, 4]. The current ISAC model holds 112 components, which are a selection of known food and inhalant allergens, as well as allergens

*Correspondence: m.a.blankestijn@umcutrecht.nl
[1] Department of Dermatology and Allergology, University Medical Center Utrecht, Utrecht University, Heidelberglaan 100, 3584 CX Utrecht, The Netherlands
Full list of author information is available at the end of the article

from others sources such as latex (see Additional file 1: Table 1).

Components can be grouped into protein families based on their biological function and structural homology [5–7]. In plant food allergy, important protein families include the pathogenesis related protein family 10 (PR-10) proteins, profilins, seed storage proteins and non-specific lipid transfer proteins (nsLTP). PR-10 proteins and profilins are considered labile proteins, and sensitization to these proteins is usually associated with mild symptoms, mostly limited to the oral cavity [8]. Storage proteins and nsLTPs on the other hand, are considered resistant to thermal processing, and pH changes, and are associated with moderate to severe symptoms upon ingestion [5, 9–13]. The amount of cross-reactivity between allergens from the same family varies between protein families. Extensive cross-reactivity is seen within the PR-10 proteins and profilins [14]. Clinical cross-reactivity between storage proteins of different plant foods appears to be limited, although (in vitro) cross-reactivity within and between specific tree nuts and legumes has been described [15–17]. Co-sensitization, also between different protein families, is a common phenomenon in daily practice [18].

The aim of this paper was to identify the most frequently recognized plant food components and protein families using sensitization data from multiplex CRD in an adult population suspected of food allergy. Additionally, we wanted to investigate (co-)sensitization patterns with regard to food protein families, focused on PR-10 and storage proteins. For this purpose, we focused on sensitization only, while also including demographic data such as age and sex.

Methods

Patient selection

A retrospective explorative study was conducted. The study population consisted of every adult patient that received diagnostic analysis using ImmunoCAP ISAC 112 in our food allergy outpatient clinic of the Dermatology/Allergology department of our tertiary hospital in Utrecht, The Netherlands, between April 2012 and September 2016. All results of the ImmunoCAP ISAC were collected, regardless of clinical parameters. In case more than one ISAC was performed in a single patient, which was the case in $n = 3$, only the first/oldest was included. The population consisted of patients referred by general practitioners and secondary care dermatology and allergy clinics because of a potential food allergy. In general, an ISAC was ordered based on the physician's judgment in case of suspicion of multiple (plant) food allergies (i.e. fruits, legumes and tree nuts). Demographic data, i.e. age at time of blood draw and sex, were acquired for each patient.

ImmunoCAP ISAC

The ImmunoCAP ISAC was performed according to the manufacturer's instructions (Thermo Fisher Scientific, Uppsala, Sweden). On the ISAC, specific IgE binds to the components spotted on the chip and is then detected by immunofluorescence. Fluorescence intensity is measured by laser scanning and reported semi-quantitatively as ISAC Standardized Units (ISU) [19]. ISU values are reported in a range of 0.3–100. A patient was considered sensitized to a component on the ISAC in case of an ISAC Standardized Units (ISU) value of 0.3 or higher as recommended by the manufacturer. Subjects with sIgE against nJug r 2 were considered truly sensitized to Jug r 2 in case of no detectable sIgE against CCD marker nMUXF3 on ISAC, excluding reactivity to known carbohydrate epitopes on nJug r 2 on ISAC [20].

Statistics

Descriptive analyses were performed and presented as percentages or median values with interquartile range (IQR). The Chi square test was performed to assess differences in sex or sensitization frequency between groups. Differences in age and ISU levels between groups were assessed by Mann–Whitney *U* test. Spearman correlation was used to analyze correlations between ISU levels. A p value < 0.05 was considered statistically significant. Where necessary, a Bonferroni correction was applied to correct for multiple testing (112 components) by using a p value of 0.0004. Analyses were performed using SPSS Statistics 21 (IBM Corporation, Armonk, NY, USA).

Ethics

All ISAC tests were performed during routine care. The local Medical Ethics Review Committee confirmed that ethical approval is not required (nr. 15-249).

Results

A total of 305 patients with ISACs performed were included. Median age of the subjects was 32 years (range 16–79, IQR 22–45) and 74% was female. Sixteen ISACs (5%) were negative for all tested components. The following analyses were done using the total population of 305 subjects, unless stated otherwise. In our population, 91% was sensitized to two or more components of the ISAC and 85% to five or more, with a median amount of components recognized of 17 out of 112.

Out of 305 subjects, 92% was sensitized to at least one inhalant component on the ISAC. The major inhalant allergens include pollen (tree, grass and weed), house dust mite (HDM) and animal dander (cat, dog, mouse or horse). Tree pollen sensitization was most common (79%), with birch, alder and hazel pollen's PR-10 proteins being the most often recognized (see Additional file 1: Table 1), followed by grass (70%) and weed pollen (32%). Of our population, 55% recognized at least one component of the common Dermatophagoides house dust mites (Der p 1, Der p 2, Der p 10, Der f 1 and Der f 2). Sensitization to animal dander was seen in 56% of all subjects, with cat dander being most often recognized (49%). Polysensitization to inhalant allergens was very common with 73% sensitized to two or more of the inhalant allergen groups (pollen, HDM, animal dander) (Fig. 1). Of all subjects, 43% was sensitized to components from all three groups (pollen, HDM, animal dander; Fig. 1).

In all subjects sensitized to at least one food component ($n = 265$; 87%), the median amount of food components recognized was 6 out of 49. Additionally, 87% of the 265 was sensitized to three or more food components and 15% to 10 or more. The top recognized components were Bet v 1, Cor a 1.04 and Mal d 1 (see Additional file 1: Table 1). Of the total population, 74% was sensitized to any food PR-10 protein, followed by 35% to any storage protein, 15% to any food nsLTP, 8% to food tropomyosin (Pen m 1) and 3% to parvalbumin (Gad c 1). Since no food components from the profilin family are present on the ISAC, sensitization to Birch pollen profilin Bet v 2 was used as an indication for profilin sensitization [21], which was observed in 15% of all subjects. The following results will focus on PR-10 and storage protein sensitization since they were the most recognized plant food allergens.

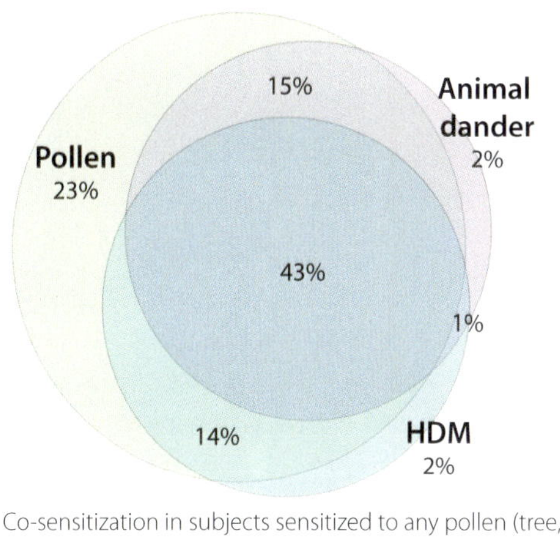

Fig. 1 Co-sensitization in subjects sensitized to any pollen (tree, grass and weed), house dust mite (HDM) and animal dander (cat, dog, mouse or horse) proteins. Of the total population ($n = 305$), 25 subjects were not sensitized to any component of the three inhalant allergen groups

Co-sensitization between protein families

Sensitization often was not limited to just pollen or non-pollen related food components. Of all patients sensitized to one or more PR-10 food components, 34% was also sensitized to one or more storage proteins. The overlap of sensitization to PR-10 proteins, storage proteins and nsLTPs, the third most recognized protein family of food components, is shown in Fig. 2.

Sensitization to food PR-10 proteins without pollen sensitization

Seven of the 228 subjects sensitized to PR-10s (3%) demonstrated sensitization to food PR-10 components without concomitant sensitization to PR-10 pollen components from birch (Bet v 1), alder (Aln g 1) or hazel (Cor a 1.01). Of these seven subjects, three were only sensitized to Cor a 1.04, three to Ara h 8 and one to both Cor a 1.04 and Ara h 8. In these subjects, titers for the positive PR-10 food components were generally low (< 2 ISU). Interestingly, all four subjects sensitized to Ara h 8 were also sensitized to Ara h 1, 2, 3 and 6, but not Ara h 9. Of the four sensitized to Cor a 1.04, only one demonstrated sensitization to other hazelnut components.

Sensitization patterns within PR-10 proteins

Subjects sensitized to PR-10 proteins ($n = 228$) were in most cases ($\geq$ 90%) sensitized to a combination of at least six PR-10 proteins: Bet v 1, Cor a 1.04, Mal d 1, Aln g 1, Pru p 1, Cor a 1.01 (Fig. 3a). Sensitization to PR-10 proteins Gly m 4, Api g 1 and Act d 8, occurred clearly less often. To assess possible explanations for this, the group of PR-10 sensitized subjects ($n = 228$) was split into two groups, based on this difference in the extent of PR-10 sensitization. Subjects that were sensitized to one or more 'less common PR-10 proteins' ($n = 147$; 64%) were compared with the ones only sensitized to one or more 'common PR-10 proteins' ($n = 81$; 36%). Several differences in sensitization patterns could be observed. In the group sensitized to the less common PR-10s, ISU values of all PR-10 proteins were significantly higher (all $p < 0.0001$; for example Bet v 1 median 28 [IQR 15–54] vs 8.0 [IQR 3.1–17.5]). Additionally, this group demonstrated more frequent sensitization to Phl p 6 (timothy grass; $p < 0.0001$) and Ole e 1 (olive pollen; $p < 0.0001$). Sensitization to the other components did not significantly differ in frequency or ISU levels but the total amount of (both food and inhalant) components recognized on the ISAC was significantly higher (median 22 vs 13 out of 112, $p < 0.0001$) in the group sensitized to uncommon PR-10s. Age and sex distribution was equal in the two groups.

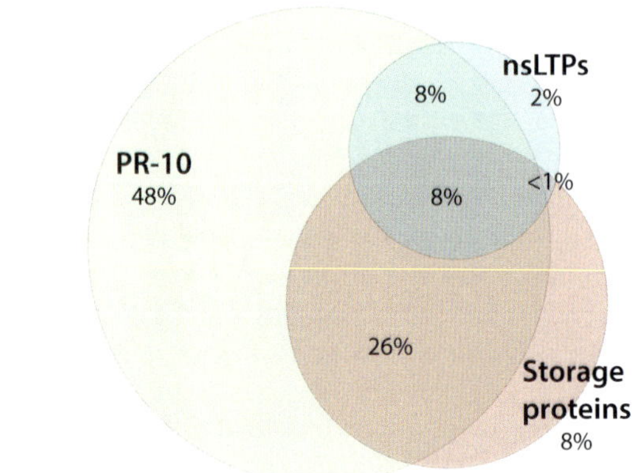

Fig. 2 Co-sensitization in subjects sensitized to at least one food PR-10 protein, storage protein or non-specific lipid transfer protein (nsLTPs) from food, present on the ImmunoCAP ISAC. Of the total population ($n = 305$), 52 subjects were not sensitized to any food component of the three protein families

Co-sensitization within PR-10 and storage proteins

Thirty-nine percent of the food sensitized subjects ($n = 265$) was solely sensitized to food components of the PR-10 protein family and not to any of the other food protein families or components. Co-sensitization to multiple components of the PR-10 protein family was common (Fig. 3a). This co-sensitization was accompanied by a high correlation between the ISU values found for these components (Fig. 3b).

Within storage proteins, co-sensitization was limited (Fig. 4a). Co-sensitization was mostly observed between the different peanut storage proteins (Ara h 1, 2, 3, and 6) and, to a lesser extent, between Ara h 1 and 3 on the one hand and Gly m 6 (soy) and Ana o 2 (cashew) on the other hand. Of the four peanut storage proteins on the ISAC, subjects were on average sensitized to 3 out of 4 and the majority was sensitized to all four (100 out of 179 sensitized to peanut storage proteins). Subjects sensitized to Cor a 9, Gly m 5 and Ses i 1 were frequently co-sensitized to peanut, soy and/or walnut storage proteins. In our cohort, we observed mostly very low correlations in ISU values between the storage proteins (Fig. 4b). A clear exception was Ara h 2 and 6 (spearman's rho 0.92; $p < 0.001$). Additionally, a strong correlation in ISU value was observed between Ara h 1 and 3, as well as Ara h 3 and Gly m 6.

Discussion

In our study, sensitization to birch pollen related (PR-10) food allergens was very common, which is as expected in our birch-endemic area. Birch pollen's Bet v 1 was overall the most recognized component with the highest median titer, supporting its assumed role as primary sensitizer [22]. Although co-sensitization to PR-10 proteins was

a

When sensitized for...		n	%	% also sensitized for Bet v 1	Cor a 1.04	Mal d 1	Aln g 1	Pru p 1	Cor a 1.01	Ara h 8	Gly m 4	Api g 1	Act d 8
Bet v 1	Birch pollen	**221**	72%		98%	94%	94%	86%	90%	72%	52%	37%	29%
Cor a 1.04	Hazelnut	**220**	72%	98%		92%	93%	85%	90%	73%	52%	36%	30%
Mal d 1	Apple	**207**	68%	100%	98%		96%	90%	94%	76%	56%	39%	31%
Aln g 1	Alder pollen	**207**	68%	100%	99%	96%		90%	96%	76%	56%	40%	31%
Pru p 1	Peach	**190**	62%	100%	99%	98%	98%		97%	78%	58%	41%	33%
Cor a 1.01	Hazel pollen	**200**	66%	100%	99%	98%	100%	93%		78%	58%	41%	33%
Ara h 8	Peanut	**164**	54%	98%	98%	96%	96%	91%	95%		66%	45%	35%
Gly m 4	Soy	**115**	38%	100%	100%	100%	100%	97%	100%	94%		50%	41%
Api g 1	Celery	**82**	27%	100%	98%	99%	100%	95%	100%	90%	70%		51%
Act d 8	Kiwi	**65**	21%	100%	100%	98%	100%	97%	100%	89%	72%	65%	

b

	Bet v 1	Cor a 1.04	Mal d 1	Aln g 1	Pru p 1	Cor a 1.01	Ara h 8	Gly m 4	Api g 1	Act d 8
Bet v 1										
Cor a 1.04	0,94									
Mal d 1	0,92	0,90								
Aln g 1	0,92	0,89	0,87							
Pru p 1	0,86	0,85	0,91	0,85						
Cor a 1.01	0,89	0,88	0,87	0,95	0,86					
Ara h 8	0,71	0,73	0,72	0,78	0,72	0,78				
Gly m 4	0,62	0,60	0,65	0,66	0,66	0,68	0,69			
Api g 1	0,51	0,51	0,52	0,59	0,49	0,59	0,56	0,46		
Act d 8	0,51	0,55	0,52	0,57	0,51	0,56	0,49	0,41	0,49	

Fig. 3 **a** Frequency of sensitization to PR-10 proteins (left) and percentage of sensitized subjects with concomitant co-sensitization to other PR-10 proteins (right). Darker shade of orange indicates higher frequency of co-sensitization. **b** Spearman correlation results of the ISU values found for the different PR-10 proteins

a

When sensitized for...		n	%	Ara h 6	Ara h 2	Jug r 1	Ara h 1	Gly m 6	Ara h 3	Ana o 2	Jug r 2	Ber e 1	Cor a 9	Gly m 5	Ses i 1	Fag e 2
				% also sensitized for												
Ara h 6	Peanut - 2S albumin	**60**	20%		88%	35%	55%	42%	45%	28%	20%	13%	23%	22%	15%	-
Ara h 2	Peanut - 2S albumin	**55**	18%	96%		36%	58%	44%	47%	29%	20%	13%	24%	24%	13%	-
Jug r 1	Walnut - 2S albumin	**36**	12%	58%	56%		42%	42%	33%	33%	33%	31%	39%	11%	25%	-
Ara h 1	Peanut - 7S globulin	**36**	12%	92%	89%	42%		67%	69%	39%	19%	19%	31%	33%	11%	-
Gly m 6	Soy - Glycicin	**30**	10%	83%	80%	50%	80%		77%	43%	23%	27%	43%	37%	17%	-
Ara h 3	Peanut - 11S globulin	**28**	9%	96%	93%	43%	89%	82%		43%	21%	25%	36%	43%	11%	-
Ana o 2	Cashew nut - 11S globulin	**20**	7%	85%	80%	60%	70%	65%	60%		25%	15%	45%	40%	30%	-
Jug r 2	Walnut - 7S globulin	**37**	12%	32%	30%	32%	19%	19%	16%	14%		22%	22%	11%	5%	-
Ber e 1	Brazil nut - 2S albumin	**19**	6%	42%	37%	58%	37%	42%	37%	16%	42%		37%	11%	16%	-
Cor a 9	Hazelnut - 11S globulin	**17**	6%	82%	76%	82%	65%	76%	59%	53%	47%	41%		29%	29%	-
Gly m 5	Soy - Beta-conglycin	**15**	5%	87%	87%	27%	80%	73%	80%	53%	27%	13%	33%		7%	-
Ses i 1	Sesame - 2S albumin	**12**	4%	75%	58%	75%	33%	42%	25%	50%	17%	25%	42%	8%		-
Fag e 2	Buckwheat - 2S albumin	**0**	0%	-	-	-	-	-	-	-	-	-	-	-	-	-

b

	Ara h 6	Ara h 2	Jug r 1	Ara h 1	Gly m 6	Ara h 3	Ana o 2	Jug r 2	Ber e 1	Cor a 9	Gly m 5	Ses i 1
Ara h 6												
Ara h 2	0,92											
Jug r 1	0,38	0,37										
Ara h 1	0,71	0,72	0,34									
Gly m 6	0,59	0,59	0,39	0,71								
Ara h 3	0,67	0,67	0,30	0,78	0,79							
Ana o 2	0,46	0,44	0,40	0,48	0,51	0,47						
Jug r 2	0,19	0,16	0,26	0,04	0,09	0,10	0,10					
Ber e 1	0,17	0,14	0,39	0,20	0,28	0,24	0,10	0,16				
Cor a 9	0,42	0,39	0,56	0,40	0,55	0,42	0,46	0,17	0,37			
Gly m 5	0,43	0,44	0,10	0,50	0,50	0,58	0,43	0,12	0,07	0,27		
Ses i 1	0,28	0,22	0,40	0,13	0,22	0,10	0,36	0,09	0,15	0,32	0,03	

Fig. 4 **a** Frequency of sensitization to storage proteins (left) and percentage of sensitized subjects with concomitant co-sensitization to other storage proteins (right). Darker shade of orange indicates higher frequency of co-sensitization. **b** Spearman correlation results of the ISU values found for the different storage proteins proteins

very prevalent, sensitization frequency differed between food PR-10 proteins. When comparing the subjects sensitized to 'uncommon PR-10 proteins' from soy (Gly m 4), celery (Api g 1) and kiwi (Act d 8) with those sensitized to only the 'common' PR-10 proteins, we observed significantly more frequent sensitization to specific grass and olive tree pollen in the group sensitized to uncommon PR10 s as well as overall more extensive sensitization to components on ISAC. An interaction or causal relationship between these allergens is unlikely. These differences in the amount of PR-10 proteins recognized, could be due to variability in allergen exposure, structural homology or allergenic properties (e.g. lability) between Bet v 1 and other PR-10 proteins [23]. For example, Cor a 1.04 (hazelnut) and Mal d 1 (apple) both have 67% amino acid sequence identity with Bet v 1 [24, 25], while for Ara h 8 (peanut) and Api g 1 (celery) this is only 46 and 42% respectively [26]. Interestingly, for Act d 8 (kiwi) the sequence identity was 53%, which would rule out sequence identity as sole explanation [27]. Also, technical issues with (the components of) the ISAC platform could play a role in explaining the found differences in sensitization frequency. Sensitization to these 'uncommon PR-10 proteins' could be an indication of more extensive polysensitization in our Western European geographic area. Interestingly, a very similar 'hierarchical order' of sensitization frequency for PR-10 proteins (i.e. Bet v 1 > Cor a 1.04 > Mal d 1 etc.) was recently described in both Swedish children and Austrian adolescents, also characterized using multiplex specific IgE testing [28, 29]. While these are all birch endemic countries, overall sensitization patterns differed, especially in Austria where grass sensitization was more prevalent [29]. This could indicate that this hierarchical order of sensitization to PR-10 proteins is not influenced by co-sensitization to other types of allergens. Additionally, in the Swedish children, all part of the BAMSE birth cohort, this hierarchical order already revealed itself at the age of 4 years old and appeared to have stabilized around 16 years old [28].

We identified seven subjects sensitized to food PR-10 proteins, without concomitant sensitization to PR-10 proteins from pollen, present on the ISAC. Birch pollen's Bet v 1 is considered the major PR-10 protein and primary sensitizer in birch pollen related food allergy [22]. Food PR-10 proteins are thought to be unable to induce primary sensitization due to their susceptibility to gastrointestinal digestion [30]. However, the co-sensitization to other peanut allergens in the Ara h 8 positive and pollen negative subjects could indicate primary sensitization to Ara h 8 via peanut ingestion or possibly skin contact [31]. Alternatively, technical aspects of the ISAC and its recombinant PR-10 components could have resulted in false positive or false negative results for food or pollen PR-10 proteins respectively. Other studies are needed to further investigate this. In literature, sensitization to PR-10s from hazelnut (Cor a 1) and peach (Pru p 1), without concomitant sensitization to Bet v 1, has been reported before [29, 32, 33]. Datema et al. [33] hypothesized that sensitization to Bet v 1-like pollen components from other *Fagales* species, such as hazel, oak, alder, or beech might be responsible for cross-reactive sensitization to Cor a 1 in their Bet v 1-negative patients. In our seven patients, alder's Aln g 1 and hazel's Cor a 1.01 were negative as well. Additionally, in our study, hazelnut Cor a 1.04 and apple Mal d 1 were recognized more frequently and with a higher median titer than alder's Aln g 1 and hazel's Cor a 1.01. Therefore, the sensitization potential of PR-10 proteins from pollen other than Bet v 1 appears limited. Still, Bet v 1-like pollen components from *Fagales* species have been identified, such as Que a 1 (*Quercus alba*; white oak), Cas s 1 (*Castanea sativa*; chestnut) and Fag s 1 (*Fagus sylvatica;* European beech), which could have played a role in these patients [34]. These components could not be tested in our population.

For storage proteins, cross-reactivity between proteins from different foods is uncommon [35]. However, we did observe some striking combinations in co-sensitization in our population. For peanut allergens, co-sensitization to multiple peanut proteins was common. While Ara h 2 and 6 are both 2S albumins, Ara h 1 and 3 belong to different subtypes of peanut storage proteins. Cross-reactivity between Ara h 2 and 6 has been demonstrated in several experiments [36–38], but there is limited data suggesting cross-reactivity between Ara h 2 on the one hand and Ara h 1 and 3 on the other hand [36]. In our data, we observed a moderately strong correlation in ISU levels between Ara h 1 and 3 and between those two and Ara h 2 and 6, which could be the result of common co-sensitization as well as cross-reactivity. Another common co-sensitization was between peanut and soy components. This was also observed before in a population of soy allergic patients from our clinic [39]. While the moderately strong correlations suggest potential cross-reactivity, inhibition experiments are needed to confirm this finding. Interestingly, sensitization to less frequently recognized allergens cashew Ana o 2, hazelnut Cor a 9, soy Gly m 5 and sesame Ses i 1 was often accompanied with co-sensitization to peanut. In the case of Cor a 9 and Ses i 1, co-sensitization to walnut Jug r 1 was common as well. While these observations could indicate distinct patterns in sensitization, they might be (partly) influenced by patient selection for ISAC testing. Different studies are needed to properly assess the clinical relevance of these co-sensitizations [18].

The ISACs in this population were ordered during routine care in outpatients with a suspected food allergy. While it is therefore an unselected outpatient group, there is a certain selection bias due to the nature of the test. The ISAC consists of a selection of food components, mostly of plant food origin. However, certain components that have been established to be clinically relevant, such as hazelnut Cor a 14 [10], are not present on the ISAC. Additionally, most components are also available separately on the ImmunoCAP platform, making it financially unfeasible to perform an ISAC in case of few suspected allergies, e.g. only peanut, a single tree nut or isolated fish or shellfish allergy. Due to the selection of components on the ISAC, together with the financial costs of the test, in our tertiary food allergy clinic, the ISAC is generally ordered for suspected multiple plant food allergies. Additionally, sensitization to nsLTPs and profilins is infrequent in our population and its role in clinical allergies in our population appears limited [10, 40, 41]. Therefore, we chose to focus this study on PR-10 and storage proteins. Another important limitation of this study is the use of sensitization data, without data on food allergy diagnosis, clinical symptoms or atopic co-morbidity. Clinically irrelevant sensitization is a known limitation of sensitization tests in (food) allergy diagnostics, especially with cross-reactive allergens such as PR-10 proteins [42, 43]. Furthermore, we did not take potential seasonal variation in (specific) IgE levels into account [44, 45], although this effect has not been studied with ISAC yet. Strength of this study is the analyses of a large adult population using a current multiplex specific IgE test with 112 components. Similar studies were mainly focused on children or adolescents [29] or performed using older test platforms with less components [46].

Conclusions

In our population of adults with a suspected food allergy, sensitization to PR-10 proteins was most frequent, often with co-sensitization to food allergens from other protein families. Within the storage proteins, sensitization to multiple peanut allergens was most common (on average 3 out of 4). Sensitization to PR-10 proteins from food, without concomitant sensitization to PR-10 proteins from pollen, occurred in a subset of subjects. Less commonly recognized PR-10 proteins appeared indicative of polysensitization to both food and inhalant allergens.

Abbreviations

CRD: component-resolved diagnostics; ISAC: ImmunoCAP ISAC; ISU: ISAC Standardized Units; PR-10: pathogenesis related protein family 10; nsLTP: non-specific lipid transfer protein; sIgE: specific IgE.

Authors' contributions

MAB: conception, design, data acquisition and interpretation, drafting manuscript. ACK, RJBK: conception, design, data interpretation, critical revision of manuscript. EFK, TL, HR, HGO: data interpretation, critical revision of manuscript. All authors read and approved the final manuscript.

Author details
[1] Department of Dermatology and Allergology, University Medical Center Utrecht, Utrecht University, Heidelberglaan 100, 3584 CX Utrecht, The Netherlands. [2] Laboratory of Translational Immunology, University Medical Center Utrecht, Utrecht University, Heidelberglaan 100, 3584 CX Utrecht, The Netherlands.

Acknowledgements
Not applicable.

Competing interests
The authors declare that they have no competing interests with regard to this research, but their institution has previously received speaker fees and research funding from ThermoFisher Scientific.

Funding
This research received no specific grant or funding.

References

1. Canonica GW, Ansotegui IJ, Pawankar R, Schmid-Grendelmeier P, van Hage M, Baena-Cagnani CE, et al. A WAO–ARIA–GA2LEN consensus document on molecular-based allergy diagnostics. World Allergy Organ J. 2013;6:17. https://doi.org/10.1186/1939-4551-6-17.
2. van Hage M, Hamsten C, Valenta R. ImmunoCAP Assays: pros and cons in allergology. J Allergy Clin Immunol. 2017. https://doi.org/10.1016/j.jaci.2017.05.008.
3. Williams P, Önell A, Baldracchini F, Hui V, Jolles S, El-Shanawany T. Evaluation of a novel automated allergy microarray platform compared with three other allergy test methods. Clin Exp Immunol. 2016;184:1–10. https://doi.org/10.1111/cei.12721.
4. Ahlgrim C, Gutermuth J, Onell A, Borres MP, Schäffner I, Darsow U, et al. Comparison of molecular multiplex and singleplex analysis of IgE to grass pollen allergens in untreated German grass pollen-allergic patients. J Investig Allergol Clin Immunol. 2015;25:190–5.
5. Breiteneder H, Radauer C. A classification of plant food allergens. J Allergy Clin Immunol. 2004;113:821–30. https://doi.org/10.1016/j.jaci.2004.01.779 **(quiz 831)**.
6. Breiteneder H, Mills ENC. Molecular properties of food allergens. J Allergy Clin Immunol. 2005;115:14–23. https://doi.org/10.1016/j.jaci.2004.10.022 **(quiz 24)**.
7. Hoffmann-Sommergruber K, Mills ENC. Food allergen protein families and their structural characteristics and application in component-resolved diagnosis: new data from the EuroPrevall project. Anal Bioanal Chem. 2009;395:25–35. https://doi.org/10.1007/s00216-009-2953-z.
8. Geroldinger-Simic M, Zelniker T, Aberer W, Ebner C, Egger C, Greiderer A, et al. Birch pollen-related food allergy: clinical aspects and the role of allergen-specific IgE and IgG4 antibodies. J Allergy Clin Immunol. 2011;127(616–622):e1. https://doi.org/10.1016/j.jaci.2010.10.027.
9. Masthoff LJ, Hoff R, Verhoeckx KCM, van Os-Medendorp H, Michelsen-Huisman A, Baumert JL, et al. A systematic review of the effect of thermal processing on the allergenicity of tree nuts. Allergy. 2013;14:983–93. https://doi.org/10.1111/all.12185
10. Masthoff LJN, Mattsson L, Zuidmeer-Jongejan L, Lidholm J, Andersson K, Akkerdaas JH, et al. Sensitization to Cor a 9 and Cor a 14 is highly specific for a hazelnut allergy with objective symptoms in Dutch children and adults. J Allergy Clin Immunol. 2013;132:393–9. https://doi.org/10.1016/j.jaci.2013.02.024.
11. Pedrosa M, Boyano-Martínez T, García-Ara MC, Caballero T, Quirce S. Peanut seed storage proteins are responsible for clinical reactivity in Spanish peanut-allergic children. Pediatr Allergy Immunol. 2012;23:654–9. https://doi.org/10.1111/j.1399-3038.2012.01337.x.
12. Asero R, Mistrello G, Roncarolo D, Amato S, Falagiani P. Analysis of the heat stability of lipid transfer protein from apple. J Allergy Clin Immunol. 2003;112:1009–11. https://doi.org/10.1016/S0091-6749(03)02006-2.
13. van der Valk JPM, Gerth van Wijk R, Dubois AEJ, de Groot H, Reitsma M, Vlieg-Boerstra B, et al. Multicentre double-blind placebo-controlled food challenge study in children sensitised to cashew nut. PLoS ONE. 2016;11:e0151055. https://doi.org/10.1371/journal.pone.0151055.
14. Santos A, Van Ree R. Profilins: mimickers of allergy or relevant allergens? Int Arch Allergy Immunol. 2011;155:191–204. https://doi.org/10.1159/000321178.
15. Bublin M, Breiteneder H. Cross-reactivity of peanut allergens. Curr Allergy Asthma Rep. 2014;14:426. https://doi.org/10.1007/s11882-014-0426-8.
16. van der Valk JPM, J Dubois AE, Gerth van Wijk R, Wichers HJ, de Jong NW. Systematic review on cashew nut allergy. Allergy. 2014;69:692–8. https://doi.org/10.1111/all.12401.
17. Sirvent S, Cantó B, Gómez F, Blanca N, Cuesta-Herranz J, Canto G, et al. Detailed characterization of Act d 12 and Act d 13 from kiwi seeds: implication in IgE cross-reactivity with peanut and tree nuts. Allergy. 2014. https://doi.org/10.1111/all.12486.
18. Masthoff LJ, van Hoffen E, Mattsson L, Lidholm J, Andersson K, Zuidmeer-Jongejan L, et al. Peanut allergy is common among hazelnut-sensitized subjects but is not primarily the result of IgE cross-reactivity. Allergy. 2015;70:265–74. https://doi.org/10.1111/all.12554.
19. van Hage M, Schmid-Grendelmeier P, Skevaki C, Plebani M, Canonica W, Kleine-Tebbe J, et al. Performance evaluation of ImmunoCAP® ISAC 112: a multi-site study. Clin Chem Lab Med. 2017;55(4):571–7. https://doi.org/10.1515/cclm-2016-0586.
20. Villalta D, Conte M, Asero R, Da Re M, Stella S, Martelli P. Isolated IgE reactivity to native walnut vicilin-like protein (nJug r 2) on ISAC™ microarray is due to cross-reactive carbohydrate epitopes. Clin Chem Lab Med. 2013;51:1991–5. https://doi.org/10.1515/cclm-2013-0027.
21. Villalta D, Asero R. Sensitization to the pollen pan-allergen profilin. Is the detection of immunoglobulin E to multiple homologous proteins from different sources clinically useful? J Investig Allergol Clin Immunol. 2010;20:591–5.
22. Jahn-Schmid B, Radakovics A, Lüttkopf D, Scheurer S, Vieths S, Ebner C, et al. Bet v 1142-156 is the dominant T-cell epitope of the major birch pollen allergen and important for cross-reactivity with Bet v 1-related food allergens. J Allergy Clin Immunol. 2005;116:213–9. https://doi.org/10.1016/j.jaci.2005.04.019.
23. Roulias A, Pichler U, Hauser M, Himly M, Hofer H, Lackner P, et al. Differences in the intrinsic immunogenicity and allergenicity of Bet v 1 and related food allergens revealed by site-directed mutagenesis. Allergy Eur J Allergy Clin Immunol. 2014;69:208–15. https://doi.org/10.1111/all.12306.
24. Vanekkrebitz M, Hoffmannsommergruber K, Machado MLD, Susani M, Ebner C, Kraft D, et al. Cloning and sequencing of Mal d 1, the major allergen from apple (*Malus domestica*), and its immunological relationship to Bet v 1, the major birch pollen allergen. Biochem Biophys Res Commun. 1995;214:538–51. https://doi.org/10.1006/bbrc.1995.2320.
25. Lüttkopf D, Müller U, Skov PS, Ballmer-Weber BK, Wüthrich B, Skamstrup Hansen K, et al. Comparison of four variants of a major allergen in hazelnut (*Corylus avellana*) Cor a 1.04 with the major hazel pollen allergen

Cor a 1.01. Mol Immunol. 2002;38:515–25. https://doi.org/10.1016/S0161-5890(01)00087-6.

26. Mittag D, Akkerdaas J, Ballmer-Weber BK, Vogel L, Wensing M, Becker W-M, et al. Ara h 8, a Bet v 1—homologous allergen from peanut, is a major allergen in patients with combined birch pollen and peanut allergy. J Allergy Clin Immunol. 2004;114:1410–7. https://doi.org/10.1016/j.jaci.2004.09.014.
27. Oberhuber C, Bulley SM, Ballmer-Weber BK, Bublin M, Gaier S, DeWitt ÅM, et al. Characterization of Bet v 1-related allergens from kiwifruit relevant for patients with combined kiwifruit and birch pollen allergy. Mol Nutr Food Res. 2008. https://doi.org/10.1002/mnfr.200800146.
28. Westman M, Lupinek C, Bousquet J, Andersson N, Pahr S, Baar A, et al. Early childhood IgE reactivity to pathogenesis-related class 10 proteins predicts allergic rhinitis in adolescence. J Allergy Clin Immunol. 2015;135:1199–206. https://doi.org/10.1016/j.jaci.2014.10.042.
29. Stemeseder T, Klinglmayr E, Moser S, Lueftenegger L, Lang R, Himly M, et al. Cross-sectional study on allergic sensitization of Austrian adolescents using molecule-based IgE profiling. Allergy. 2017;72:754–63. https://doi.org/10.1111/all.13071.
30. Bohle B, Zwölfer B, Heratizadeh A, Jahn-Schmid B, Antonia YD, Alter M, et al. Cooking birch pollen-related food: divergent consequences for IgE- and T cell-mediated reactivity in vitro and in vivo. J Allergy Clin Immunol. 2006;118:242–9. https://doi.org/10.1016/j.jaci.2006.03.011.
31. Tordesillas L, Goswami R, Benedé S, Grishina G, Dunkin D, Järvinen KM, et al. Skin exposure promotes a Th2-dependent sensitization to peanut allergens. J Clin Invest. 2014;124:4965–75. https://doi.org/10.1172/JCI75660.
32. Flinterman AE, Akkerdaas JH, den Hartog Jager CF, Rigby NM, Fernandez-Rivas M, Hoekstra MO, et al. Lipid transfer protein-linked hazelnut allergy in children from a non-Mediterranean birch-endemic area. J Allergy Clin Immunol. 2008;121(423–428):e2. https://doi.org/10.1016/j.jaci.2007.10.009.
33. Datema MR, Zuidmeer-Jongejan L, Asero R, Barreales L, Belohlavkova S, de Blay F, et al. Hazelnut allergy across Europe dissected molecularly: a EuroPrevall outpatient clinic survey. J Allergy Clin Immunol. 2015. https://doi.org/10.1016/j.jaci.2014.12.1949.
34. Search results for "Bet v 1-like." Allergome.org 2017. http://allergome.org/. Accessed 16 May 2017.
35. Moreno FJ, Clemente A. 2S albumin storage proteins: what makes them food allergens? Open Biochem J. 2008;2:16–28. https://doi.org/10.2174/1874091X00802010016.
36. Bublin M, Kostadinova M, Radauer C, Hafner C, Szépfalusi Z, Varga E-M, et al. IgE cross-reactivity between the major peanut allergen Ara h 2 and the nonhomologous allergens Ara h 1 and Ara h 3. J Allergy Clin Immunol. 2013;132:118–24. https://doi.org/10.1016/j.jaci.2013.01.022.
37. Lehmann K, Schweimer K, Reese G, Randow S, Suhr M, Becker W-M, et al. Structure and stability of 2S albumin-type peanut allergens: implications for the severity of peanut allergic reactions. Biochem J. 2006;395:463–72. https://doi.org/10.1042/BJ20051728.
38. Koppelman SJ, de Jong GAH, Laaper-Ertmann M, Peeters KABM, Knulst AC, Hefle SL, et al. Purification and immunoglobulin E-binding properties of peanut allergen Ara h 6: evidence for cross-reactivity with Ara h 2. Clin Exp Allergy. 2005;35:490–7. https://doi.org/10.1111/j.1365-2222.2005.02204.x.
39. Klemans RJB, Knol EF, Michelsen-Huisman A, Pasmans SGMA, de Kruijf-Broekman W, Bruijnzeel-Koomen CAFM, et al. Components in soy allergy diagnostics: Gly m 2S albumin has the best diagnostic value in adults. Allergy. 2013;68:1396–402. https://doi.org/10.1111/all.12259.
40. Blankestijn MA, Blom WM, Otten HG, Baumert JL, Taylor SL, Bruijnzeel-Koomen CAFM, et al. Specific IgE to Jug r 1 has no additional value compared with extract-based testing in diagnosing walnut allergy in adults. J Allergy Clin Immunol. 2017;139(688–690):e4. https://doi.org/10.1016/j.jaci.2016.07.026.
41. Klemans RJB, Broekman HCHP, Knol EF, Bruijnzeel-Koomen CAFM, Otten HG, Pasmans SGMA, et al. Ara h 2 is the best predictor for peanut allergy in adults. J Allergy Clin Immunol Pract. 2013;1:632–8. https://doi.org/10.1016/j.jaip.2013.07.014.
42. Werfel T, Asero R, Ballmer-Weber BK, Beyer K, Enrique E, Knulst AC, et al. Position paper of the EAACI: food allergy due to immunological cross-reactions with common inhalant allergens. Allergy Eur J Allergy Clin Immunol. 2015;70:1079–90. https://doi.org/10.1111/all.12666.
43. Ebo DG, Bridts CH, Verweij MM, De Knop KJ, Hagendorens MM, De Clerck LS, et al. Sensitization profiles in birch pollen-allergic patients with and without oral allergy syndrome to apple: lessons from multiplexed component-resolved allergy diagnosis. Clin Exp Allergy. 2010;40:339–47. https://doi.org/10.1111/j.1365-2222.2009.03345.x.
44. Skamstrup Hansen K, Vieths S, Vestergaard H, Skov PS, Bindslev-Jensen C, Poulsen LK. Seasonal variation in food allergy to apple. J Chromatogr B Biomed Sci Appl. 2001;756:19–32. https://doi.org/10.1016/S0378-4347(01)00068-8.
45. Somville MA, Machiels J, Gilles JG, Saint-Remy JM. Seasonal variation in specific IgE antibodies of grass-pollen hypersensitive patients depends on the steady state IgE concentration and is not related to clinical symptoms. J Allergy Clin Immunol. 1989;83:486–94. https://doi.org/10.1016/0091-6749(89)90138-3.
46. Scala E, Alessandri C, Bernardi ML, Ferrara R, Palazzo P, Pomponi D, et al. Cross-sectional survey on immunoglobulin E reactivity in 23,077 subjects using an allergenic molecule-based microarray detection system. Clin Exp Allergy. 2010;40:911–21. https://doi.org/10.1111/j.1365-2222.2010.03470.x.

18

Impaired health-related quality of life in adolescents with allergy to staple foods

Jennifer Lisa Penner Protudjer[1,2], Sven-Arne Jansson[1,3], Roelinde Middelveld[1,2], Eva Östblom[1,4,5], Sven-Erik Dahlén[1,2], Marianne Heibert Arnlind[6,7], Ulf Bengtsson[8], Ingrid Kallström-Bengtsson[9], Birgitta Marklund[10], Georgios Rentzos[8], Ann-Charlotte Sundqvist[4], Johanna Åkerström[8] and Staffan Ahlstedt[1,2*]

Abstract

Background: Cow's milk, hen's egg and wheat are staple foods in a typical western diet. Despite the ubiquity of these foods, the impact of staple food allergy on health-related quality of life (HRQL) amongst adolescents is incompletely understood. The aims of this study were to make use of the Swedish version of EuroPrevall's disease-specific food allergy quality of life questionnaire-teenager form (FAQLQ-TF) and to investigate the association between objectively-diagnosed staple food allergy and HRQL amongst adolescents.

Methods: In this cross-sectional study, 58 adolescents aged 13–17 years [n = 40 (69 %) boys] with objectively-diagnosed allergy to the staple foods cow's milk, hen's egg and/or wheat and living in Stockholm, Sweden were included. Adolescents completed the FAQLQ-TF, which has a corresponding scale of 1 = best HRQL, and 7 = worst HRQL. Overall HRQL and domain-specific HRQL were established. Adolescents also reported symptoms, adrenaline auto injector (AAI) prescription and presence of other food allergies. A history of anaphylaxis was defined among those reporting difficulty breathing, inability to stand/collapse, and/or loss of consciousness. Clinically different HRQL was set at a mean difference of ≥ 0.5.

Results: Overall mean HRQL was poorer than average [mean: 4.70/7.00 (95 % CI 4.30–5.01)]. The domain risk of accidental exposure was significantly associated with clinically better HRQL than the domain allergen avoidance and dietary restrictions (mean difference = 0.76; $p < 0.001$). Girls had clinically worse, but not statistically significantly different mean HRQL than boys (mean difference = 0.71; $p < 0.07$). HRQL tended to be worse amongst those with allergies to more than three foods or an AAI prescription. The number and types of symptoms, including a history of anaphylaxis were not associated with worse HRQL.

Conclusions: As ascertained via a food allergy-specific questionnaire, adolescents with staple food allergy report poorer than average HRQL, specifically in relation to emerging independence and the need for support. Girls have clinically worse HRQL than boys. The number and type of previous symptoms and history of anaphylaxis were not associated with worse HRQL.

Keywords: Adolescents, Food allergy, Health-related quality of life

Background

Food allergy affects 2–8 % of adolescents [1, 2]. In this group, health-related quality of life (HRQL) or 'the effects of an illness and its consequent therapy upon a patient, as perceived by the patient [3], may be impacted [4–6], particularly in relation to social well-being and independence [7]. Further, adolescents with food allergy report worse overall HRQL compared to matched non-food allergic controls [4, 5], or to adolescents with other chronic conditions [4, 8]. Notably, these studies involved the use of generic HRQL questionnaires [4, 5, 8], which may not identify the subtleties of food allergy or issues specific to the disease [9]. To address this limitation, EuroPrevall's

*Correspondence: staffan.ahlstedt@ki.se
[1] The Centre for Allergy Research, Karolinska Institutet, P.O. Box 287, 17177 Stockholm, Sweden
Full list of author information is available at the end of the article

food allergy-specific HRQL questionnaires were specifically developed and validated to glean insights into food allergy that cannot be ascertained by generic questionnaires [9, 10]. The self-reported adolescent version of this questionnaire, the food allergy quality of life questionnaire-teenager form (FAQLQ-TF), presents a unique means by which to capture perceptions of HRQL of adolescents with food allergy. Self-reported data for this age group is important given the disagreement between adolescent- and parent-reported HRQL [6].

Previous studies on HRQL amongst adolescents with food allergy have focused on a wide range [4, 6] or unspecified [5] foods, as well as reported, rather than objectively diagnosed food allergies [5]. However, we believe that objectively diagnosed allergies to certain foods warrant particular attention. For example, allergies to the staple foods cow's milk, hen's egg [11] and wheat [12], typically present in infancy and often exist concomitantly [12]. Although these allergies often resolve by school age [11, 12], those with more severe symptoms or multiple food allergies may experience persistence of staple food allergy through later ages [11, 12]. As staple foods are ubiquitous in a typical western diet and are consequently difficult to avoid, the HRQL of adolescents experiencing disease persistence is likely to be impacted. Thus, we hypothesised that adolescents with staple food allergies would have poor HRQL, and that adolescents with a history of severe symptoms would have the worst HRQL. To this end, the aims of this study were to make use of the Swedish version of EuroPrevall's FAQLQ-TF and to investigate the association between objectively-diagnosed staple food allergy and HRQL amongst adolescents.

Methods

Study design and participants

In this cross-sectional study, adolescents aged 13–17 years with paediatric allergist-diagnosed allergy to one or more staple foods (cow's milk, hen's egg and/or wheat) were identified from medical records and recruited in 2010–2012 by a paediatric nurse from the outpatient allergy clinic at Sachs' Children and Youth Hospital, Södersjukhuset, in Stockholm, Sweden.

Inclusion criteria were a convincing history of allergy to one or more of the above-mentioned staple foods ascertained either by a positive food challenge with evident symptoms, or by levels of food specific Immunoglobulin E (IgE) antibodies levels associated with a 95 % probability of a positive result in a double-blind placebo controlled food challenge [13]. Exclusion criteria were an unclear allergy diagnosis to staple food(s), poor understanding of the Swedish language, or presence of coeliac disease, diabetes and/or a malignancy. Information on concomitant allergic disease (asthma, allergic rhinitis, allergic conjunctivitis, eczema) was also obtained. A total of 87 adolescents were eligible and invited to participate. These adolescents were mailed the FAQLQ-TF (described below, English version available as an Additional file 1), as well as an information letter and a postage-paid return envelope. Parents were mailed an information letter and consent form. Completed FAQLQ-TF and signed parental consent forms were received from 58 adolescents (67 % of those eligible; Fig. 1). Adolescents received two movie tickets following receipt of completed questionnaires. This study was approved by the Regional Ethical Review Board in Stockholm, Sweden (Dnr 2009/84-31/5). Personal data were treated according to the Swedish Personal Data Act.

Exposures

Both the number of staple food allergies, as well as the number of offending foods (at least one staple food allergy and, participant-reported allergies to other foods) were considered as exposures.

Adolescents responded to 36 closed-ended questions on food allergy symptoms, from which we generated specific symptoms:

Gastrointestinal: stomach upset; vomiting; diarrhoea.

Oral: itchy tongue, mouth or lips; swollen tongue or lips.

Upper respiratory: runny or blocked nose; sneezing.

Lower respiratory: itchy or tight throat; difficulty swallowing; shortness of breath; wheeze; cough.

Cardiovascular/neurological: dizziness; tachycardia; blurred vision; inability to stand/collapse; loss of consciousness.

The most severe symptoms, including difficulty breathing, inability to stand/collapse, and/or loss of consciousness, involved the respiratory- and/or cardiovascular/neurological systems. In keeping with our previous publications on children [27] and adults [26], and approximating as best as possible the criteria outlined by Sampson et al. [14], such symptoms are collectively referred to as anaphylaxis. Adolescents were asked if they had been prescribed an adrenaline auto injector (AAI).

Outcome

Food allergy quality of life questionnaire-teenager form (FAQLQ-TF)

The FAQLQ-TF [9] was translated into Swedish as per World Health Organization guidelines [15], and was piloted in 10 Swedish-speaking adolescents to ascertain comprehension. Following minor linguistic adjustments, the translation was deemed adequate. The FAQLQ-TF contains 28 questions on HRQL, each of which has corresponding closed-ended answers on a 7-point scale where 1 is best HRQL and 7 is worst HRQL [9]. Overall HRQL established by taking the mean of the 28 questions. These

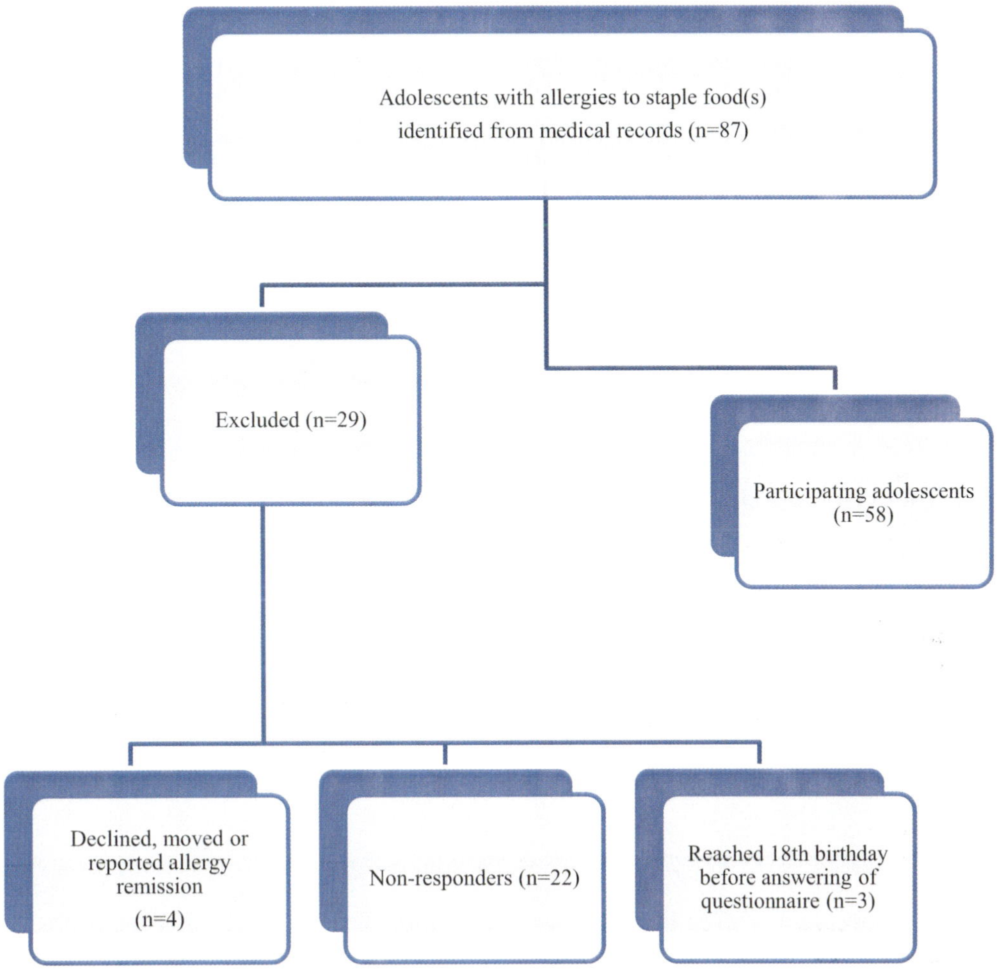

Fig. 1 Flow chart detailing enrolment of adolescents with objectively-diagnosed staple food allergy

questions were also designed to address three domains: allergen avoidance and dietary restrictions (AADR), emotional impact (EI) and risk of accidental exposure (RAE). The first domain, AADR, describes adolescents' perceptions of limitations, hesitations and refusals of foods that they purchase or are offered in social situations. The second domain, EI, reflects adolescents' fears of an allergic reaction or accidental consumption of the food(s) to which they are allergic and their disappointment when others do not take their food allergy seriously. The third domain, RAE, captures adolescents' assessments of needing to be cautious about purchasing food or eating out in relation to changes in ingredients, incorrect disclosure of ingredients and touching certain foods.

Statistics

Floor and ceiling effects (percentages of patients with minimal and maximum scores, respectively) of the FAQLQ-TF were calculated to verify discriminative capacity. These effects were considered present if >15 % of a sample of a minimum of 50 individuals achieved the lowest or highest possible scores, respectively. Absence of these effects demonstrates the efficacy of the questionnaire.

Descriptive statistics included sample sizes (n), percentages, means, parametric two-sample t-tests and 95 % CI. Statistical significance was set at $p < 0.05$. Overall and domain-specific HRQL scores were calculated for the entire study population and stratified by gender. To permit statistical comparisons, the number of staple food allergies was classified into 2 dichotomous groups: 1 vs. 2–3. The number of offending foods was classified into 4 groups: 1, 2, 3 or >3. As described above, adolescents reported on symptoms. Adolescents may forget or inaccurately report their symptoms. Thus, we performed intraclass correlations of adolescent-reported symptoms with those reported by their parents as part of a parallel study [32] to measure reliability. These analyses showed modest correlations between adolescent- and parent-reported symptoms, with increasing reliability with increasingly severe symptoms (results not shown). As such, we present the results herein based on adolescent-reported symptoms.

Univariable and multivariable linear regression analyses were performed to identify predictors of HRQL. Potential covariates were identified based on prior knowledge of the exposures and outcome. The covariates gender, number of symptoms, history of anaphylaxis, AAI prescription and concomitant allergic disease were included in the final model as they statistically and independently altered the prediction model. The same models were used for overall and domain-specific HRQL. In keeping with previous publications on HRQL assessed via the FAQLQ, a score of $\geq \pm 0.5$ was considered to be clinically relevant [9, 16]. Analysis was performed with STATA Statistical Software (release 13.1; StataCorp, College Station, Texas, USA).

Results

The discriminant capacity of the FAQLQ-TF was confirmed as domain-specific floor and ceiling effects were below 15 % (results not shown).

Our study population included 58 adolescents, of whom 40 (69 %) were boys (Table 1). Most (62 %) of participants were allergic to only one staple food, although 7 % were allergic to all three staple foods. The most common staple food allergy was to hen's egg (79 %). Other participant-reported allergies to other foods, particularly to tree nuts (60 %) and peanuts (53 %), were also common. Nearly all adolescents reported lower respiratory (95 %) and dermatological (90 %) symptoms. Gastrointestinal symptoms were also common (68 %). Although symptoms involving the cardiovascular/neurological system were the least common, they were nonetheless reported by 27 % of adolescents.

Table 1 Descriptive allergy characteristics of adolescents with objectively-diagnosed staple food allergy

	n	%
Sex		
Boys	40	69.0
Girls	18	31.0
Number of staple food allergies		
1	36	62.1
2	18	31.0
3	4	6.9
Offending staple foods[a]		
Hen's egg	46	79.3
Cow's milk	29	50.0
Wheat	5	8.6
Participant-reported allergies to other foods[a]		
Tree nuts	35	60.3
Peanuts	31	53.4
Fruit	17	29.3
Vegetables	8	13.8
Fish	9	15.5
Shellfish	12	20.7
Soy	6	10.3
Sesame seeds	2	3.4
Number of offending foods[b]		
1	8	13.8
2	10	17.2
3	13	22.4
>3	27	46.6
Symptoms resulting from staple foods[a]		
Gastrointestinal	28	68.3
Dermatological	37	90.2
Oral cavity	32	39.0
Upper respiratory	16	39.0
Lower respiratory	39	95.1
Cardiovascular	11	26.8
Anaphylaxis	23	56.1
Concomitant allergic disease[c]		
None or one	11	19.0
Two or more	47	81.0

[a] Not mutually exclusive

[b] Includes at least 1 objectively-diagnosed staple food, as well as any participant-reported allergies to other foods

[c] Asthma, allergic rhinitis, allergic conjunctivitis and/or eczema

Overall HRQL and domain-specific HRQL are presented in Fig. 2. The overall HRQL mean score was 4.70/7.00 (95 % CI 4.30–5.01). Girls had clinically worse, but not statistically significantly different HRQL than boys (5.12 ± 1.01 vs. 4.51 ± 1.23, respectively; mean difference = 0.71; $p < 0.07$).

With consideration to the different domains, the mean scores for AADR and EI were comparable (Fig. 2). In contrast, RAE was significantly associated with clinically better HRQL compared to the reference domain, AADR (mean 4.19/7.00; 95 % CI 3.82–4.56 vs. mean 4.95/7.00; 95 % CI 4.65–5.25, respectively; mean difference = 0.76; $p < 0.001$). Only the domain, EI, differed significantly between the sexes, with clinically worse HRQL amongst girls than boys (5.38 ± 1.4 vs. 4.50 ± 0.24; mean difference = 0.88; $p < 0.04$).

Investigation to the individual questions of each domain revealed further insights into the fine tuning of the HRQL of the different domains. For example, in the domain AADR, compared to the question with the highest mean score (i.e. worst HRQL), 'How troublesome

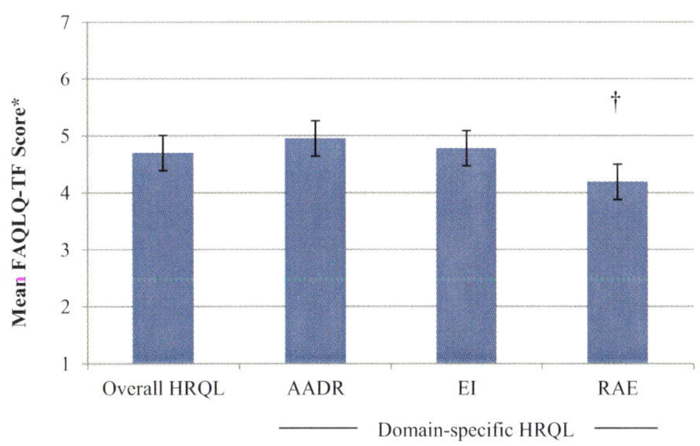

Fig. 2 Overall- and domain-specific HRQL mean scores and 95 % CI for adolescents with objectively-diagnosed staple food allergy. *Asterisk* FAQLQ-TF on a scale of 1–7, where 1 corresponds to best HRQL and 7 corresponds to worst HRQL; based on self-report. † Compared to AADR ($p < 0.001$). *HRQL* health-related quality of life, *AADR* allergen avoidance and dietary restrictions, *EI* emotional impact, *RAE* risk of accidental exposure

do you find it, because of your food allergy, that you must check yourself whether you can eat something when eating out', factors that were associated with significantly better HRQL included limitations on eating, buying or refusing foods, or spontaneously accepting invitations to a meal. Within the domain, EI, compared to the reference question, 'How disappointed are you when people don't take your food allergy into account?,' factors associated with significantly better HRQL included feeling discouraged, carrying an AAI, or fears related to eating something 'wrong' or something new. Within the domain, RAE, compared to the reference question, 'How troublesome do you find it, because of your food allergy, that you have to explain to people around you that you have a food allergy?,' the only factor associated with significantly better HRQL related to labelling discrepancies between bulk and individual packaging (Table 2).

In linear regression analyses adjusted for sex, number of symptoms, history of anaphylaxis, AAI prescription and concomitant allergic disease (excluding the predictor), girls had clinically worse and but not statistically significant HRQL than boys ($B = -0.58$; 95 % CI -1.34; 0.19; $p = 0.13$; Table 3). Similarly, allergies to >3 staple food allergies and AAI prescription reached the threshold of ≥ 0.5 for clinical relevance but only trended towards significance ($p = 0.13$ and $p = 0.06$, respectively).

Consideration to the presence vs. absence of specific symptoms including anaphylaxis attributable to staple foods yielded no statistically significant associations. Only previous lower respiratory symptoms reached the threshold for clinically better HRQL ($B = 0.67$; 95 % CI -1.37; 2.70, $p = 0.51$; Table 4).

Discussion

In this cross-sectional study of adolescents with objectively-diagnosed staple food allergies to cow's milk, hen's egg and/or wheat, overall HRQL, as ascertained by a food allergy specific questionnaire, was poorer than average. The domain risk of accidental exposure was significantly associated with clinically better HRQL than the domain allergen avoidance and dietary restrictions. Girls had clinically worse, but not statistically significantly different HRQL than boys. HRQL tended to be worse amongst adolescents with allergies to more than three foods or those who had been prescribed an AAI. In contrast, the number and type of previous symptoms and history of anaphylaxis were not associated with worse HRQL.

We highlight the key strengths of this study we used a food allergy-specific questionnaire that is robust for adolescents with food allergies [9, 17] that provided insights into associations between food allergy and HRQL that could not have been gleaned via a generic questionnaire [9]. Similarly, this work presents the first results of the Swedish version of the FAQLQ-TF. In our study, participants had objectively-diagnosed allergies, thus providing insight into the impact of true, rather than perceived, food allergy on HRQL. Amongst children, HRQL does not differ between these two phenotypes [18]. However, consideration of the association between objectively-diagnosed allergy and adolescent-reported HRQL warrants consideration as this age group is increasingly responsible for their own food choices, and thus the potential consequences of inappropriate food choices. Although adolescents' food choices are influenced by their allergies, they also make choices based on peers and sensory preferences [19]. We believe that we are the first group to report on HRQL amongst adolescents with allergies to foods that are ubiquitous in a typical western diet, but which also receive less attention in relation to HRQL than other common food allergens, such as peanuts or tree nuts.

We also acknowledge the limitations of our study. Our study was cross-sectional in design, thereby precluding establishment of a causal relationship between staple food allergy and HRQL. As well, our study population included more boys than girls. As evidenced in the general adolescent population [20], and amongst food hypersensitive adolescents for whom HRQL was established using a generic questionnaire [5], boys generally have better HRQL than girls. Thus, we surmise that, had adolescent boys and girls been equally represented, overall HRQL may have been even worse.

The FAQLQ-TF is specifically designed to capture adolescents' perceptions of HRQL [9]. Elsewhere, responses from Dutch adolescent-parent pairs to the FAQLQ have been compared [6]. In that study, adolescents were

Table 2 Mean scores for individual questions used to calculate domain-specific HRQL

	Mean	*p* value†
Allergen avoidance and dietary restrictions		
How troublesome do you find it, because of your food allergy, that you:		
Must check yourself whether you can eat something when eating out?	5.76	
Must read labels?	5.74	0.95
Hesitate eating a product when you have doubts about it?	5.67	0.75
Must always be alert to what you are eating?	5.66	0.70
Are less able to taste or try various products when eating out?	5.36	0.15
Are able to eat fewer products?	5.21	<0.05
Are limited as to the products that you can buy?	4.47	<0.001
Are less able to spontaneously accept an invitation to stay for a meal?	4.09	<0.001
Must be careful about touching certain foods?	3.47	<0.001
Must refuse treats at school or work?	2.58	<0.001
Emotional impact		
Answer the following:		
How disappointed are you when people don't take your food allergy into account?	5.50	
How discouraged do you feel during an allergic reaction?	4.74	<0.05
How troublesome do you find it, because of your food allergy, that you:		
Have the feeling that you have less control of what you eat when eating out?	5.40	0.86
Must carry an EpiPen®?	4.36	<0.01
How frightened are you because of your food allergy:		
Of accidentally eating something wrong?	4.59	<0.05
Of an allergic reaction?	4.53	<0.05
To eat something that you have never eaten before?	4.31	<0.05
Risk of accidental exposure		
How troublesome do you find it, because of your food allergy, that you:		
That you have to explain to people around you that you have a food allergy?	5.00	
That during social activities others can eat the food to which you are allergic?	4.95	0.88
That during social activities your food allergy is not taken into account enough?	4.47	0.17
That the ingredients of a food change?	4.45	0.10
That the label states: "May contain (traces of)…."?	4.43	0.15
That the labelling of the bulk packaging (e.g. box or bag) is different than the individual packages?	3.27	<0.001

FAQLQ-TF on a scale of 1–7, where 1 corresponds to best HRQL and 7 corresponds to worst HRQL; based on self-report

† Compared to the individual question with the highest mean score (i.e. worst HRQL) within each domain

allergic to a wide range of common food allergens, but staple food allergy did not predominate. Amongst these adolescent-parent pairs, adolescents reported clinically worse, but not statistically significant differences in HRQL. This finding underscores the need to specifically query adolescents' perceptions of HRQL and address not only statistical differences but consideration to the magnitude of the differences. Interestingly, our domain-specific scores exceeded the clinically relevant difference of $\geq$0.5 compared to the Dutch study [6], as well as other studies in which the FAQLQ-TF was used [6, 9, 17, 21]. Collectively, these studies suggest that staple food allergy is associated with worse HRQL than allergies to other foods. One can speculate that this may be due to the ubiquity of staple foods in a typical western diet, making them challenging to avoid. This challenge may be compounded by the fact that, although many countries have regulatory frameworks for allergens contained in processed foods [22], such labelling most commonly identifies non-staple foods [23] and may contribute to confusion and complacency amongst food allergic individuals [24, 25].

We identified that staple food allergy impacted on adolescents' lifestyles, as underscored by poorer than average overall HRQL mean score [i.e. better HRQL], as well as within the domain, AADR. Others have reported similar findings on the impact of food allergy on adolescents' lifestyles [6]. The similarities between these findings are

Table 3 Linear regression analyses of HRQL for adolescents with objectively-diagnosed staple food allergy

	n	*B*	95 % CI for *B*	p value
Sex				
Boys	18	Ref		
Girls	40	−0.58	−1.34; 0.19	0.13
Number of staple food allergies				
1	36	Ref		
2–3	22	0.37	−0.31; 1.06	0.28
Number of offending foods[a]				
1	10	Ref		
2	9	0.79	−0.43; 2.01	0.20
3	13	0.03	−1.11; 1.17	0.95
>3	26	0.82	−0.24; 1.89	0.13
Number of symptoms resulting from staple foods				
0–3	15	Ref		
4–6	26	0.10	−0.87; 1.07	0.83
Adrenaline auto injector possession				
No	14	Ref		
Yes	44	0.78	−0.02; 1.57	0.06

Adjusted for the covariates: sex, number of symptoms, history of anaphylaxis, adrenaline auto injector prescription and concomitant allergic disease, excluding predictor

[a] Includes at least 1 objectively-diagnosed staple food, as well as participant-reported allergies to other foods

Table 4 Linear regression analyses for presence vs. absence of specific symptoms resulting from staple foods in adolescents with objectively-diagnosed staple food allergy

	n	*B*	95 % CI for *B*	p value
Gastrointestinal				
No	13	Ref		
Yes	28	0.02	−1.04; 1.08	0.97
Dermatological[a]				
No	4	Ref		
Yes	37	0.41	−1.86; 2.68	0.72
Oral				
No	9	Ref		
Yes	32	0.41	−0.98; 1.80	0.57
Upper respiratory				
No	25	Ref		
Yes	16	0.29	−0.88; 1.44	0.62
Lower respiratory[a]				
No	2	Ref		
Yes	39	0.67	−1.37; 2.70	0.51
Cardiovascular				
No	30	Ref		
Yes	11	0.29	−0.88; 1.45	0.62
History of anaphylaxis				
No	18	Ref		
Yes	23	−0.33	−1.23; 0.58	0.46

Adjusted for the covariates: sex, number of symptoms, history of anaphylaxis, adrenaline auto injector prescription and concomitant allergic disease, excluding predictor

Non-mutually exclusive symptoms

[a] Interpret with caution due to small counts

not surprising, as adolescents spend increasing amounts of time in social settings away from home. However, our findings extend those of previous studies, as we were able to disentangle the specific factors that contributed most to worse HRQL.

In the present study, adolescents reported worse HRQL related to emerging independence and the need for support, as evidenced by domain-specific mean scores which were highest for the questions relating to needing to check for themselves if they can eat a food whilst dining out, expressing disappointment when their food allergies are not taken into account, or explaining to others about their food allergy. Previously, we reported that differences between the domains were present amongst adults [26], but not children [27] with staple food allergy. As with adults [26] and children [27], adolescents with staple food allergy reported significantly worse HRQL if they had multiple food allergies or possessed an AAI. Likewise, both adolescents and adults [26] reported worse HRQL within the domain AADR. As different domains were defined for children, a comparison of the domains between children and adolescents is not possible. In contrast to both adults [26] or children [27], adolescents did not report worse HRQL in association with a history of anaphylaxis or the number and type of symptoms. Taken together, it could be speculated that children may not feel burdened by the dietary restrictions imposed by staple food allergy, likely as the responsibility for safe food choices is assumed by their parents/guardians, whereas adolescents and adults do have to assume this responsibility. The burden of dietary restrictions and safe food choices has also been qualitatively explored amongst adolescents. Unlike non-food allergic adolescents, those with food allergies feel safe under parental control and thus do not necessarily want to make food-related decisions independently [19]. Adolescents with food allergy describe themselves as being very mature for their age, yet dependent on others in the event of a reaction [28]. One can speculate that these opposing characteristics may result in worse food allergy-specific HRQL.

Unlike other chronic conditions which adolescents may neglect or be non-compliant [29], food allergy cannot be ignored for longer than an interval between meals or snacks. But given that food is an integral part of social events, feelings of exclusion and 'being different' may ensue [7]. This may begin to explain why food allergy is strongly associated with worse HRQL. This may also explain why neither the number of allergies or symptoms, nor AAI prescription is a predictor of clinically worse HRQL. Further, adolescents often base their food choices primarily on enjoyment and secondarily on content [19], thereby engaging in risk taking behaviours [30] that may potentially lead to severe reactions. Yet, like others [9], we found no difference in HRQL between those with vs. without a history of anaphylaxis.

The financial burden of food allergy on healthcare systems [31] and on households [32] is high, and allergy-related hospitalisations are increasing [33]. Worse HRQL also predicts greater healthcare costs [34]. Thus, addressing HRQL amongst adolescents, as well as children [27] and adults [26] with staple food allergy warrants considerable attention.

Conclusions

As ascertained via a food allergy-specific questionnaire, adolescents with staple food allergy report poorer than average HRQL, specifically in relation to emerging independence and the need for support. Girls have clinically worse HRQL than boys. The number and type of previous symptoms and history of anaphylaxis were not associated with worse HRQL (Additional file 1.).

Abbreviations

AADR: allergen avoidance and dietary restrictions; AAI: adrenaline auto-injector; EI: emotional impact; FAQLQ-TF: food allergy quality of life questionnaire-teenager form; HRQL: health-related quality of life; RAE: risk of accidental exposure; 95 % CI: 95th percent confidence interval.

Authors' contributions

JP contributed to the design of this manuscript, performed the data analyses and formulated the draft manuscripts. SAJ contributed to the study design, and provided critical comments on the results as well as on the draft manuscripts. RM contributed to the study design, scrutinized the questionnaires and letters, contributed to the interpretation of the data analyses and provided critical comments on the draft manuscripts. EÖ contributed to the study design and collection of the patients, and provided critical comments on the draft manuscripts. SED contributed to the study design, was instrumental for the grant applications for the study, scrutinized the results and their interpretation and critiqued the draft manuscripts. MHA contributed to the study design, formulation of the questionnaires and provided comments on the draft manuscripts. UB contributed to the study design, formulation of the questionnaires and provided comments on the draft manuscripts. IK-B contributed to the study design, formulation of the questionnaires and provided comments on the draft manuscripts. BM contributed to the study design, formulation of the questionnaires and provided comments on the draft manuscripts. GR contributed to the study design, formulation of the questionnaires and provided comments on the draft manuscripts. A-CS contributed to the selection of the patients and their diagnosis, formulation of the questionnaires as well as interpretation of the analysis of the results. JÅ contributed to the formulation of the questionnaires as well as interpretation of the analysis of the results. SA headed the project, contributed to the study design, contributed to the formulation of the questionnaires, contributed to the interpretation and presentation of the results and provided critical comments on the draft manuscripts. All authors read and approved the final manuscript.

Author details

[1] The Centre for Allergy Research, Karolinska Institutet, P.O. Box 287, 17177 Stockholm, Sweden. [2] Institute of Environmental Medicine, Karolinska Institutet, Stockholm, Sweden. [3] Department of Public Health and Clinical Medicine, Umeå University, Umeå, Sweden. [4] Sachs' Children and Youth Hospital, Södersjukhuset, Stockholm, Sweden. [5] Department of Clinical Research and Education, Södersjukhuset, Karolinska Institutet, Stockholm, Sweden. [6] Swedish Council on Health Technology Assessment, SBU, Stockholm, Sweden. [7] Department of Learning, Informatics, Management and Ethics, and Medical Management Centre, Karolinska Institutet, Stockholm, Sweden. [8] Allergy Unit, Sahlgrenska University Hospital, Gothenburg, Sweden. [9] The Swedish Asthma and Allergy Foundation, Stockholm, Sweden. [10] Department of Health and Caring Sciences, Linnaeus University, Kalmar, Sweden.

Acknowledgements

We acknowledge Ms. Margareta Andersson for help with organising questionnaire postage and data entry.

Competing interests

The authors declare that they have no competing interests.

Funding

This study was funded by The Centre for Allergy Research (CfA) at the Karolinska Institutet, the EU project EuroPrevall (FP6 contract number FOOD-CT-2005-514000), the Swedish Asthma and Allergy Foundation and the Sahlgrenska University Hospital. Jennifer LP Protudjer is a postdoctoral researcher funded by the Karin and Sten Mörtstedt Initiative on Anaphylaxis and the Swedish Allergy and Asthma Foundation.

References

1. Rona RJ, Keil T, Summers C, Gislason D, Zuidmeer L, Sodergren E, et al. The prevalence of food allergy: a meta-analysis. J Allergy Clin Immunol. 2007;120(3):638–46.
2. Sicherer SH, Sampson HA. Food allergy: epidemiology, pathogenesis, diagnosis, and treatment. J Allergy Clin Immunol. 2014;133(2):291–307.
3. de Blok BMJ, Dubois AE, Hourihane JO. The impact of food allergy on quality of life. In: Mills ENC, Wichers H, Hoffmann-Sommergruber K, editors. Managing allergens in food. Cambridge: Woodhead Publishing; 2006.
4. Flokstra-de Blok BM, Dubois AE, Vlieg-Boerstra BJ, Oude Elberink JN, Raat H, DunnGalvin A, et al. Health-related quality of life of food allergic patients: comparison with the general population and other diseases. Allergy. 2010;65(2):238–44.

5. Marklund B, Ahlstedt S, Nordström G. Health-related quality of life among adolescents with allergy-like conditions—with emphasis on food hypersensitivity. Health Qual Life Outcomes. 2004;2:65.
6. van der Velde JL, Flokstra-de Blok BM, Hamp A, Knibb RC, Duiverman EJ, Dubois AE. Adolescent-parent disagreement on health-related quality of life of food-allergic adolescents: who makes the difference? Allergy. 2011;66(12):1580–9.
7. DunnGalvin A, Dubois AE, Flokstra-de Blok BM, Hourihane JO. The effects of food allergy on quality of life. Chem Immunol Allergy. 2015;101:235–52.
8. Mo F, Choi BC, Li FC, Merrick J. Using health utility index (HUI) for measuring the impact on health-related quality of life (HRQL) among individuals with chronic diseases. Sci World J. 2004;4:746–57.
9. Flokstra-de Blok BM, DunnGalvin A, Vlieg-Boestra BJ, Oude Elbernik JN, Duiverman EJ, Hourihane JO, et al. Development and validation of the self-administered food allergy quality of life questionnaire for adolescents. J Allergy Clin Immunol. 2008;122(1):139–44.
10. Salvilla SA, Dubois AEJ, Flokstra-de Blok BM, Panesar SS, Worth A, Patel S, et al. Disease-specific health-related quality of life instruments for IgE-mediated food allergy. Allergy. 2014;69:834–44.
11. Burks AW, Land MH. Long-term follow-up of IgE-mediated food allergy: determining persistence versus clinical tolerance. Ann Allergy Asthma Immunol. 2014;112:200–6.
12. Keet CA, Matsui EC, Dhillon G, Lenehan P, Paterakis M, Wood RA. The natural history of wheat allergy. Ann Allergy Asthma Immunol. 2009;2009(102):5.
13. Boyce JA, Assa'ad A, Burks AW, Jones SM, Sampson HA, Wood RA, et al. Guidelines for the diagnosis and management of food allergy in the United States: report of the NIAID-sponsored expert panel. J Allergy Clin Immunol. 2010;126(6 Suppl):S1–58.
14. Sampson HA, Muñoz-Furlong A, Campbell RL, Adkinson NF Jr, Bock SA, Branum A, et al. Second symposium on the definition and management of anaphylaxis: summary report—second National Institute of Allergy and Infectious Disease/Food Allergy and Anaphylaxis Network symposium. Ann Emerg Med. 2006;47(4):373–80.
15. World Health Organization. Process of translation and adaptation of instruments. 2013. http://www.who.int/substance_abuse/research_tools/translation/en/. Accessed 4 Nov 2013.
16. Saleh-Langenberg J, Goossens NJ, Flokstra-de Blok BM, Kollen BJ, van der Meulen GN, Le TM, et al. Predictors of health-related quality of life of European food-allergic patients. Allergy. 2015;70(6):616–24.
17. van der Velde JL, Flokstra-de Blok BM, Vlieg-Boerstra BJ, Oude Elberink JNG, Schouten JP, DunnGalvin A, et al. Test-retest reliability of the food allergy quality of life questionnaires (FAQLQ) for children, adolescents and adults. Qual Life Res. 2009;18(2):245–51.
18. Venter C, Sommer I, Moonesinghe H, Grundy J, Glasbey G, Dean T. Health-related quality of life in children with perceived and diagnosed food hypersensitivity. Pediatr Allergy Immunol. 2015;26(2):126–32.
19. Sommer I, MacKenzie H, Venter C, Dean T. An exploratory investigation of food choice behavior of teenagers with and without food allergies. Ann Allergy Asthma Immunol. 2014;112(5):446–52.
20. Group K, Michel G, Bisegger C, Fuhr DC, Abel T. Age and gender differences in health-related quality of life of children and adolescents in Europe: a multilevel analysis. Qual Life Res. 2009;18(9):1147–57.
21. Flokstra-de Blok BM, van der Velde JL, Vlieg-Boerstra BJ, Oude Elberink JNG, DunnGalvin A, Hourihane JO, et al. Health-related quality of life of food allergic patients measured with generic and disease-specific questionnaires. Allergy. 2010;65(8):1031–8.
22. Taylor SL, Baumert JL. Worldwide food allergy labeling and detection of allergens in processed foods. Chem Immunol Allergy. 2015;101:27–34.
23. Zurzolo GA, Mathai ML, Koplin JJ, Allen KJ. Precautionary allergen labelling following new labelling practice in Australia. J Paediatr Child Health. 2013;49(4):E306–10.
24. Barnett J, Muncer K, Leftwich J, Shepherd R, Raats MM, Gowland MH, et al. Using 'may contain' labelling to inform food choice: a qualitative study of nut allergic consumers. BMC Public Health. 2011;11:734.
25. Zurzolo GA, Koplin JJ, Mathai ML, Tang MK, Allen KJ. Perceptions of precautionary labelling among parents of children with food allergy and anaphylaxis. Med J Aust. 2013;198(11):621–3.
26. Jansson SA, Heibert-Arnlind M, Middelveld RJ, Bengtsson UJ, Sundqvist AC, Kallström-Bengtsson I, et al. Health-related quality of life, assessed with a disease-specific questionnaire, in Swedish adults suffering from well-diagnosed food allergy to staple foods. Clin Transl Allergy. 2013;3(1):21.
27. Protudjer JLP, Jansson SA, Östblom E, Heibert Arnlind M, Bengtsson U, Dahlen S-E, et al. Health-related quality of life in children with objectively-diagnosed staple food allergy assessed with a disease-specific questionnaire. Acta Paediatr. 2015;104(10):1047–54.
28. Stjerna ML. Food, risk and place: agency and negotiations of young people with food allergy. Soc Health Illness. 2015;37(2):284–97.
29. Protudjer JLP, Dumontet J, McGavock JM. My Voice: a grounded theory analysis of the lived experience of type 2 diabetes in adolescence. Can J Diabetes. 2014;38(4):229–36.
30. Monks H, Gowland MH, MacKenzie H, Erlewyn-Lajeunesse M, King R, Lucas JS, et al. How do teenagers manage their food allergies? Clin Exp Allergy. 2010;40(10):1533–40.
31. Patel DA, Holdford DA, Edwards E, Carroll NV. Estimating the economic burden of food induced allergic reactions and anaphylaxis in the United States. J Allergy Clin Immunol. 2011;128(1):110–5.
32. Protudjer JLP, Jansson SA, Arnlind Heibert M, Bengtsson U, Kallström-Bengtsson I, Marklund B, et al. Household costs associated with objectively-diagnosed allergy to staple foods in children and adolescents. J Allergy Clin Immunol. 2015;3(1):68–75.
33. Kivistö J, Protudjer JLP, Karjalainen J, Wickman M, Bergström A, Mattila V. Hospitalizations due to allergic reactions in Finnish and Swedish children between 1999 and 2011. Allergy. 2016;71(5):677–83.
34. Seid M, Varni JW, Segall D, Kurtin PS. Health-related quality of life as a predictor of pediatric healthcare costs: a two-year prospective cohort analysis. Health Qual Life Outcomes. 2004;2:48.

Exploratory analysis of CD63 and CD203c expression in basophils from hazelnut sensitized and allergic individuals

Bianca Lötzsch[1†], Sabine Dölle[1†], Stefan Vieths[2] and Margitta Worm[1*]

Abstract

Background: Sensitization to hazelnut (HN) is frequent and requires clarification to determine whether this sensitization is clinically relevant. The aim of this study was to investigate basophil activation profiles in HN-sensitized and allergic subjects.

Methods: Basophil activation was determined by flow cytometric analyses of CD63 and CD203c expression using several HN allergen concentrations. Depending on their clinical reaction pattern, an oral allergy symptom group (OAS, n = 20), a systemic reaction group (n = 12) and a sensitized group without clinical symptoms (n = 20) were identified. Additionally, 10 non-allergic and non-sensitized individuals served as controls.

Results: CD63 and CD203c expression differed between allergic (OAS and systemic group) and sensitized subjects. The HN concentration required to activate 30% of CD203c$^+$ basophils [effective concentration (EC)30] was significantly higher in sensitized versus the allergic group (p = 0.0089). This was more pronounced when the basophil allergen threshold sensitivity (CD-sens) was calculated (CD63: p = 0.018; CD203c: p = 0.009).

Conclusion: Our data indicate that the basophil activation test may provide information to better distinguish between sensitized and allergic subjects if several allergen concentrations are considered. CD203c expression displayed a better discrimination compared to CD63; therefore, its diagnostic value might be superior compared with CD63.

Keywords: Food allergy, Hazelnut, Basophil activation test, CD63, CD203

Background

In Europe, hazelnut (*Corylus avellana*) is a frequent cause of food allergy [1] with a prevalence of 0.1–0.5% [2]. In adults, hazelnut (HN) allergy is often associated with a pre-existing birch pollen allergy that can develop after inhalant sensitization with the major birch pollen allergen Bet v 1, a pathogenesis-related protein of family 10 [3]. Homologous immunoglobulin (Ig)E-binding epitopes of the pollen-related major HN allergen Cor a 1 are responsible for cross reactivity to Bet v 1 [4, 5]. In Central Europe, sensitization to Bet v 1 is the major cause of pollen-associated food allergies [1]. Up to 50–90% of birch-pollen-allergic patients develop sensitivity to food such as HN, apple, and others [3].

In addition to Cor a 1, other HN allergens, namely, Cor a 2 (profilin), Cor a 8 (lipid transfer protein), Cor a 9 (legumin-like protein), Cor a 11 (vicilin-like protein) and Cor a 14 (2S albumin), have been described to cause HN sensitization [6–8].

Although, HN allergy frequently leads to oral allergic symptoms (OAS), it can also cause severe and even life-threatening reactions [9, 10].

The diagnosis of food allergy mainly includes a detailed case history, skin prick testing (SPT) and the measurement of food-specific IgE (sIgE) [11, 12]. However, the low specificity of SPT and sIgE may cause over-diagnosis, which leads to unnecessary diet restrictions resulting in

*Correspondence: margitta.worm@charite.de
†Bianca Lötzsch and Sabine Dölle contributed equally to this work.
[1] Department of Dermatology and Allergology, Allergy-Center-Charité, Charité - Universitätsmedizin Berlin, Charitéplatz 1, 10117 Berlin, Germany
Full list of author information is available at the end of the article

a lower quality of life [13]. Thus, the diagnosis of a food allergy should be proven by double-blind, placebo-controlled oral food challenges (DBPCFC) [11, 12]. Although, DBPCFC is the gold standard in diagnosing food allergies, it is not often included in daily evaluation for several reasons such as limited time and resources [14, 15].

Diagnostic tests that may support the discrimination between sensitized and symptomatic subjects without the high risk of developing an anaphylactic reaction are desirable. The basophil activation test (BAT) is an in vitro test that determines the expression of defined basophil markers (CD63 and CD203c) after allergen activation. The BAT has been suggested as a useful tool for the diagnosis of different IgE-mediated allergies [16].

The aim of this study was to investigate the CD63 and CD203c activation profiles in sensitized and symptomatic HN-allergic subjects considering several HN allergen concentrations. Moreover, we correlated the data from these surface markers with diagnostic parameters (SPT and sIgE), which are the most frequently used.

Methods

Subjects

Subjects were recruited from the Allergy-Centre-Charité (Berlin, Germany). Four groups (control, sensitized, OAS, systemic) were stratified based on case history including a detailed questionnaire about their symptoms after ingesting HN and the SPT data. Symptoms like itching or swelling of the oral mucosa (lips, tongue, palate), as well as throat tightness and dysphagia were counted for OAS. The following symptoms were considered as systemic: dyspnea, vomiting, emesis, diarrhea, generalised urticaria, general erythema, angioedema, as well as cardio-vascular symptoms, and rhinitis/rhinoconjunctivitis. Exclusion criteria were pregnancy, lactation, the use of antihistamines, and immunomodulating or immunosuppressive drugs. The study was approved by the local ethics committee of Charité (EA-No.: 1832/Si.258). All subjects gave written informed consent to participate in the study.

Skin prick test (SPT)

A SPT was performed (according to the recommendations [17]) with birch extract (Alk-Abelló, Wedel, Germany) and with fresh food (HN, apple, celery, carrot) by using the prick-to-prick method. Histamine dihydrochloride (10 mg/ml, ALK-Abelló) and sodium chloride (0.9% NaCl, ALK-Abelló) served as positive and negative controls. SPT was considered positive if the wheal diameter was $\geq$3 mm after 15 min.

Total and specific immunoglobulin E

The serum samples were stored at −20 °C until use. The measurement of the total and sIgE to rBet v 1, rCor a 1.04 (hereina ter referred to as rCor a 1) and rCor a 8 were determined with the ImmunoCAP System (Thermo Fisher Scientific, Uppsala, Sweden) according to the manufacturer's instructions. In addition, Cor a 9, Cor a 11 and Cor a 14 were measured by the Paul-Ehrlich-Institute (Langen, Germany).

Basophil activation test (BAT)

For measurement of basophil activation, heparinized blood samples were taken from subjects and analyzed within 24 h. The blood samples were stimulated with increasing concentrations (10^{-6}–10 µg/ml) of HN extract (European hazelnut extract, Greer Labs, Lenoir, NC, USA) and incubated for 15 min at 37 °C. Anti-human IgE (BIOZOL HP6029/HP6061, Eching, Germany) was used as positive, and RPMI 1640 medium (Bio Chrom AG, Berlin, Germany) was used as a negative control. Cells were stained with anti-CD63-FITC (BD Biosciences, Franklin Lakes, NJ, USA), anti-CD203c-PE (Immunotech Inc., Canada), anti-CD3-VioBlue (Myltenyi Biotec GmbH, Bergisch-Gladbach, Germany) and anti-CCR3-APC (R&D Systems, Minneapolis, MN, USA). After adding lysing solution (BD Biosciences, Franklin Lakes, NJ, USA), the basophils were analyzed by flow cytometry (Miltenyi MACS Quant Flow Cytometer, Bergisch-Gladbach, Germany). $CD3^-/CCR3^+$ cells were gated as basophils, $CD3^-/CCR3^+/CD203^{high+}$ cells were analyzed for basophil activation, and $CD3^-/CCR3^+/CD63^+$ cells were defined as degranulated basophils. The data were analyzed using the MACSQuantify Software™ program (Miltenyi Biotec GmbH). Expression values were normalized for basophil activation induced by anti-IgE. The analysis of CD203c expression was based on the allergen concentration, which activated 30% of $CD203c^+$ basophils [effective concentration (EC)30] as previously performed [18]. For CD63, the maximal percentage of CD63 up-regulation at one allergen dose (CD-max) was measured. Additionally, the basophil allergen threshold sensitivity (CD-sens) and EC50 (the effective concentration giving 50% of maximum up-regulation) were calculated as described by Glaumann et al. [19]. Subjects with less than 15% change in $CD3^-/CCR3^+/CD203^{high+}$ or $CD3^-/CCR3^+/CD63^+$ expression between negative and positive control were regarded as non-responders and excluded from further analysis (n = 5).

Statistical analysis

Statistical analysis was performed with IBM SPSS Statistics (Chicago, IL, USA) and Prism (GraphPad Software, San Diego, CA, USA). All results are shown as medians with ranges (min–max, unless otherwise stated). Differences between the groups were verified with the Kruskal–Wallis test or Mann–Whitney U test for non-Gaussian

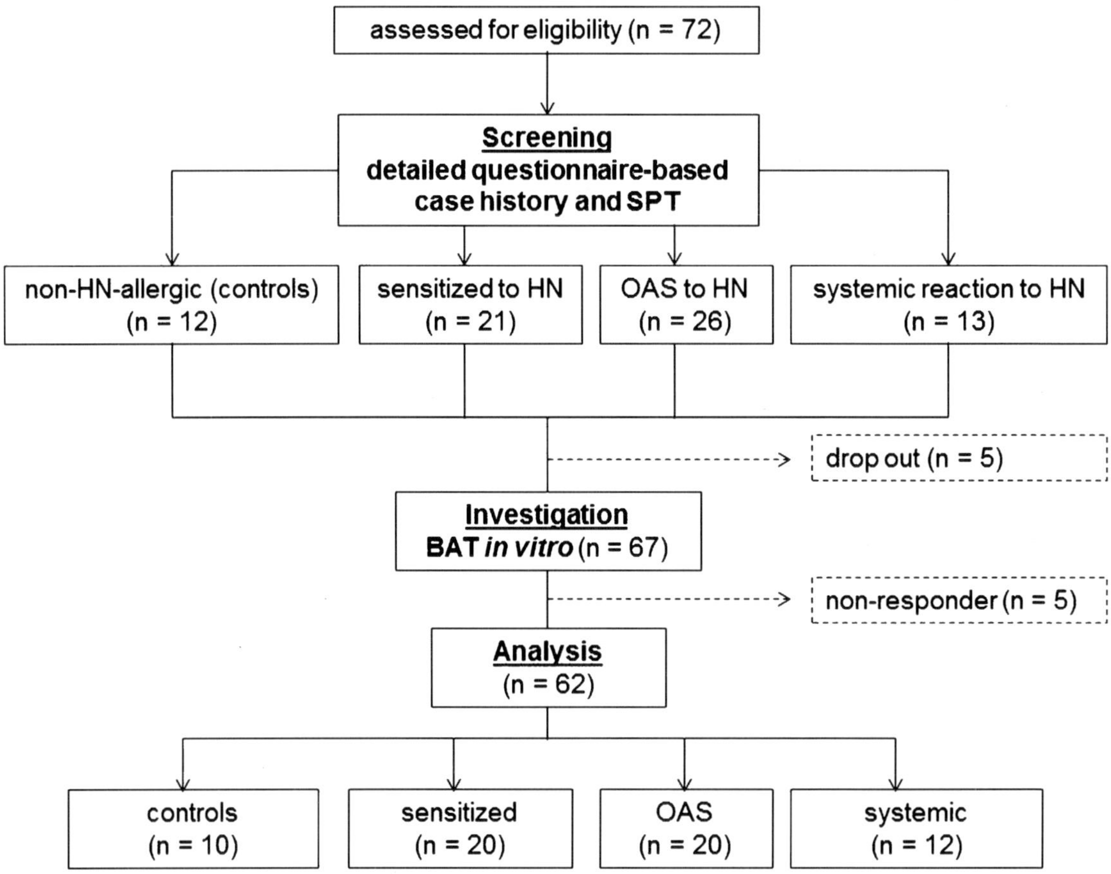

Fig. 1 Study flow chart and classification of subjects. *HN* hazelnut, *SPT* skin prick test, *OAS* oral allergic symptoms, *BAT* basophil activation test

distribution. The Spearman correlation coefficient was used for comparison between the diagnostic tests. p values <0.05 were considered to be statistically significant. Significant results should be regarded as descriptive and explorative due to the small sample size in this study.

Results

Identification of subjects

In total, 72 subjects were screened, and the BAT was performed in 67 individuals; of these, 62 were analyzed [median age: 31 (19–62) years, n = 40 (65%) females and n = 22 (35%) males; Fig. 1; Table 1]. Table 1 summarizes the subjects' characteristics. In this study, 10 subjects had a negative SPT for HN and birch and no symptoms when consuming HN (controls) and 20 subjects showed no symptoms but had a positive SPT for HN (sensitized). In addition, 32 subjects had a positive SPT for HN and according to their clinical symptoms, these were divided into subjects with OAS (n = 20) and subjects with systemic reactions (n = 12).

Sensitization profile

SPT and sIgE were used to assess the sensitization status. All subjects from the sensitized, OAS and systemic groups had a positive SPT to HN (inclusion criteria). The wheal diameters for HN were not significantly different between the sensitized and symptomatic groups (Table 1). A similar pattern was observed when the birch pollen extract was used. In the symptomatic group, all 32 subjects, and in the sensitized group, 15 of 20 subjects, had a positive SPT to birch pollen extract (Table 1).

Total IgE levels were comparable among the sensitized, OAS and systemic groups and as expected, significantly higher compared to the control group (Table 1). In the sensitized group, the sIgE level against rCor a 1 [1.9 (0.0–7.4) kU/l] was significantly lower compared to the sIgE level from the OAS group [6.7 (0.0–63.8) kU/l], but not compared to the systemic group [3.5 (0.1–28.1 kU/l)]. For both symptomatic groups, higher ratios of sIgE to total IgE levels were calculated for Cor a 1 in comparison to the sensitized group. The ratios for rBet v 1 were comparable between the sensitized and symptomatic groups (Table 1). No sensitization to Cor a 9, Cor a 11 or Cor a 14 were found.

Basophil activation profiles

The BAT was performed in 67 screened subjects; among these, 5 (3.35%) were non-responders (Fig. 1).

The CD63 expression measured as basophil reactivity (maximal reactivity, CD-max) showed differences between clinically symptomatic (OAS/systemic) and sensitized subjects (Fig. 2a). The median CD63 expression in the sensitized group was lower for all HN extract concentrations than the median of CD63 expression of the subjects with symptomatic HN allergy. However, no significant differences were detected by comparing CD-max, which was measured at a concentration of 0.1 μg/ml of HN extract in the groups (sensitized, OAS, systemic) (Fig. 2c). Additionally, EC50 and CD-sens for CD63 were calculated (Table 2). We detected a significant higher CD-sens in the symptomatic group: 44.73 (13.01–96.72; $p = 0.018$) compared to the sensitized group: 6.59 (0.07–57.84). However, we could not differentiate between the OAS and systemic groups.

For CD203c, the effective concentration by which 30% of basophils were activated (EC30) was calculated. Higher HN concentrations were required to achieve an increase of CD203c expression in sensitized subjects (Fig. 2b), which was significant when calculated for EC30 ($p = 0.0089$, Fig. 2d). In order to better compare, we calculated EC50 and CD-sens for CD203c too (Table 2). The measured differences between CD-sens of the symptomatic group: 80.33 (14.64–267.87) and the sensitized group: 10.03 (3.55–82.90) were significant ($p = 0.009$). Again, we could not differentiate between the OAS and systemic group.

Correlations between SPT, sIgE and BAT

We identified statistical correlations ($p < 0.001$) between the CD63 and CD203c expression values at single HN concentration versus SPT, sIgE to rCor a 1, and sIgE to rBet v 1. The highest correlation was detected for 0.01 μg/ml and is summarized in Table 3. A correlation between

Table 1 Subjects' characteristics

	Controls (n = 10)	Sensitized (n = 20)	OAS (n = 20)	Systemic (n = 12)	p values
Age (median [min–max] in years)	30 [20–57]	26 [19–60]	32 [21–51]	40 [24–62]	NS
Male sex (%)	2 (20%)	12 (60%)	6 (30%)	2 (17%)	0.041[c]
Atopic history [number (%)]					
Allergic rhinitis	3[a] (30%)	14 (70%)	16 (75%)	9 (75%)	
Atopic dermatitis	2 (20%)	5 (25%)	9 (50%)	5 (33%)	
Allergic asthma	–	9 (35%)	10 (55%)	8 (58%)	
SPT (median [min–max] in mm)					
Birch	0*	6 [0–12]	7 [0–11]	9 [3–11]	NS
Hazelnut	0*	4 [3–8]	5 [3–10]	6 [4–14]	NS
Celery	0*	0 [0–7]	3 [0–10]	4 [0–7]	NS
Apple	0*	3 [0–8]	4 [0–7]	5 [0–20]	NS
Carrot	0*	0 [0–10]	3 [0–15]	4 [0–14]	NS
IgE (median [min–max] in kU/l)					
Total-IgE	16 [3–34]*	184 [20–2097]	178 [24–6861]	59 [26–4801]	NS
sIgE Bet v 1	0.0 [0.0–0.1]*	3.5 [0.0–16.2]	10.2 [0.0–72.4]	5.9 [0.1–43.6]	NS
sIgE Cor a 1	0.0 [0.0–0.1]*	1.9 [0.0–7.4]	6.7 [0.0–63.8]	3.5 [0.1–28.1]	0.0254[d]
sIgE Cor a 8	n.d.	n.d.	0.2 [0.0–1.3]	0.0 [0.0–0.0]	NS
Ratio[b] (median [min–max])					
rBet v 1/total-IgE	0.00*	0.04 [0.00–4.19]	0.07 [0.00–13.0]	0.04 [0.00–11.9]	NS
rCor a 1/total-IgE	0.00*	0.02 [0.00–0.80]	0.20 [0.00–4.36]	0.18 [0.00–4.77]	0.0226[e]

Statistical significances were analyzed with Kruskal–Wallis test

* Significant difference of the control group versus the other groups

[a] According to case history, not caused by birch pollen

[b] Calculated as sIgE * sIgE/total IgE

[c] Sensitized versus control and systemic group

[d] Sensitized versus OAS group

[e] Sensitized versus OAS and systemic group

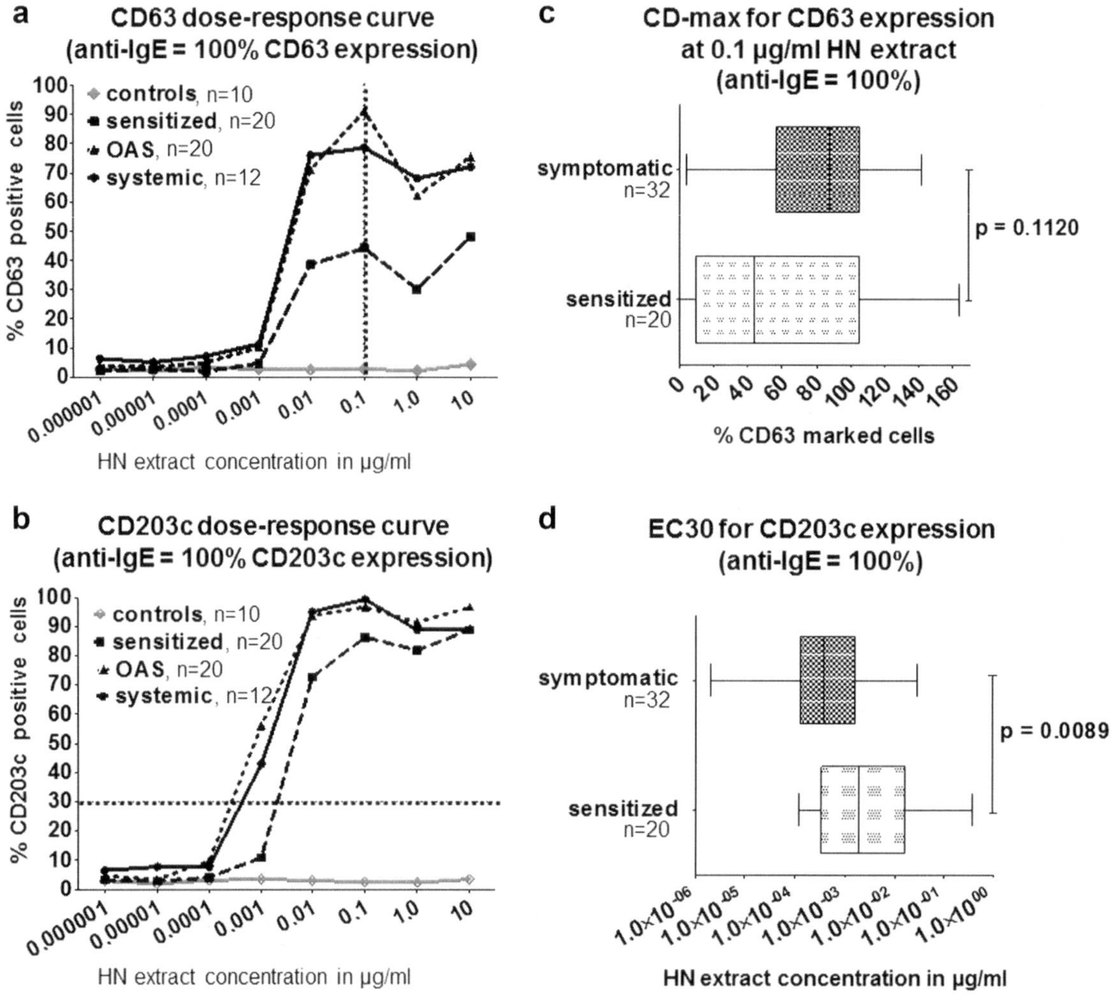

Fig. 2 Expression of CD63 and CD203c normalized for basophil activation induced by the positive control (anti-IgE). **a**, **b** The dose–response curves for CD63 (**a**) and CD203c (**b**). The values are shown as medians. For a clear picture, the ranges are not shown in **a** and **b**. The net values are depicted in Additional file 1: Figure S1 as medians with interquartile ranges for the four groups. The *vertical dotted line* indicates the maximum CD63 expression (CD-max) at the hazelnut (HN) concentration of 0.1 µg/ml (**a**), and the *horizontal dotted line* gives the concentration required to activate 30% of $CD203c^+$ basophils [effective concentration (EC)30] (**b**). **c**, **d** The comparison between the sensitized (n = 20) and symptomatic (OAS and systemic, n = 32) groups by **c** Maximum CD63 expression (CD-max) at 0.1 µg/ml of hazelnut (HN) extract and **d** HN extract concentrations that activated 30% of basophils (EC30). Statistical significances were analyzed with Mann–Whitney U test

CD-sens versus the other diagnostic measurements was only detected for CD203c (Table 3).

Discussion

Our results show that the BAT is a useful tool to determine biological activity against a food allergen such as HN. The correlation between CD203c/CD63 expression and the sensitization results measured by sIgE and SPT indicates basophil activity can be linked to sensitization status. Moreover, the CD203c-based BAT may distinguish between sensitized and symptomatic individuals but only if a careful dose–response analysis is performed.

The literature is controversial about the advantages and disadvantages of basophil surface markers [20]. CD63, compared to CD203c, is not a basophil-specific marker and has been shown to be less specific and less sensitive (in grass pollen and house dust mite allergy, latex allergy, wasp venom hypersensitivity, peanut allergy) [21–23]. On the other hand, the up-regulation of CD63 expression has been reported to provide similar results to CD203c expression in cat-allergic subjects [24] and to be more sensitive and specific in egg-allergic children [23]. All these data suggest a high variability of sensitivity and specificity depending on the allergen and cohort that was studied.

Table 2 Basophil allergen threshold sensitivity (CD-sens) and half-maximal effective concentration (EC50)

Subject group	No. of subjects	CD63			CD203c		
		EC50 (ng/ml)	CD-sens	p values	EC50 (ng/ml)	CD-sens	p values
Sensitized	20	15.18 (1.73–1336)	6.59 (0.07–57.84)		10.09 (1.21–33.38)	10.03 (3.55–82.90)	
OAS	20	2.24 (1.05–7.12)	44.73 (14.07–96.38)	0.028	0.97 (0.17–6.95)	104.55 (14.92–602.48)	0.006
Systemic	12	2.61 (0.98–9.94)	40.40 (10.23–104.61)	NS	1.74 (0.55–7.95)	59.35 (13.27–190.12)	NS
Symptomatic (OAS + systemic)	32	2.24 (1.04–7.70)	44.73 (13.01–96.72)	0.018	1.27 (0.37–7.02)	80.33 (14.64–267.87)	0.009

Values are given as median with interquartile range (IQR). Statistical significances were analyzed with Mann–Whitney U test compared to the sensitized group

Table 3 Correlation of basophil activation test (BAT) with different diagnostic tests

	Expression values at 0.01 μg/ml HN		CD-sens	
	CD63	CD203c	CD63	CD203c
...with SPT (HN)	0.561; $p < 0.001$	0.620; $p < 0.001$	0.064; NS	0.389; $p = 0.003$
...with IgE values				
Total-IgE	0.203; $p = 0.113$	0.245; NS	−0.262; NS	−0.020; NS
sIgE rBet v 1	0.689; $p < 0.001$	0.777; $p < 0.001$	0.203; NS	0.539; $p < 0.001$
sIgE rCor a 1	0.690; $p < 0.001$	0.754; $p < 0.001$	0.208; NS	0.541; $p < 0.001$

Correlation between CD63 and CD203c expression values at 0.01 μg/ml: 0.784; $p < 0.001$ and CD-sens: 0.561; $p < 0.001$

Spearman correlation coefficient (r; p value) of BAT values at 0.01 μg/ml HN concentration and CD-sens for CD63 and CD203c with skin prick test (SPT) for hazelnut (HN), total and sIgE levels

In this study, measuring CD203c expression was superior to CD63 when sensitized and symptomatic groups were considered (Fig. 2c, d; Table 2). However, with the BAT, we were not able to distinguish a patient with systemic reactions from a patient with OAS. The ability to differentiate between the symptom severities was limited either by the diagnostic assessment, which was based on clinical history, or by the Cor-a-1-based HN allergy in our cohort. It is known that Cor a 1 can induce severe allergic symptoms but may require the intake of larger amounts of the Bet v 1 homologues such as it is the case for Gly m 4 in soy-containing dietary food products, or it may need allergen-protective matrix effects [12]. The biological activity of Cor a 1 might be very high in birch pollen endemic regions, [25] thus, the difference between OAS and more severe allergic reactions are not detected in the BAT.

CD203c as well as CD63 expression values at a HN concentration of 0.01 μg/ml correlated with the SPT and sIgE results (Table 3). Considering CD-sens, a correlation was detected for CD203c but not CD63. Thus, the BAT can be used as a functional assay to detect sensitization status, which had been shown previously [26]. However, in our hands, CD203c seems to be superior compared to CD63. Moreover, the BAT has the potential to more closely resemble the clinical phenotype of patients [27]. In previous studies, we have shown the usefulness of CD203c expression in demonstrating differences of the allergenicity between native and roasted HN extracts [2] and between two different tomato cultivars [18]. Previous reports, where CD63 and CD203c expression were analyzed in combination, support our findings [28–30]. The data of Wanich et al. [28] indicate less basophil activity in tolerant versus symptomatic cow's milk-allergic subjects. The BAT could also differentiate between tolerant and symptomatic peanut-sensitized subjects [30]. Santos et al. [29] demonstrated the utility of basophils as biomarkers for severity and threshold of allergic reaction in a pediatric cohort suffering from peanut allergy. Whether a combined analysis is suitable is a matter of discussion due to different expression kinetics [16, 31].

Differences regarding kinetics might be a reason for the findings when comparing CD63 and CD203c in our cohort. The maximal up-regulation of CD63 occurs within 25–30 min, whereas CD203c requires only 10–20 min [32]. The stimulation time used in this study averaged 15 min to capture both markers.

For practical reasons, basophil activation experiments should be restricted to a single allergen concentration [16, 32]. However, an individual, highly heterogeneous basophil response has been described previously [33] and was also present in our cohort. Thus, a single allergen concentration is not sufficient to analyze basophil responses.

The BAT offers many advantages in food allergy. In contrast to sIgE, the BAT provides a biological readout [34]. A wide range of food, raw material, purified or recombinant allergens can be analyzed [35]. Unspecific positive reactions are less frequent in BAT compared to SPT. In addition, SPT bears the risk of sensitization [36]. Moreover, basophils can be analyzed even when the subject receives anti-allergic treatment [37]. However, other studies demonstrated an inhibitory effect of immunosuppressants such as cyclosporin A [38] or other drugs (statins) [39]. Therefore, a careful history regarding a possible drug intake is mandatory if a BAT is considered.

The diagnosis of food allergy is mainly based on patient history, analysis of IgE and/or SPT, ideally combined with DBPCFC, which is still the gold standard in the diagnosis of food allergy [11, 12]. However, DBPCFC is expensive and time-consuming for both the physician and the patient and is often refused by the patient. Additionally, there is a risk for patients to experience severe allergic reactions. Thus, in this study, a detailed case history including allergy-focused diet history assessment was used to define the status of HN allergy, which had previously been shown to have a high diagnostic values [40, 41].

However, an ex vivo but highly diagnostic method to reliably predict clinical reactivity is desirable. Neither the presence of sIgE in the circulation nor the presence of biologically active IgE on mast cells are suitable to differentiate between sensitization and clinical allergy [35], with perhaps the exception of Cor a 9 and Cor a 14 in children cohorts [41, 42]. For both allergens, an age-dependent variability seems to exist, as allergic adults are less sensitized to both components [43]. In our cohort, no sensitization to Cor a 9, Cor a 11 or Cor a 14 was found. Thus, in our cohort Cor a 1 is the predominate allergen. The sIgE to Cor a 1 was lower in the sensitized group compared to the symptomatic groups (significant for OAS group), which was more pronounced when calculated as a sIgE/total-IgE-ratio. Glaumann et al. [19] investigated the utility of BAT in an Ara h 8-sensitized cohort. Ara h 8 is a Bet v 1 homologue in peanut like Cor a 1 in HN. They could show that the BAT adds safety information if sIgE and DBPCFC results were controversial. Thus, the BAT might be useful if clinical history, SPT and/or sIgE measurement are inconsistent or in addition an oral food challenge is not possible [42]. Furthermore, the use of recombinant allergens in the BAT might have added value in discriminating between clinically relevant and mere sensitization [44, 45] and should be considered in future studies.

Most BAT protocols are not standardized. For the future, protocol optimization is required and should consider preanalytical conditions and well-defined flow cytometry gating protocols [46]. The timeframe of analysis is relevant as well; ideally, the BAT should be performed immediately after a blood draw [37, 46] but at least within 24 h, as longer storage time can lead to a loss of basophil reactivity and false negative results [37].

A weakness of this study is the small number of analyzed subjects and the results should be regarded explorative. However, we were able to differentiate between non-allergic, sensitized and symptomatic subjects. The inclusion of HN-sensitized subjects is a strength of the study, as such a group is essential to validate a diagnostic test in allergy [33]. Still, due to the small sample size, necessary diagnostic parameters (sensitivity, specificity, positive and negative predictive value) were not calculated. Furthermore, the diagnosis of a symptomatic HN allergy was based on clinical history, as mentioned above. Moreover, we did not prove that the activation of the basophils with the HN extract was exclusively via cross-linking surface-bound sIgE against HN (Cor a 1) or via cross-reaction of surface-bound sIgE against birch homologues (Bet v 1).

The sensitivity and specificity of the BAT is influenced by the rate of non-responders. These patients do not show activation after anti-IgE stimulation [33]. The reason for this non-responsiveness of the basophils is a selective decrease in Syk expression, which is a downstream event of FcεRI activation [33]. The proportion of non-responders depends on the BAT protocol and varies between 5 and 25% [32, 33]. In this study, 3.25% of patients when considering both expression markers and up to 6.5% of patients when considering only CD63 expression were non-responders.

Conclusion

In summary, the CD203c-based BAT differentiates between sensitization and clinically relevant allergy in HN-sensitized individuals. The use of a given allergen extract at several concentrations is required, and the development of standardized protocols are needed to compare results obtained from different cohorts and allergens.

Abbreviations

BAT: basophil activation test; CD-max: the maximal percentage of surface marker up-regulation at one allergen dose; CD-sens: basophil allergen threshold sensitivity; DBPCFC: double-blind, placebo-controlled oral food challenges; EC: effective concentration; HN: hazelnut; IgE: immunoglobulin E; sIgE: specific immunoglobulin E; OAS: oral allergy symptom; SPT: skin prick test.

Authors' contributions

MW and SD designed the study; BL and SD performed the statistical analyses; BL performed the basophil activation test and wrote the first draft of the manuscript; SD and MW provided laboratory assistance; SV performed sIgE testing for Cor a 9, Cor a 11 and Cor a 14; SV and MW critically reviewed the analyses and edited the manuscript; SD edited and formatted the final version of the manuscript. All authors read and approved the final manuscript.

Author details
[1] Department of Dermatology and Allergology, Allergy-Center-Charité, Charité - Universitätsmedizin Berlin, Charitéplatz 1, 10117 Berlin, Germany. [2] Paul-Ehrlich-Institut, Langen, Germany.

Acknowledgements
We thank Thermo Fisher Scientific for performing the sIgE-testing. The authors also thank Dennis Ernst (technician) for supporting our lab work and for his assistance and help in conducting the flow cytometric measurements.

Competing interests
The authors declare that they have no competing interests.

References

1. Burney PG, Potts J, Kummeling I, Mills EN, Clausen M, Dubakiene R, et al. The prevalence and distribution of food sensitization in European adults. Allergy. 2014;69:365–71.
2. Worm M, Hompes S, Fiedler EM, Illner AK, Zuberbier T, Vieths S. Impact of native, heat-processed and encapsulated hazelnuts on the allergic response in hazelnut-allergic patients. Clin Exp Allergy. 2009;39:159–66.
3. Katelaris CH. Food allergy and oral allergy or pollen-food syndrome. Curr Opin Allergy Clin Immunol. 2010;10:246–51.
4. Flinterman AE, Akkerdaas JH, Knulst AC, van Ree R, Pasmans SG. Hazelnut allergy: from pollen-associated mild allergy to severe anaphylactic reactions. Curr Opin Allergy Clin Immunol. 2008;8:261–5.
5. Le TM, van Hoffen E, Lebens AF, Bruijnzeel-Koomen CA, Knulst AC. Anaphylactic versus mild reactions to hazelnut and apple in a birch-endemic area: different sensitization profiles? Int Arch Allergy Immunol. 2013;160:56–62.
6. Schocker F, Luttkopf D, Scheurer S, Petersen A, Cistero-Bahima A, Enrique E, et al. Recombinant lipid transfer protein Cor a 8 from hazelnut: a new tool for in vitro diagnosis of potentially severe hazelnut allergy. J Allergy Clin Immunol. 2004;113:141–7.
7. Lauer I, Foetisch K, Kolarich D, Ballmer-Weber BK, Conti A, Altmann F, et al. Hazelnut (*Corylus avellana*) vicilin Cor a 11: molecular characterization of a glycoprotein and its allergenic activity. Biochem J. 2004;383:327–34.
8. Roux KH, Teuber SS, Sathe SK. Tree nut allergens. Int Arch Allergy Immunol. 2003;131:234–44.
9. Worm M, Moneret-Vautrin A, Scherer K, Lang R, Fernandez-Rivas M, Cardona V, et al. First European data from the network of severe allergic reactions (NORA). Allergy. 2014;69:1397–404.
10. Grabenhenrich LB, Dölle S, Moneret-Vautrin A, Kohli A, Lange L, Spindler T, et al. Anaphylaxis in children and adolescents: the European Anaphylaxis Registry. J Allergy Clin Immunol. 2016;137:1128–37.
11. Muraro A, Werfel T, Hoffmann-Sommergruber K, Roberts G, Beyer K, Bindslev-Jensen C, et al. EAACI food allergy and anaphylaxis guidelines: diagnosis and management of food allergy. Allergy. 2014;69:1008–25.
12. Worm M, Reese I, Ballmer-Weber B, Beyer K, Bischoff SC, Claßen M, et al. Guidelines on the management of IgE-mediated food allergies. S2K-Guidelines of the German Society for Allergology and Clinical Immunology (DGAKI) in collaboration with the German Medical Association of Allergologists (AeDA), the German Professional Association of Pediatricians (BVKJ), the German Allergy and Asthma Association (DAAB), German Dermatological Society (DDG), the German Society for Nutrition (DGE), the German Society for Gastroenterology, Digestive and Metabolic Diseases (DGVS), the German Society for Oto-Rhino-Laryngology, Head and Neck Surgery, the German Society for Pediatric and Adolescent Medicine (DGKJ), the German Society for Pediatric Allergology and Environmental Medicine (GPA), the German Society for Pneumology (DGP), the German Society for Pediatric Gastroenterology and Nutrition (GPGE), German Contact Allergy Group (DKG), the Austrian Society for Allergology and Immunology (ÖGAI), German Professional Association of Nutritional Sciences (VDOE) and the Association of the Scientific Medical Societies Germany (AWMF). Allergo J Int. 2015;24:256–93.
13. Muraro A, Dubois AE, DunnGalvin A, Hourihane JO, de Jong NW, Meyer R, et al. EAACI food allergy and anaphylaxis guidelines. Food allergy health-related quality of life measures. Allergy. 2014;69:845–53.
14. Lieberman JA, Sicherer SH. Diagnosis of food allergy: epicutaneous skin tests, in vitro tests, and oral food challenge. Curr Allergy Asthma Rep. 2011;11:58–64.
15. Le TM, Lindner TM, Pasmans SG, Guikers CL, van Hoffen E, Bruijnzeel-Koomen CA, et al. Reported food allergy to peanut, tree nuts and fruit: comparison of clinical manifestations, prescription of medication and impact on daily life. Allergy. 2008;63:910–6.
16. Ebo DG, Sainte-Laudy J, Bridts CH, Mertens CH, Hagendorens MM, Schuerwegh AJ, et al. Flow-assisted allergy diagnosis: current applications and future perspectives. Allergy. 2006;61:1028–39.
17. Heinzerling L, Burbach G, van Cauwenberge P, Papageorgiou P, Carlsen KH, Lodrup Carlsen KC, et al. Establishing a standardized quality management system for the European Health Network GA2LEN. Allergy. 2010;65:743–52.
18. Dölle S, Lehmann K, Schwarz D, Weckwert W, Scheler C, George E, et al. Allergenic activity of different tomato cultivars in tomato allergic subjects. Clin Exp Allergy. 2011;41:1643–52.
19. Glaumann S, Nilsson C, Johansson SG, Asarnoj A, Wickman M, Borres MP, et al. Evaluation of basophil allergen threshold sensitivity (CD-sens) to peanut and Ara h 8 in children IgE-sensitized to Ara h 8. Clin Mol Allergy. 2015;13:5.
20. Abuaf N, Rostane H, Rajoely B, Gaouar H, Autegarden JE, Leynadier F, et al. Comparison of two basophil activation markers CD63 and CD203c in the diagnosis of amoxicillin allergy. Clin Exp Allergy. 2008;38:921–8.
21. Potapinska O, Gorska E, Zawadzka-Krajewska A, Kulus M, Wasik M, Demkow U. The usefulness of CD203c expression measurement on basophils after activation with grass pollen and *Dermatophagoides pteronyssinus* antigens. Preliminary study. Pneumonol Alergol Pol. 2009;77:138–44.
22. Boumiza R, Monneret G, Forissier MF, Savoye J, Gutowski MC, Powell WS, et al. Marked improvement of the basophil activation test by detecting CD203c instead of CD63. Clin Exp Allergy. 2003;33:259–65.
23. Ocmant A, Mulier S, Hanssens L, Goldman M, Casimir G, Mascart F, et al. Basophil activation tests for the diagnosis of food allergy in children. Clin Exp Allergy. 2009;39:1234–45.
24. Ocmant A, Peignois Y, Mulier S, Hanssens L, Michils A, Schandene L. Flow cytometry for basophil activation markers: the measurement of CD203c up-regulation is as reliable as CD63 expression in the diagnosis of cat allergy. J Immunol Methods. 2007;320:40–8.
25. Blanc F, Bernard H, Ah-Leung S, Przybylski-Nicaise L, Skov PS, Purohit A, et al. Further studies on the biological activity of hazelnut allergens. Clin Transl Allergy. 2015;5:26.
26. Nilsson N, Nilsson C, Hedlin G, Johansson SG, Borres MP, Nopp A. Combining analyses of basophil allergen threshold sensitivity, CD-sens, and IgE antibodies to hydrolyzed wheat, omega-5 gliadin and timothy grass enhances the prediction of wheat challenge outcome. Int Arch Allergy Immunol. 2013;162:50–7.
27. Santos AF, Lack G. Basophil activation test: food challenge in a test tube or specialist research tool? Clin Transl Allergy. 2016;6:10.
28. Wanich N, Nowak-Wegrzyn A, Sampson HA, Shreffler WG. Allergen-specific basophil suppression associated with clinical tolerance in patients with milk allergy. J Allergy Clin Immunol. 2009;123(789–94):e20.
29. Santos AF, Du Toit G, Douiri A, Radulovic S, Stephens A, Turcanu V, et al. Distinct parameters of the basophil activation test reflect the severity and threshold of allergic reactions to peanut. J Allergy Clin Immunol. 2015;135:179–86.
30. Santos AF, Douiri A, Becares N, Wu SY, Stephens A, Radulovic S, et al. Basophil activation test discriminates between allergy and tolerance in peanut-sensitized children. J Allergy Clin Immunol. 2014;134:645–52.

31. MacGlashan D Jr. Expression of CD203c and CD63 in human basophils: relationship to differential regulation of piecemeal and anaphylactic degranulation processes. Clin Exp Allergy. 2010;40:1365–77.
32. De Week AL, Sanz ML, Gamboa PM, Aberer W, Bienvenu J, Blanca M, et al. Diagnostic tests based on human basophils: more potentials and perspectives than pitfalls. II. Technical issues. J Investig Allergol Clin Immunol. 2008;18:143–55.
33. Kleine-Tebbe J, Erdmann S, Knol EF, MacGlashan DW Jr, Poulsen LK, Gibbs BF. Diagnostic tests based on human basophils: potentials, pitfalls and perspectives. Int Arch Allergy Immunol. 2006;141:79–90.
34. Falcone FH, Knol EF, Gibbs BF. The role of basophils in the pathogenesis of allergic disease. Clin Exp Allergy. 2011;41:939–47.
35. Asero R, Ballmer-Weber BK, Beyer K, Conti A, Dubakiene R, Fernandez-Rivas M, et al. IgE-mediated food allergy diagnosis: current status and new perspectives. Mol Nutr Food Res. 2007;51:135–47.
36. Ruëff F, Bergmann KC, Brockow K, Fuchs T, Grübl A, Jung K, et al. Hauttests zur Diagnostik von allergischen Soforttypreaktionen. Allergo J. 2010;19:402–15.
37. Sturm EM, Kranzelbinder B, Heinemann A, Groselj-Strele A, Aberer W, Sturm GJ. CD203c-based basophil activation test in allergy diagnosis: characteristics and differences to CD63 upregulation. Cytom B Clin Cytom. 2010;78:308–18.
38. Majlesi Y, Samorapoompichit P, Hauswirth AW, Schernthaner GH, Ghannadan M, Baghestanian M, et al. Cerivastatin and atorvastatin inhibit IL-3-dependent differentiation and IgE-mediated histamine release in human basophils and downmodulate expression of the basophil-activation antigen CD203c/E-NPP3. J Leukoc Biol. 2003;73:107–17.
39. Hauswirth AW, Natter S, Ghannadan M, Majlesi Y, Schernthaner GH, Sperr WR, et al. Recombinant allergens promote expression of CD203c on basophils in sensitized individuals. J Allergy Clin Immunol. 2002;110:102–9.
40. Skypala IJ, Calderon MA, Leeds AR, Emery P, Till SJ, Durham SR. Development and validation of a structured questionnaire for the diagnosis of oral allergy syndrome in subjects with seasonal allergic rhinitis during the UK birch pollen season. Clin Exp Allergy. 2011;41:1001–11.
41. Masthoff LJ, van Hoffen E, de Reus A, Boonacker CW, Bruijnzeel-Koomen CA, Pasmans SG, et al. Hazelnut allergy differs between children and adults in frequency of severity, aetiology and relevance of diagnostic parameters. Clin Exp Allergy. 2014;44:1539–45.
42. Brandström J, Nopp A, Johansson SG, Lilja G, Sundqvist AC, Borres MP, et al. Basophil allergen threshold sensitivity and component-resolved diagnostics improve hazelnut allergy diagnosis. Clin Exp Allergy. 2015;45:1412–8.
43. Masthoff LJ, Mattsson L, Zuidmeer-Jongejan L, Lidholm J, Andersson K, Akkerdaas JH, et al. Sensitization to Cor a 9 and Cor a 14 is highly specific for a hazelnut allergy with objective symptoms in Dutch children and adults. J Allergy Clin Immunol. 2013;132:393–9.
44. van Erp FC, Knol EF, Pontoppidan B, Meijer Y, van der Ent CK, Knulst AC. The IgE and basophil responses to Ara h 2 and Ara h 6 are good predictors of peanut allergy in children. J Allergy Clin Immunol. 2016. doi:10.1016/j.jaci.2016.06.041.
45. Faber MA, Van Gasse AL, Decuyper II, Uyttebroek A, Sabato V, Hagendorens MM, et al. IgE-reactivity profiles to nonspecific lipid transfer proteins in a northwestern European country. J Allergy Clin Immunol. 2016. doi:10.1016/j.jaci.2016.06.016.
46. Chirumbolo S. Basophil activation test in allergy: time for an update? Int Arch Allergy Immunol. 2012;158:99–114.

20

Better recognition, diagnosis and management of non-IgE-mediated cow's milk allergy in infancy: iMAP—an international interpretation of the MAP (Milk Allergy in Primary Care)

Carina Venter[1†], Trevor Brown[2†], Rosan Meyer[3], Joanne Walsh[4], Neil Shah[5], Anna Nowak-Węgrzyn[6], Tong-Xin Chen[7], David M. Fleischer[1], Ralf G. Heine[8], Michael Levin[9], Mario C. Vieira[10] and Adam T. Fox[11,12*]

Abstract

Cow's milk allergy (CMA) is one of the most common presentations of food allergy seen in early childhood. It is also one of the most complex food allergies, being implicated in IgE-mediated food allergy as well as diverse manifestations of non-IgE-mediated food allergy. For example, gastrointestinal CMA may present as food protein induced enteropathy, enterocolitis or proctocolitis. Concerns regarding the early and timely diagnosis of CMA have been highlighted over the years. In response to these, guideline papers from the United Kingdom (UK), Australia, Europe, the Americas and the World Allergy Organisation have been published. The UK guideline, 'Diagnosis and management of non-IgE-mediated cow's milk allergy in infancy—a UK primary care practical guide' was published in this journal in 2013. This Milk Allergy in Primary Care (MAP) guideline outlines in simple algorithmic form, both the varying presentations of cow's milk allergy and also focuses on the practical management of the most common presentation, namely mild-to-moderate non-IgE-mediated allergy. Based on the international uptake of the MAP guideline, it became clear that there was a need for practical guidance beyond the UK. Consequently, this paper presents an international interpretation of the MAP guideline to help practitioners in primary care settings around the world. It incorporates further published UK guidance, feedback from UK healthcare professionals and affected families and, importantly, also international guidance and expertise.

Background

Over the last 2 decades, many countries have seen a significant rise in the number of children suffering from food allergy, defined as an adverse health effect arising from a specific immune response that occurs reproducibly on exposure to a given food [1]. The impact on quality of life for families with food allergy has been shown to be significantly worse than for those with chronic pain disorders [2] or diabetes [3]. For most infants with suspected cow's milk allergy (CMA) this can be clinically subdivided into either immediate-onset *IgE-mediated,* where the adverse effects appear usually within minutes following ingestion or delayed onset *non-IgE-mediated* where the effects develop usually after ≥2 h [4]. It is difficult to define IgE-mediated food allergy into milder and more severe forms as external factors often determine the severity of reaction, with anaphylaxis being the most severe presentation [5]. The spectrum of non-IgE-mediated CMA is broad; encompassing symptoms that range in severity from mild rectal bleeding in milk protein induced proctocolitis to the severe vomiting and collapse that can be seen in food protein induced enterocolitis syndrome (FPIES). Evidence from the United Kingdom

*Correspondence: adam.fox@gstt.nhs.uk
†Carina Venter and Trevor Brown are joint first authors.
[11] Department of Paediatric Allergy, Guys and St Thomas' Hospitals NHS Foundation Trust, London, UK
Full list of author information is available at the end of the article

(UK) [6] shows that the majority of infants presenting with suspected CMA fall into a 'mild-to-moderate' [7] clinical expression of non-IgE-mediated allergy. Although the severities of the non-IgE-mediated reactions were not clearly defined, data from the EuroPrevall study indicates the presence of milder forms of non-IgE-mediated food allergy in Europe, particularly in the Netherlands, Italy and Poland [8].

Whilst attempting to monitor this overall rise in suspected food allergy in children, some controversy has arisen over the true incidence of this 'mild-to-moderate' non-IgE-mediated sub-group presenting characteristically in infancy with mostly gastrointestinal-related symptoms such as abdominal discomfort, gastro-oesophageal reflux and abnormal bowel frequency and consistency. In 2015 Schoemaker et al. [8] reported, as part of the EuroPrevall project that the national incidences of CMA in Europe vary across countries with the majority of children with CMA in the UK and the Netherlands suffering from the non-IgE-mediated form. However, the very low incidences reported in some countries have become the subject of debate. Nowak-Wegrzyn et al. [9] and Koletzko et al. [10] argued that the children with non-IgE-mediated CMA in 4 out of the 9 EuroPrevall countries were selectively missed due to clinical unawareness of gastro-intestinal symptoms and their relation to possible CMA. Non-IgE-mediated food allergy is also often reported in Latin America [11]. In line with the previously published MAP (Milk Allergy in Primary Care) guideline [7], the diagnosis of mild-to-moderate non-IgE-mediated CMA requires the strict avoidance of all cow's milk containing foods for an agreed trial period, i.e. an elimination diet, followed by clinical improvement and then subsequent relapse coincident with reintroduction. This elimination-reintroduction sequence is the only way of reliably diagnosing gastrointestinal manifestations of non-IgE-mediated CMA in infants such as infantile allergic proctocolitis, mild-to-moderate allergic enteropathy and cow's milk-induced gastro-oesophageal reflux or constipation because there is no allergy skin or blood test for non-IgE-mediated food allergy.

This paper, whilst acknowledging all the possible clinical presentations of CMA in infancy (IgE and non-IgE with their differing diagnostic approaches), will focus primarily on the better recognition, confirmation and management of these infants presenting with suspected mild-to-moderate non-IgE-mediated CMA. The actual management of IgE-mediated CMA and the more severe presentations of non-IgE-mediated CMA, such as FPIES, Eosinophilic Esophagitis and food protein induced enteropathy with faltering growth will not be addressed. This iMAP guideline builds on the strengths of the previous UK MAP guideline, designed with a UK primary care focus, which has been demonstrated to effectively improve the recognition and earlier diagnosis of mild-to-moderate non-IgE-mediated CMA [12] but has now been reviewed with an international focus. The guideline does not represent the views of, nor is it endorsed by, any professional organisation, nor was it supported by any commercial entity at any point in the development process.

Considerations behind the publication of the 2013 UK MAP guideline [7]

A UK birth cohort study published in 2008 showed that 2–3% of 1–3 year olds suffer from confirmed CMA [13]. Worldwide this prevalence ranges between 1.9 and 4.9% [14], making it one of the most common food allergies in the first years of life. In 2010 a review of 1000 infants with CMA randomly chosen from a UK primary care database [6] showed that 86% were first diagnosed in primary care and that the majority remained there for their care. 42% of the infants were referred on, usually to the care of a general paediatrician. Only a few were seen at a specialist level multidisciplinary paediatric allergy service. The majority presented clinically with mild-to-moderate symptoms of suspected non-IgE-mediated CMA. Significantly smaller numbers could have been categorised as either severe non-IgE-mediated CMA or immediate-onset IgE-mediated CMA. The review highlighted evidence of under-recognition, misdiagnosis, significant delay in diagnosis and sub-optimal management of the infants especially in choosing the most appropriate initial alternative formula suitable for the management of CMA, when breast milk is not available. Fewer than 1 in 5 families had received support from a dietitian [6]. The problem of over and under diagnosis of CMA with its inherent undesirable nutritional management is not unique to the UK. Van den Hooge et al. [15] and Vieira et al. [11] report similar problems in the Netherlands and Latin America respectively. To address the need for better diagnosis of food allergy, six international guideline papers were published from the: United States (US) [1], World Allergy Organization (WAO) [14], European Academy of Allergy, Asthma and Clinical Immunology (EAACI) [16], UK, National Institute of Health and Care Excellence (NICE) [17], British Society for Allergy and Clinical Immunology (BSACI) [18] and European Society for Paediatric Gastroenterology Hepatology and Nutrition (ESPGHAN) [19].

The UK NICE 2011 clinical guideline on the 'Diagnosis and assessment of food allergy in children and young people in primary care and community settings', Clinical Guideline 116 (CG116) [17], addressed within its given scope only the presentation and initial assessment of any suspected food allergy. As part of the initial assessment, it particularly emphasised the need to clinically differentiate between non-IgE-mediated and IgE-mediated expressions of food allergy.

Subsequently, a subgroup of the clinicians on the NICE guideline development group published the MAP guideline in 2013 [7]. It addressed in a simple algorithm-based pathway the initial presentation of the differing clinical expressions of CMA in infancy (both non-IgE and IgE) and the on-going management in primary care of those children with confirmed mild-to-moderate non-IgE-mediated CMA.

Considerations behind the publication of this 2017 updated version of MAP

Evidence showing the effectiveness of the MAP guideline [7] in positively changing UK prescribing patterns has been published [12]. Since 2013, frequent citations and use of MAP across the world have indicated that it is of practical clinical relevance not only for the UK but also for healthcare professionals working in other national healthcare systems. The important early healthcare contacts where the possibility of CMA needs to be explored between parents and a 'first contact' clinician do not essentially change from one healthcare system to another.

Significantly, UK NICE has now produced two further publications; in 2015 a NICE Clinical Knowledge Summary (CKS) on the diagnosis and management in primary care of 'cow's milk protein allergy in children' [20], and in 2016 the NICE Quality Standard for food allergy [21]. Since the publication of the MAP guideline in 2013, the BSACI also published their specialist guidelines on cow's milk allergy [18]. Since then, to our knowledge no other CMA guidelines have been published internationally.

This growing number of guidelines with clinical relevance to CMA gives rise to the very real potential for 'guideline overload'. A recent UK paper surveyed over 400 general practitioners (GPs) and 300 parents looking at the current 'journey from diagnosis to management of milk allergy' for parents and the doctors in primary care [22]. The authors suggested an ideal pathway for the better identification and management of CMA by healthcare professionals should include improved education focusing on the current guidelines and the development of simple tools from the guidelines, such as algorithms, to aid diagnosis and management. A required action highlighted by the parents was the development of a simple tool centred on their recording of possible symptoms that they could take to the appointment with their healthcare professional. Meeting such requests will be of practical clinical relevance for healthcare professionals and families in all healthcare systems.

These NICE primary care guidelines are UK focused and were not intended to be accessed and interpreted by clinicians based outside of the UK. However, the guidance was widely adopted outside of the UK, suggesting the need for an updated non-UK focused interpretation. The aim of this paper is therefore to both incorporate these recent UK publications and to adapt MAP into a more internationally suited version. Management of Milk Allergy in Primary Care (iMAP), to act as both a UK and international guideline with amended algorithms (Figs. 2, 3), supported by other practical tools for both families and healthcare professionals in primary care (Additional files 1, 2, 3, 4).

Clinicians recognise the important role families and carers have in supporting children with food allergy and that 'family members and carers should be involved in the decision-making process about investigations, treatment and care' [20]. This iMAP version aims to facilitate that important role.

Presentation and recognition of CMA

Revisiting CMA nomenclature

The UK NICE guidelines along with other national and international guidelines clearly indicate that CMA is broadly divided into IgE-mediated and non-IgE-mediated disease. Although they acknowledge that the non-IgE-mediated presentation can be divided into mild-to-moderate and more severe presentations, there is currently no international consensus with clearly agreed definitions of these presentations. Indeed even in terms of Eosinophilic Oesophagitis (EoE), experts and international bodies disagree about whether this is a disease that is primarily non-IgE-mediated [23] or in fact a mixed IgE and non-IgE-mediated disease [1].

The allergy-focused clinical history

The allergy-focused clinical history continues to form the 'cornerstone of diagnosis' in food allergy and 'children and young people with suspected food allergy should have an allergy-focused clinical history taken' [21]. EAACI also recently published a task force report on how to take an allergy-focused diet history to aid with the diagnosis of a food allergy [24].

This process will support the clinician to distinguish between IgE-mediated and non-IgE-mediated reactions, based primarily on the information provided by the family. This will then inform the healthcare professional with the appropriate competencies/clinical expertise to decide which other tests, if any, are needed to confirm the diagnosis and then how the food allergy should be managed.

- Any family history of atopic disease in parents or siblings.
- Any history of early atopic disease in the infant.
- The infant's feeding history including growth.

The iMAP Allergy-focused Clinical History

for **Suspected Cow's Milk Allergy** in **Infancy**

'The Cornerstone of the Diagnosis'

Ask about:

- A family history of atopic disease (atopic dermatitis, asthma, allergic rhinitis or food allergy) in parents or siblings
  – a reported history along with symptoms of suspected cow's milk allergy makes the diagnosis more likely; this applies to both IgE-mediated and non-IgE-mediated
- Sources of cow's milk protein and how much is being or was ingested:
  Exclusive breast feeding - when cow's milk protein from maternal diet comes through in the breast milk (low risk of clinical allergy)
  Mixed feeding - when cow's milk protein is given to the breast feeding infant e.g. top-up formulas, on weaning with solids
  Formula-feeding infant - the commonest presentation, particularly in countries where there is poor adherence with the WHO guidance (14) of exclusive breastfeeding for 6 months
- Presenting symptoms, to include:
  - if more than one symptom, the sequence of clinical presentation of each one
  - age of first onset
  - timing of onset following ingestion (atopic dermatitis - such 'timing' can be very variable)
    IgE-mediated - usually within minutes, but can be up to 2 hours
    Non-IgE-mediated - usually after ≥2 hours or even days
  - duration, severity and frequency
  - reproducibility on repeated exposure
  - amount and form of milk protein that may be causing symptoms
- Details of any concern with feeding difficulties and/or poor growth
- Details of any changes in diet and any apparent response to such changes
- Details of any other previous management, including medication, for the presenting symptoms and any apparent response to this

Fig. 1 Taking and allergy focussed clinical history: Adapted from the UK NICE guideline CG116 on food allergy

- Presenting symptoms and signs that may be indicating possible CMA.
- Details of previous management, including any medication and the perceived response to any treatment or dietary change.

Figure 1 provides a list of questions to ask during the allergy-focused history, but in short such a history will focus on the following questions [7].

The symptoms of the infant at first presentation are a key feature in the diagnostic process. It is important to consider that possible symptoms (Fig. 2) can be variable and overlap with common infant health issues such as irritability (colic), gastro-oesophageal reflux and atopic dermatitis that may not necessarily be CMA-related. There is also often confusion between immediate-onset IgE-mediated allergy and delayed-onset non-IgE-mediated allergy symptoms.

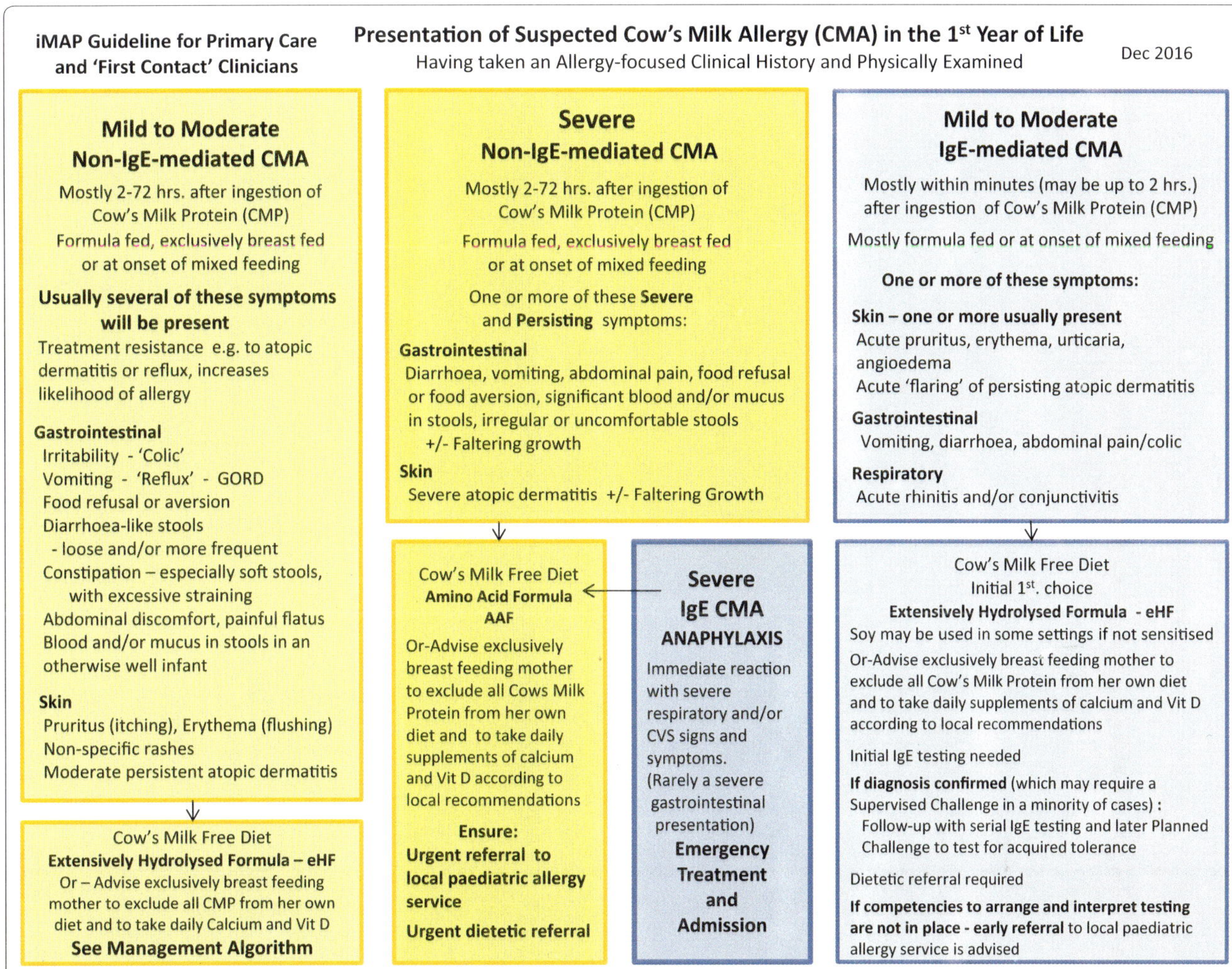

Fig. 2 Presentation of suspected cow's milk allergy (CMA) in the 1st year of Life

An attempt should therefore be made to elicit a history of all symptoms, assess which are significantly out of the range of normal, and classify them as indicating suspected IgE-mediated or non-IgE-mediated disease. The 4 possible symptom complexes of: IgE-mediated disease (mild-to-moderate or severe) and non-IgE-mediated disease (mild-to-moderate or severe) serve as an entry point for an initial dietary management strategy (Fig. 2).

Recognising the importance of the first contact consultation between the family and the healthcare professional, the iMAP guideline team are in the process of developing a symptom tool. There is currently just one published Cow's milk related symptom score (CoMiSS) and this needs further validation [25]. Initial data however, indicates that a change in CoMiSS from baseline to month 1 after milk exclusion, can be used to predict CMA [26] (Fig. 2).

As part of the allergy-focused healthcare consultation, it is important to carry out a physical examination [20], particularly looking for signs indicating any allergy-related comorbidities such as atopic dermatitis and, in addition, performing weight, length and head circumference measurements.

Diagnosis

Diagnosis of non-IgE-mediated CMA

If the clinical history suggests non-IgE-mediated CMA and the child 'has not had a severe delayed reaction', it is recommended to offer a trial elimination of the suspected allergen and subsequent reintroduction [21] (Fig. 3).

We have previously described indications for the different formulas for the diagnosis and management of the varying expressions of CMA based on a consensus of national and international guidelines [7]. As the iMAP guideline focuses on the diagnosis and management of mild-to-moderate CMA, we wish to highlight here the following points:

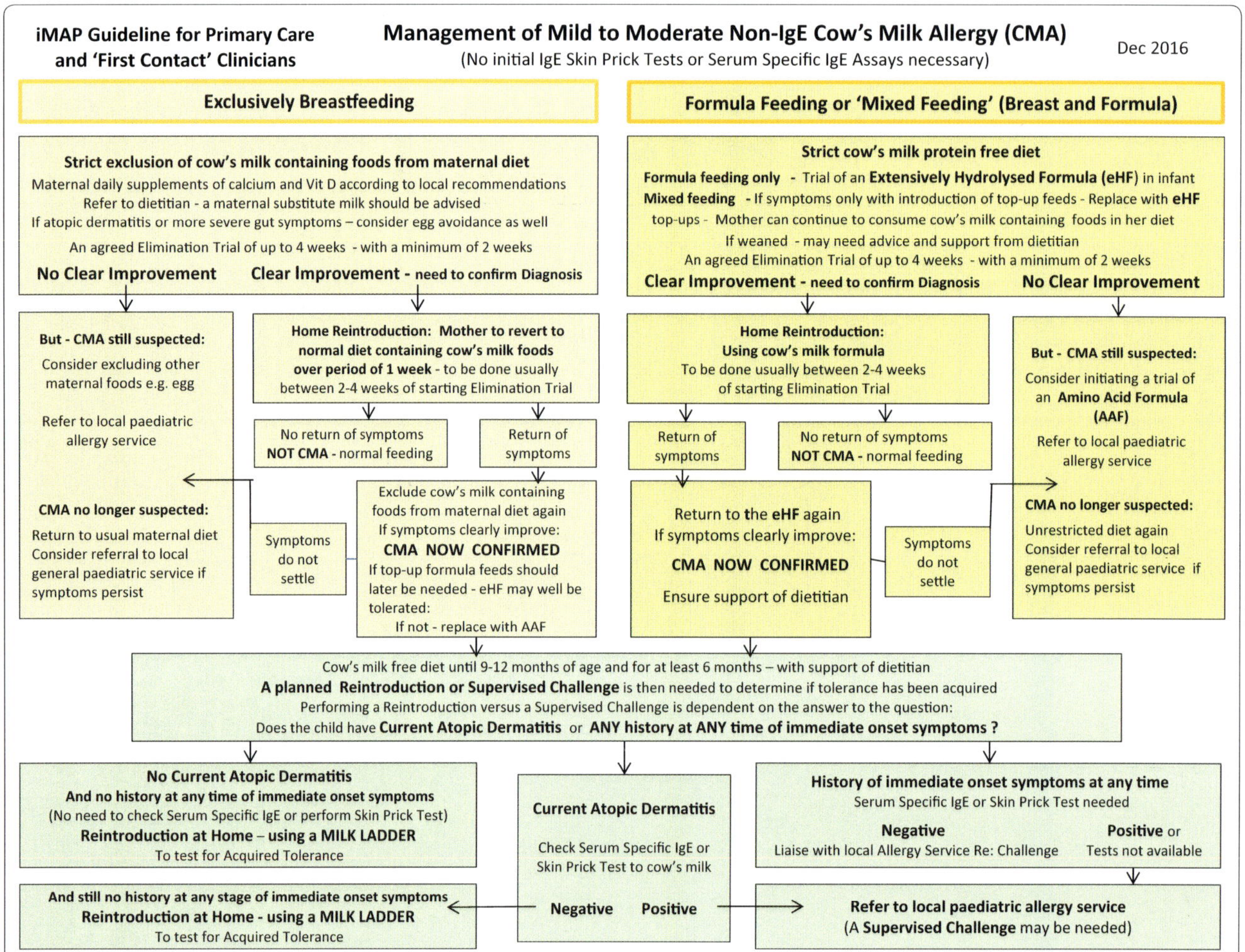

Fig. 3 Management of mild to moderate non-IgE cow's milk allergy (CMA)

Extensively hydrolysed formulas (eHFs) continue to be recommended as the initial prescribed formulas for most infants presenting with suspected mild-to-moderate CMA. However, worldwide, there is at least one example of national practice where an amino acid-based formula (AAF) is commonly chosen as the initial diagnostic trial formula in all suspected cases of CMA, e.g. China. Therefore, the authors acknowledge that practice varies and in some countries an AAF is used as the initial diagnostic trial formula for CMA. It is however important to note that such practice is based on local services, reimbursements of formulas and not born out of clinical evidence based indications for AAF [27].

When an infant reacts to the amount of milk protein passed on from maternal consumption during breastfeeding, it is recommended to avoid cow's milk from the maternal diet as the first priority. If a supplemental formula is required, an eHF or AAF may be utilised [28]. This decision needs to be taken on an individualised basis, as this depends on whether full symptom resolution has occurred on a maternal elimination diet, the nutritional status of the infant and the underlying CMA diagnosis.

In view of the international focus of the iMAP guidelines, we want to acknowledge that soy formula may be used as the first line alternative to cow's milk formula in some countries, e.g. South Africa. It is however not recommended under 6 months of age in the USA, Europe, UK, Brazil and Australia and not as the first line of treatment except for Australia where soy may be recommended as first line treatment in infants over 6 months of age in certain CMA conditions [14, 29].

Therefore, local interpretation of the iMAP guidelines may be required in some clinical scenarios.

The reintroduction step, following clear improvement of symptoms during the elimination trial, is of ultimate importance to confirm the diagnosis. In the absence of such a planned reintroduction step to confirm the return of symptoms and their subsequent resolution on recommencing the elimination diet, the risk of a significant number of infants continuing unnecessarily on an expensive and nutritionally demanding diet will remain. The optimum time to explain and agree on the need for the planned early reintroduction is when the trial elimination diet is first started. At that consultation it can be helpful to allow the family to take away with them a factsheet explaining why such a trial elimination diet is needed, followed by a planned reintroduction (Additional file 1).

The iMAP Management Algorithm for mild-to-moderate non-IgE-mediated CMA (Fig. 3) provides guidance on the length and type of the initial elimination diet; for up to 4 weeks (with a minimum of 2 weeks) in conjunction with optimal dietary advice. It is important to emphasise that we are looking for a clear improvement and not necessarily a complete resolution of symptoms [22].

There is an accompanying iMAP written protocol for both the parent and healthcare professional, setting out how cow's milk protein can then be gradually, simply and safely reintroduced into either the mother's or infant's diet at home to confirm or exclude the diagnosis (Additional file 2).

Diagnosis of IgE-mediated CMA

If the clinical history suggests IgE-mediated CMA, then 'further testing is recommended' [21]. This can be done as 'either a skin prick test or blood test for specific IgE antibodies to the suspected food allergens...' [21] (Fig. 2).

It is important to recognise that a positive skin prick test or a positive serum specific IgE blood test simply shows sensitisation (i.e. presence of IgE antibodies) to a food allergen, but, on its own, does not confirm an allergy. The final diagnosis of clinical allergy depends on the interpretation of the results in the context of the clinical history and made by a clinician with the appropriate training and skills [21]. The ability of primary care-based clinicians to perform and interpret these tests will differ from country to country. In many cases these tests should ideally be performed in secondary care or allergy referral centers [20]. Additionally, in some cases the history and the allergy test results will not be sufficient to confirm the diagnosis. A supervised food challenge will then be required, and must only be performed under the care of medical providers with the relevant training and skills [17].

It should be emphasised that the iMAP early Home Reintroduction to confirm diagnosis and then the iMAP Home Milk Ladder to test for later acquired tolerance should only be used in children with mild-to-moderate non-IgE-mediated CMA and not in other presentations such as IgE-mediated CMA or severe non-IgE-mediated CMA (e.g. FPIES).

Whilst waiting for a specialist assessment, the iMAP Presentation Algorithm (Fig. 2) guides as to the necessary change to either the maternal diet or infant formula. It may also be helpful to direct parents to national patient support websites.

Management of mild-to-moderate confirmed non-IgE-mediated CMA within primary care or by the 'first contact' clinician (Fig. 3)

When the diagnosis of mild-to-moderate non-IgE-mediated CMA is confirmed, iMAP provides guidance on the on-going management in primary care and recommends dietetic support. The management will include continuation of treatment with a suitable alternative formula or, if indicated, maternal allergen avoidance. Most importantly, milk free weaning advice should be provided by the dietitian not only to ensure that cow's milk is avoided in the infant's complementary diet, but also to address growth [11], nutritional [30] and feeding problems in the short [31] and long term [32].

The on-going management includes a second planned reintroduction of milk protein when the time comes to test for acquired tolerance. The iMAP Management Algorithm guides on the timing of this as well. It is usually carried out in the form of a graduated 'Milk Ladder' (Additional file 3). Ideally at this stage a dietitian will be taking the lead.

In the development of this new iMAP Milk Ladder, a number of factors were taken into account such as the dose of cow's milk protein provided, the timing and temperature of heating, as well as the matrix effect of wheat and fat [5]. Healthy eating, general feeding practices across the world and other food allergies have also been taken into account. The dietitians involved in developing the Ladder have therefore reduced the number of Steps in the Ladder. Many of the high sugar foods have been removed as a necessary step, but are still offered as an option, once a certain Step has been passed, e.g. milk chocolate/candy can be given once Step 5 (yoghurt) is passed. Foods eaten by only certain cultural groups have been removed, such as Shepherd's pie.

Suspected severe non-IgE mediated CMA

In the uncommon situation of the infant presenting with more severe symptoms leading to a suspected severe expression of non-IgE-mediated CMA, the iMAP Presentation Algorithm (Fig. 2) identifies these infants, advises on the need for early onward referral to a specialist allergy service. For most of these infants the severity of the symptoms and their significant improvement on commencing the elimination diet will be enough to confirm the diagnosis. However, should they still need an early food challenge to confirm or exclude the diagnosis that will need to be done under the careful supervision of a specialist allergy team [21].

Referral

Any specialist allergy service for children should be led by a paediatrician or other appropriately trained physician, supported by a multidisciplinary team made up of specialist dietitians, nurses and ideally a clinical psychologist all with the necessary expertise in childhood food allergy. Due to the multisystem involvement of CMA, other medical specialities may also need to be readily accessible, including gastroenterology and dermatology.

Conclusion

CMA is one of the most common food allergies affecting children worldwide and, with few exceptions, presents in the first months of life. Clinically it is complex due to its differing possible presentations making it challenging to diagnose. These factors have underscored the need for UK NICE guidance as well as the MAP primary care CMA guideline written by a group of the clinicians who were part of the NICE food allergy guideline development group. Most infants who present with suspected CMA have non-IgE-mediated manifestations with mild-to-moderate and delayed-onset symptoms. However, those infants who present with either immediate-onset IgE-mediated symptoms or those who progress to more severe non-IgE-mediated symptoms need to be promptly and reliably identified in order to allow early referral.

There is evidence that there are significant care issues for these young infants with any expression of CMA and also for their families. Evidence showing the effectiveness of the earlier MAP guideline in positively changing UK prescribing patterns has been published. This newer MAP guideline version, iMAP (based now on a wider range of relevant UK NICE publications and the input of international clinical experts) with its amended algorithms and growing portfolio of accompanying practical tools should help both primary care or 'first contact' clinicians work better with the families to further improve the quality of care. Hopefully this will lead to better health outcomes including: the earlier identification of CMA, early referral of children requiring specialist allergy review and identification of those remaining children who can be effectively and safely managed in primary care. This approach will be of practical clinical relevance not only for the UK but also for healthcare professionals working in other national healthcare systems.

Abbreviations

MAP: Milk Allergy in Primary Care; CMA: cow's milk allergy; FPIES: food protein induced enterocolitis syndrome; UK: United Kingdom; US: United States; WAO: World Allergy Organization; EAACI: European Academy of Allergy, Asthma and Clinical Immunology; NICE: National Institute of Health and Care Excellence; BSACI: British Society for Allergy and Clinical Immunology; ESPGHAN: European Society for Paediatric Gastroenterology Hepatology and Nutrition; CG116: Clinical Guideline 116; CKS: NICE Clinical Knowledge Summary; GPs: general practitioners; iMAP: International version: Management of Milk Allergy in Primary Care; CoMISS: cow's milk related symptom score; eHFs: extensively hydrolysed formulas; AAF: amino acid-based formula.

Authors' contributions

CV was actively involved in developing the algorithms; she led the development of the Milk Ladder with RM prepared and edited the manuscript. TB initially set up this guideline development group and subsequently has continued to contribute to the on-going development of this UK primary care-focused CMA guideline and in the preparation of this manuscript. RM was actively involved in developing the Milk Ladder and edited the manuscript and advised on the formula milk aspects of this paper. AN helped in preparation of the manuscript and advised on the non-IgE components of this publication. JW has helped in development of the algorithms and preparation of the manuscript. NS helped in preparation of the manuscript and advised on the non-IgE components of this publication. ATF helped in development of the algorithms and preparation of the manuscript. T-XC, DMF, RGH, ML and MCV each suggested how the manuscript could be further improved. All authors read and approved the final manuscript.

Author details

[1] Section of Allergy and Immunology, University of Colorado Denver School of Medicine, Children's Hospital Colorado , Box B518, 13123 East 16th Avenue, Anschutz Medical Campus, Aurora, CO 80045, USA. [2] Children's Allergy Service, Ulster Hospital, Belfast BT16 1RH, Northern Ireland, UK. [3] Department Paediatrics, Imperial College, London, London W2 1NY, UK. [4] Gurney Surgery, Castle Partnership, 101-103 Magdalen Street, Norwich NR3 1LN, UK. [5] Gastroenterology Department, Great Ormond Street Hospital, London WC1N 3JH, UK. [6] Jaffe Food Allergy Institute, Icahn School of Medicine at Mount Sinai, New York, NY 10029, USA. [7] Department of Allergy and Immunology, Shanghai Children's Medical Center, Shanghai Jiao Tong University School of Medicine, 1678 Dongfang Road, Shanghai 200127, China. [8] Royal Children's Hospital Melbourne, Murdoch Children's Research Institute, Parkville, VIC 3052, Australia. [9] Division of Paediatric Allergy and Asthma, Red Cross War Memorial Children's Hospital, University of Cape Town, Room 516, ICH Building, Cape Town, South Africa. [10] Centro de Gastroenterologica Pediatrica, Department of Paediatrics, Hospital Pequeno Principe, Pontificia Universidade Catolica do Parana, Curitiba, Brazil. [11] Department of Paediatric Allergy, Guys and St Thomas' Hospitals NHS Foundation Trust, London, UK. [12] Division of Asthma, Allergy and Lung Biology, King's College, London, London, UK.

Acknowledgements

We would like to acknowledge the help of Rosemary Martin and Alison Cassin for their valuable input in reviewing the Milk Ladder. We would like to acknowledge the help of the Wessex UK Allergy Dietitians for their help with the development of the initial Milk Ladder published in 2013.

Competing interests

Carina Venter has received educational lecture fees from Mead Johnson, Nestle and Danone. Trevor Brown has received educational lecture fees from

Mead Johnson, Danone and Abbott. Rosan Meyer has received research funding from Danone and educational lecture fees from Danone, Mead Johnson, Mead Johnson Scientific Advisory Board for Food Allergy UK, Nestle and Cow and Gate and Abbott. Joanne Walsh has received educational lecture fees from Mead Johnson and Danone and acted as a consultant for educational material for both these companies and also for Abbott and Nestle. Neil Shah has received lecture and consultancy fees from Nestle, Nutricia and Mead Johnson. Anna Nowak-Wegrzyn has received educational lecture fees from Mead Johnson, Nestle and Danone. Tong-Xin Chen has received has received lecture fees from Nestle and Danone. David Fleischer has received grant support and lecture fees from Nestle Nutrition Institute. Ralf Heine is a member of the Nestlé Nutrition Institute Scientific Advisory Board, Australia/Oceania, and the Nutricia Scientific Advisory Board, Australia, and has received educational lecture fees/honoraria from Nestlé and Nutricia/Danone. Michael Levin has received research funding from Cipla, support for educational activities from Cipla and Nutricia and educational lecture fees from Cipla. Mario Vieira has received research funding from Danone and educational lecture fees from Danone, Mead Johnson and Nestle. Adam Fox has received research funding from Danone and consultancy and/or educational lecture fees from Mead Johnson, Nestle, Danone and Abbott.

References

1. Boyce JA, Assa'a A, Burks AW, Jones SM, Sampson HA, Wood RA, et al. Guidelines for the diagnosis and management of food allergy in the United States: summary of the NIAID-sponsored expert panel report. Nutrition. 2011;27(2):253–67.
2. Godwin H, et al. The quality of life of children with food protein induced gastrointestinal allergies. Abstract presented at European Society for Paediatric Gastroenterology, Hepatology and Nutrition ESPGHAN 2013.
3. Flokstra-de Blok BM, van der Velde JL, Vlieg-Boerstra BJ, Oude Elberink JN, DunnGalvin A, Hourihane JO, et al. Health-related quality of life of food allergic patients measured with generic and disease-specific questionnaires. Allergy. 2010;65(8):1031–8.
4. Johansson SG, Bieber T, Dahl R, Friedmann PS, Lanier BQ, Lockey RF, et al. Revised nomenclature for allergy for global use: report of the Nomenclature Review Committee of the World Allergy Organization, October 2003. J Allergy Clin Immunol. 2004;113(5):832–6.
5. Turner PJ, Baumert JL, Beyer K, Boyle R, Chan CH, Clark A, et al. Can we identify patients at risk of life-threatening allergic reactions to food? Allergy. 2016;71:1241–55.
6. Sladkevicius E, Nagy E, Lack G, Guest JF. Resource implications and budget impact of managing cow milk allergy in the UK. J Med Econ. 2010;13(1):119–28.
7. Venter C, Brown T, Shah N, Walsh J, Fox AT. Diagnosis and management of non-IgE-mediated cow's milk allergy in infancy—a UK primary care practical guide. Clin Transl Allergy. 2013;3(1):23.
8. Schoemaker AA, Sprikkelman AB, Grimshaw KE, Roberts G, Grabenhenrich L, Rosenfeld L, et al. Incidence and natural history of challenge-proven cow's milk allergy in European children–EuroPrevall birth cohort. Allergy. 2015;70(8):963–72.
9. Nowak-Wegrzyn A, Fiocchi A. Is oral immunotherapy the cure for food allergies? Curr Opin Allergy Clin Immunol. 2010;10(3):214–9.
10. Koletzko S, Heine RG. Non-IgE mediated cow's milk allergy in EuroPrevall. Allergy. 2015;70(12):1679–80.
11. Vieira MC, Morais MB, Spolidoro JV, Toporovski MS, Cardoso AL, Araujo GT, et al. A survey on clinical presentation and nutritional status of infants with suspected cow' milk allergy. BMC Pediatr. 2010;10:25.
12. Wauters L, Brown T, Venter C, Dziubak R, Meyer R, Brogan B, et al. Cow's milk allergy prescribing is influenced by Regional and National Guidance. J Pediatr Gastroenterol Nutr. 2016;62(5):765–70.
13. Venter C, Pereira B, Voigt K, Grundy J, Clayton CB, Higgins B, et al. Prevalence and cumulative incidence of food hypersensitivity in the first 3 years of life. Allergy. 2008;63(3):354–9.
14. Fiocchi A, Schunemann HJ, Brozek J, Restani P, Beyer K, Troncone R, et al. Diagnosis and rationale for action against cow's milk allergy (DRACMA): a summary report. J Allergy Clin Immunol. 2010;126(6):1119–28.
15. van den Hoogen SC, van de Pol AC, Meijer Y, Toet J, van Klei C, de Wit NJ. Suspected cow's milk allergy in everyday general practice: a retrospective cohort study on health care burden and guideline adherence. BMC Res Notes. 2014;7:507.
16. Muraro A, Werfel T, Hoffmann-Sommergruber K, Roberts G, Beyer K, Bindslev-Jensen C, et al. EAACI food allergy and anaphylaxis guidelines: diagnosis and management of food allergy. Allergy. 2014;69(8):1008–25.
17. Diagnosis and assessment of food allergy in children and young people in primary care and community settings. 2011. http://www.nice.org.uk/CG116. Cited Aug 2016.
18. Luyt D, Ball H, Makwana N, Green MR, Bravin K, Nasser SM, et al. BSACI guideline for the diagnosis and management of cow's milk allergy. Clin Exp Allergy. 2014;44(5):642–72.
19. Koletzko S, Niggemann B, Arato A, Dias JA, Heuschkel R, Husby S, et al. Diagnostic approach and management of cow's-milk protein allergy in infants and children: ESPGHAN GI Committee practical guidelines. J Pediatr Gastroenterol Nutr. 2012;55(2):221–9.
20. Excellence NIfHaC. Cow's milk protein allergy in children. NICE: Clinical Knowledge Summaries. http://www.cks.nice.org.uk/cows-milk-protein-allergy-in-children.
21. Excellence NIfHaC. NICE: quality standard for food allergy. NICE Quality Standard 118. 2016. http://www.nice.org.uk/guidance/qs118.
22. Lozinsky AC, Meyer R, Anagnostou K, Dziubak R, Reeve K, Godwin H, et al. Cow's milk protein allergy from diagnosis to management: a very different journey for general practitioners and parents. Children. 2015;2(3):317–29.
23. Simon D, Cianferoni A, Spergel JM, Aceves S, Holbreich M, Venter C, et al. Eosinophilic esophagitis is characterized by a non-IgE-mediated food hypersensitivity. Allergy. 2016;71:611–20.
24. Skypala IJ, Venter C, Meyer R, deJong NW, Fox AT, Groetch M, et al. The development of a standardised diet history tool to support the diagnosis of food allergy. Clin Transl Allergy. 2015;5:7.
25. Vandenplas Y, Dupont C, Eigenmann P, Host A, Kuitunen M, Ribes-Koninckx C, et al. A workshop report on the development of the Cow's Milk-related Symptom Score awareness tool for young children. Acta Paediatr. 2015;104(4):334–9.
26. Vandenplas Y, Steenhout P, Jarvi A, Garraeauc A, Mukherjee R. Pooled analysis of the Cow's Milk Symptom Score (CoMiSS) as a predictor for the diagnosis of cow's milk allergy. In: World congress on pediatric gastroenterology, hepatology and nutrition, October 2016, Montreal. 2016.
27. Morais MB, Spolidoro JV, Vieira MC, Cardoso AL, Clark O, Nishikawa A, et al. Amino acid formula as a new strategy for diagnosing cow's milk allergy in infants: is it cost-effective? J Med Econ. 2016;19(12):1207–14.
28. Host A, Halken S. Hypoallergenic formulas—when, to whom and how long: after more than 15 years we know the right indication! Allergy. 2004;59(Suppl 78):45–52.
29. Allen KJ, Davidson GP, Day AS, Hill DJ, Kemp AS, Peake JE, Prescott SL, Shugg A, Sinn JK, Heine RG. Management of cow's milk protein allergy in infants and young children: an expert panel perspective. J Paediatr Child Health. 2009;45(9):481–6.
30. Meyer R, De Koker C, Dziubak R, Godwin H, Dominguez-Ortega G, Shah N. Dietary elimination of children with food protein induced gastrointestinal allergy—micronutrient adequacy with and without a hypoallergenic formula? Clin Transl Allergy. 2014;4(1):31.
31. Maslin K, Dean T, Arshad SH, Venter C. Fussy eating and feeding difficulties in infants and toddlers consuming a cows' milk exclusion diet. Pediatr Allergy Immunol. 2015;26(6):503–8.
32. Maslin K, Grundy J, Glasbey G, Dean T, Arshad SH, Grimshaw K, et al. Cows' milk exclusion diet during infancy: is there a long-term effect on children's eating behaviour and food preferences? Pediatr Allergy Immunol. 2016;27(2):141–6.

Body mass index and physical activity in early childhood are associated with atopic sensitization, atopic dermatitis and asthma in later childhood

Kristine Kjer Byberg[1*], Geir Egil Eide[2,3], Michele R. Forman[4], Pétur Benedikt Júlíusson[5,6] and Knut Øymar[1,6]

Abstract

Background: The results of studies on the associations of childhood excessive weight/obesity and physical activity with atopic sensitization and atopic diseases are inconsistent. We studied the associations of anthropometry and physical activity in childhood with atopic sensitization and atopic diseases in late childhood.

Methods: In a cohort study including cases exposed to preeclampsia during pregnancy and controls, anthropometry and physical activity were assessed at several ages in 617 children. Associations with atopic sensitization and atopic diseases in late childhood were analysed using multiple logistic regression.

Results: Body mass index standard deviation score (BMI SDS) at 1 year and low physical activity at 3–6 years were positively associated with atopic sensitization at 12.8 years [adjusted odds ratio (OR) 1.22; 95 % confidence interval (1.00, 1.49) and OR 2.36; (1.15, 4.81), respectively]. Change in BMI SDS from 1 to 4 years, BMI SDS at 4 years, and high physical activity at 6–10 years were positively associated with atopic dermatitis by 10.8 years [OR 1.46; (1.11, 1.92); OR 1.32; (1.06, 1.65) and OR 1.94; (1.16, 3.24); respectively]. Low physical activity at 3–6 and 6–10 years were positively associated with asthma by 10.8 years [OR 3.61; (1.56, 8.36) and OR 2.52; (1.24, 5.12), respectively].

Conclusions: BMI and physical activity in early childhood were associated with atopic sensitization, atopic dermatitis and asthma in later childhood. Larger cohorts with repeated measurements of both predictors and outcomes are required to further elucidate this issue.

Trial registration Our study was observational without any clinical intervention on the participants. Therefore, no trial registration number is available

Keywords: Allergic rhinitis, Anthropometry, Asthma, Atopic dermatitis, Child

Background

The prevalence of obesity, allergy and asthma has increased worldwide during the last decades [1, 2]. An association between obesity and asthma has been suggested both in early and late childhood [3], where obesity precedes asthma in prospective studies [4]; the association between obesity and allergy is inconsistent [5].

High birth weight or body mass index (BMI; kg/m^2) in early childhood is associated with obesity into later childhood [6]. Atopic sensitization and atopic disease commonly start in early childhood [7], and associations between accelerated weight gain in early childhood and subsequent atopic sensitization, allergic rhinitis [8] and asthma [9], have been suggested, but not for atopic dermatitis. Physical activity during childhood may also be associated with atopy, either directly or due to an influence on body composition [10].

Many of these associations of childhood obesity and physical activity with atopy appear in cross-sectional

*Correspondence: Kristine.kjer.byberg@sus.no
[1] Department of Pediatrics, Stavanger University Hospital, POB 8100, 4068 Stavanger, Norway
Full list of author information is available at the end of the article

studies [5, 10, 11]. Few longitudinal studies exist, mainly from registers [4, 5, 11].

It is unknown if an accelerated weight gain from birth is associated with an increased risk of atopy. Furthermore, it is unknown if a positive association between BMI and asthma in children is limited to those with atopy.

The present cohort study was derived from a case control study nested within three birth cohorts that focused on preeclampsia, that had repeated anthropometric measurements, linked information across childhood, and measures of atopic disease at clinical follow-ups. The aim was to study whether weight-related anthropometrics, changes in BMI SDS and physical activity at different ages in childhood are associated with atopic sensitization and atopic disease by late childhood. We hypothesized that childhood excessive weight/obesity or accelerated weight gain is positively associated and physical activity negatively associated with atopic sensitization and atopic diseases.

Methods

Study population and design

The study was a part of "the Stavanger study" described in detail previously [12]. From a population-based cohort, a nested case–control study was conducted, where offspring exposed to maternal preeclampsia and unexposed offspring were identified from all births delivered in Stavanger University hospital in 1993–1995. For each exposed offspring, two matched unexposed offspring were selected: one as the next born in the hospital (i.e. a birth match) and one as the next born matched on maternal age (i.e. a risk factor for preeclampsia). 1025 children, 366 in the preeclampsia and 659 in the control group, were invited to participate in a first follow-up study at 10.8 years (girls) and 11.8 years (boys), and a second follow-up at 12.8 years (both sexes) [13]. The ages at follow-up were selected to coincide with the ages of pubertal onset and menarche of the children. Our analyses disregarded the matched pairs due to missing participants. Therefore, in our study, data were analysed as a historical cohort adjusting for preeclampsia and maternal age, including all the children who participated in both follow-ups, with predictors as listed.

The study was approved by the Norwegian Data Inspectorate, the Regional Committee for Ethics in medical research Western Norway, and the Institutional Review Boards of the National Cancer Institute and University of Texas at Austin, United States. Mothers and children signed an informed consent/assent form at follow-up.

Outcomes

The outcomes allergic rhinoconjunctivitis, atopic dermatitis, asthma ever (evaluated at first follow-up), atopic sensitization and current asthma (evaluated at second follow-up) were defined as follows:

Atopic sensitization Blood specific immunoglobulin E (IgE) $\geq$ 0.35 kU/l for at least one common allergen. Blood was drawn at second follow-up and analysed by Phadiatop®, fx5E® and by specific IgE when positive [13]. Included allergens are shown in Fig. 1. The levels of specific IgE $\geq$ 0.35 were added, and high grade sensitization was defined as a sum >3.9 kU/l: above the lower quartile of all children being sensitized. The ordinal outcome variable atopic sensitization was categorized as: no, low grade and high grade sensitization.

Atopic disease: Asthma ever, allergic rhinoconjunctivitis or atopic dermatitis At first follow-up, questions on atopic disease of the child were asked to the mothers: "Has your child ever had doctor-diagnosed asthma or ever diagnosed with allergy in nose/eyes (hay fever) or atopic dermatitis (childhood eczema)?" Response of "yes" was classified as having the respective diagnosis.

Current asthma At second follow-up, the children answered a questionnaire on reported asthma symptoms and medication during the last year according to the International Study of Asthma and Allergies in Childhood (ISAAC) and asthma ever was recorded [14]. Current asthma at second follow-up was defined as asthma ever, in addition to asthma symptoms or the use of asthma medication the last 12 months (Additional file 1).

Predictors

Birthweight and gestational age were abstracted from hospital records. Recordings of length/height and weight measurements were collected from well-baby clinics at the target ages of 3, 6 and 12 months and 4 years. Trained nurse researchers measured height, weight, triceps skinfold and waist circumference twice in offspring at both

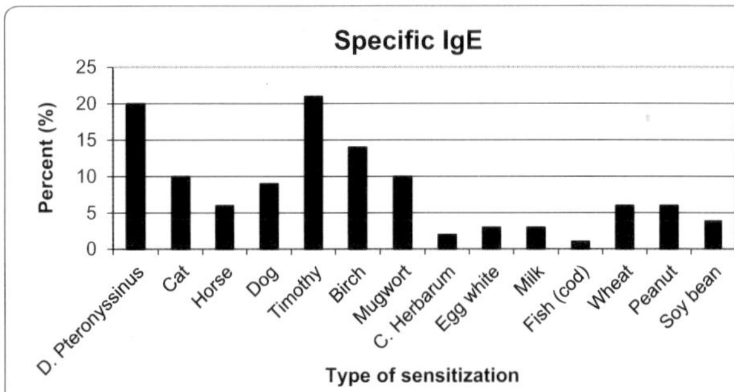

Fig. 1 Percent of children with sensitization (specific IgE > 0.35 kU/l) to common allergens, measured at 12.8 years (n = 388). *D: dermatophagoides, C: cladosporium*

follow-ups, and subscapular skinfold was measured twice at second follow-up; the average of each was used in the analysis [12]. Skinfolds were measured with Harpenden Skinfold Calliper®.

Change in weight and BMI SDS was calculated as the difference between weight and BMI SDS from each target age to the next.

At the first follow-up, the "Stanford Brief Activity Survey", a questionnaire validated for adults, was administered to the mothers requesting responses about physical activity of the child. Specifically the answers to the following questions were extracted: "How active was your child at 3–6 years?" and "How active was your child at 6–10 years?" The response categories were categorized as: passive and/or not so active = low activity, active = normal, very active = high activity [15].

Confounders

Potential confounders included categorical and continuous variables, i.e. sex; gestational age; birth order (firstborn or not); duration of breastfeeding (categories: none; <3; >3 months. This information was extracted from maternal questionnaire, and used in analyses for predictors at target ages ≥6 months); mother's preeclampsia (none, mild/moderate, severe) [16]; mother's BMI (weight at first antenatal visit and height at first follow-up); mother's smoking (at first antenatal visit); mother's doctor-diagnosed asthma [13]; mother's education (from maternal questionnaire: <9; 9–12; >12 years) and mother's age. This is illustrated in a Directed Acyclic Graph (Additional file 1: Figure S1) [17].

Statistical methods

Descriptive statistics were analysed as means, standard deviations, numbers and percentages for the main predictors and outcomes.

There was a wide range of gestational ages at birth due to the inclusion of offspring of preeclampsia and normotensives and a wide age range at later well-child visits, analysing actual values for anthropometrics as predictors would therefore not be appropriate. Instead, standard deviation scores (SDS) based on anthropometric values and actual ages were computed from validated references [18–21]. Conversions into SDS were done using R version 2.6.2 (R Development Core Team, Vienna, Austria).

The associations between anthropometrics and physical activity for each target age (see predictors), and outcomes of atopic sensitization and atopic diseases in late childhood were analysed using multiple binary and ordinal logistic regression analyses (the latter for outcome of atopic sensitization). Separate analyses of the predictors were done for each follow-up time.

Each variable was entered separately into simple regression models. Next, all potential confounders were included in fully adjusted models. Backward stepwise selections were performed to remove non-significant confounders, unless there was ≥15 % change in effect size upon removal of the confounder. Last, final models for each target age included anthropometrics, physical activity, sex of the child and all remaining confounders.

For each predictor, odds ratios with p-values from likelihood ratio tests and 95 % confidence intervals are reported. Interactions between anthropometrics and physical activity with potential confounders were tested. The significance level was 0.05 for all tests.

Also, to study possible non-straight-line associations between BMI SDS and the outcomes, multiple fractional polynomial regression (MFPR) was used with the conservative requirement of $p \leq 0.01$ for non-straight-line terms.

Due to missing values the number of participants varied between the different analyses.

IBM SPSS for windows (version 22.0.0, Chicago, Ill., USA) was used for descriptive statistics and logistic regression, and Stata SE 14 for MFPR.

Results

Characteristics of the participants

The numbers of participants in each follow-up have been published previously [13]. Briefly, 617 children assented to participate at the first follow-up and 470 at the second follow-up. There were more girls with high BMI in the first than second follow-up, and more children with atopic dermatitis in the first than the second follow-up. Otherwise, baseline characteristics were similar between those who assented to the first follow-up only and those who assented to both follow-ups [13]. The percentages of children sensitized to different allergens appear in Fig. 1. Clinical characteristics of the participants appear in Table 1.

Impact of anthropometrics (Tables 2, 3, 4)

BMI SDS at 1 year was positively associated with atopic sensitization at 12.8 years with a borderline significance (Table 2). Change in BMI SDS from 1 to 4 years and BMI SDS at 4 years were positively associated with atopic dermatitis ever at the first follow-up (Tables 2, 3).

Birthweight/BMI SDS and changes in weight or BMI SDS were not associated with allergic rhinoconjunctivitis (Tables 2, 3) or asthma (Table 4 and Additional file 2: Table S1). Skinfolds, waist circumference and waist-to-height ratio at the follow-ups were not associated with atopic sensitization or atopic disease (Additional file 2: Table S2).

Table 1 Descriptive statistics for predictors and outcomes for 617[a] children included in a matched cohort study with follow-up from birth to 12–13 years in the Stavanger area, Norway

Predictors	n	Mean	SD
Birthweight (kg)	606	3.37	0.71
BMI 3 months	541	16.4	1.52
BMI 6 months	559	17.2	1.53
BMI 1 year	559	17.2	1.49
BMI 4 years	477	15.9	1.43
BMI first follow-up[b]	610	18.0	2.91
BMI second follow-up[c]	466	18.8	3.00
Waist circumference (cm) first follow-up	610	63.5	7.80
Waist circumference (cm) second follow-up	466	68.0	7.72
Triceps skinfold (mm) first follow-up	605	11.7	4.63
Triceps skinfold (mm) second follow-up	465	12.1	4.81
Waist-to-height ratio first follow-up	610	0.42	0.04
Waist-to-height ratio second follow-up	466	0.43	0.05
Subscapular skinfold (mm) second follow-up	450	8.21	3.24

	n	%
Physical activity 3-6 years	601	
Low	72	12
Normal	370	62
High	159	26
Physical activity 6–10 years	596	
Low	99	17
Normal	376	63
High	121	20
Outcome		
Atopic sensitization at second follow-up[d]	133/388	34
Allergic rhinoconjunctivitis ever by first follow-up	131/595	22
Atopic dermatitis ever by first follow-up	149/596	25
Asthma ever by first follow-up	53/590	9
Current asthma at second follow-up	37/458	8

SD standard deviation, *BMI* body mass index (kg/m^2)

[a] Due to missing values and variation in response, the number of participants varied between the different predictors and outcomes

[b] First follow-up: 10.8 years (girls), 11.8 years (boys)

[c] Second follow-up: 12.8 years

[d] 99 (25.5 %) had high grade atopic sensitization (sum of specific IgE $\geq$ 3.9 kU/l)

Impact of physical activity (Tables 2, 4)

Low physical activity at 3–6 years was positively associated with atopic sensitization at 12.8 years (Table 2). High physical activity at 6–10 years was positively associated with atopic dermatitis ever at the first follow-up (Table 2). Low physical activity at 3–6 and 6–10 years were positively associated with asthma ever at the first follow-up (Table 4). Physical activity was not associated with allergic rhinoconjunctivitis.

In the MFPR analyses, no non-straight-line associations were found for anthropometrics or physical activity with atopic sensitization or atopic diseases (data not shown).

Discussion

In this cohort study of children followed from birth to 12.8 years, after adjusting for potential confounders, BMI in childhood was positively associated with atopic sensitization and atopic dermatitis in late childhood. High and

Table 2 The adjusted odds ratios of atopic sensitization and atopic disease in adolescence in 617 Norwegian children by weight/BMI SDS and physical activity after backward stepwise selection of potential confounders (one model for each predictor variable)

Predictor	Outcome variable (final analyses)											
	Atopic sensitization[a,b]				Allergic rhinoconjunctivitis[a]				Atopic dermatitis[c]			
Age	n	OR	95 % CI	LR-p	n	OR	95 % CI	LR-p	n	OR	95 % CI	LR-p
Weight SDS												
Birth	380	1.05	(0.87, 1.26)	0.609	580	0.92	(0.77, 1.10)	0.338	544	1.04	(0.88, 1.22)	0.638
BMI SDS												
3 months	353	1.13	(0.90, 1.41)	0.315	521	0.91	(0.73, 1.14)	0.427	487	1.04	(0.84, 1.30)	0.694
6 months	363	1.15	(0.93, 1.42)	0.205	537	0.91	(0.74, 1.12)	0.390	503	1.05	(0.86, 1.28)	0.654
1 year	363	*1.22*	*(1.00, 1.49)*	*0.050*	537	0.97	(0.80, 1.18)	0.795	503	1.06	(0.87, 1.28)	0.557
4 years[d]	320	1.01	(0.80, 1.27)	0.934	456	0.86	(0.69, 1.08)	0.191	427	*1.32*	*(1.06, 1.65)*	*0.012*
First follow-up[e]	358	0.95	(0.79, 1.15)	0.612	562	0.87	(0.73, 1.04)	0.126	527	1.11	(0.93, 1.33)	0.225
Second follow-up[e]	354	0.96	(0.79, 1.17)	0.680				N.A.				N.A.
Physical activity												
At 3–6 years[f]	320			*0.039*	456			0.157	427			0.519
Normal	192	1.00	Reference		277	1.00	Reference		259	1.00	Reference	
Low	40	*2.36*	*(1.15, 4.81)*		57	1.60	(0.83, 3.09)		57	1.30	(0.65, 2.61)	
High	88	0.90	(0.50, 1.61)		122	0.77	(0.44, 1.35)		111	1.34	(0.78, 2.30)	
At 6–10 years[g]	358			0.773	562			0.126	527			*0.033*
Normal	234	1.00	Reference		353	1.00	Reference		333	1.00	Reference	
Low	57	1.05	(0.57, 1.96)		93	1.67	(0.97, 2.87)		89	1.49	(0.87, 2.56)	
High	67	0.82	(0.45, 1.49)		116	1.15	(0.68, 1.93)		105	*1.94*	*(1.16, 3.24)*	

First follow-up: 10.8 years (girls) and 11.8 years (boys); Second follow-up: 12.8 years (both sexes)

Italics numbers indicate statistically significant results

n number of participants, *OR* odds ratio, *CI* confidence interval, *LR-p* (likelihood ratio-test p-value) refers to predictor only, *BMI* body mass index (kg/m^2), *SDS* standard deviation score, *N.A.* not applicable

[a] Adjusted for sex, preeclampsia and gestational age

[b] n = 388. Ordinal response: none, low grade, high grade (sum of specific IgE $\geq$ 3.9 kU/l; above the lower quartile of all children being sensitized)

[c] Adjusted for sex, mother's asthma and mother's smoking

[d] Also adjusted for physical activity at 3–6 years

[e] Also adjusted for physical activity at 6–10 years

[f] Also adjusted for BMI SDS at 4 years

[g] Also adjusted for BMI SDS at the first follow-up

low physical activity during childhood was differentially associated with atopic sensitization, atopic dermatitis and asthma assessed in late childhood. BMI and physical activity were not associated with allergic rhinoconjunctivitis.

Anthropometrics and outcomes

In this cohort BMI at 1 year was positively associated with atopic sensitization at 12.8 years with borderline significance. As recently reviewed by Boulet [5], some studies are consistent with and others conflict our results, which may be due to differences in the study design. Studies showing an association have been cross-sectional and therefore unable to assess whether obesity precedes sensitization [5]. In our study, the majority of children were sensitized to airborne allergens. Sensitization to airborne allergens is uncommon in Scandinavian children before the age of 1 year [22]. It is therefore probable that the high BMI at 1 year preceded airborne sensitization. However, sensitization to food allergens may have been present in the first year of life, which we did not assess. In mice, obesity lowered the threshold for atopic sensitization, suggesting that obesity causes atopy [23].

Several mechanisms explaining the association between obesity and atopic sensitization have been suggested [5]. In addition to hormonal and genetic factors, a high BMI is associated with higher body fat and altered adipokines, and in turn might predispose to atopic sensitization through inflammatory changes [24]. Our results could indicate that a high BMI at the age of 1 year is of importance.

Table 3 The adjusted odds ratios of atopic sensitization and atopic disease in adolescence in 617 Norwegian children by changes in weight/BMI SDS after backward stepwise selection of potential confounders (one model for each predictor variable)

Predictor	Outcome variable (final analyses)											
	Atopic sensitization[a,b]				Allergic rhinoconjunctivitis[a]				Atopic dermatitis[c]			
Age	n	OR	95 % CI	LR-p	n	OR	95 % CI	LR-p	n	OR	95 % CI	LR-p
Weight SDS												
Birth to 3 months	361	1.10	(0.87, 1.38)	0.408	534	0.90	(0.74, 1.09)	0.292	500	0.98	(0.80, 1.17)	0.835
BMI SDS												
3–6 months	351	1.15	(0.83, 1.60)	0.413	519	0.96	(0.71, 1.30)	0.794	485	1.15	(0.85, 1.56)	0.363
6 months to 1 year	360	1.30	(0.95, 1.76)	0.100	534	1.11	(0.83, 1.48)	0.470	500	1.07	(0.81, 1.42)	0.638
1–4 years	325	0.82	(0.62, 1.09)	0.173	456	0.82	(0.63, 1.07)	0.150	427	*1.46*	*(1.11, 1.92)*	*0.005*
4 years to first follow-up[d]	315	0.99	(0.78, 1.26)	0.940	450	1.01	(0.80, 1.28)	0.917	422	0.87	(0.70, 1.09)	0.223
First to second follow-up[e]	349	0.96	(0.65, 1.43)	0.843	N.A.	N.A.	N.A.	N.A.	N.A.	N.A.	N.A.	N.A

First follow-up: 10.8 years (girls) and 11.8 years (boys); Second follow-up: 12.8 years (both sexes)

Italics numbers indicate statistically significant results

n number of participants, *OR* odds ratio, *CI* confidence interval, *LR-p* likelihood ratio-test p-value refers to predictor only, *BMI* body mass index (kg/m^2), *SDS* standard deviation score, *N.A.* not applicable

[a] Adjusted for sex, weight/BMI SDS at start of interval, gestational age, preeclampsia (none/mild or moderate/severe)

[b] n = 388. Ordinal response: none, low grade, high grade (sum of specific IgE $\geq$ 3.9 kU/l; above the lower quartile of all children being sensitized)

[c] Adjusted for sex, weight/BMI SDS at start of interval, mother's asthma and mother's smoking

[d] Also adjusted for physical activity at 3–6 years

[e] Also adjusted for physical activity at 6–10 years

In this cohort, change in BMI SDS from 1 to 4 years and BMI at 4 years were positively associated with atopic dermatitis ever at first follow-up. In the ISAAC 3 study, overweight and obesity at 13–14 years was associated with current atopic dermatitis [10]. In a meta-analysis, mainly of cross-sectional studies, a high BMI in childhood, adolescence and adulthood was also associated with atopic dermatitis [25].

Atopic dermatitis usually has its debut in the first years of life and normally precedes any potential overweight or obesity [7]. Therefore, there may be reverse causality, but it may also be possible that overweight/obesity causes atopic dermatitis. Firstly, obesity is associated with an increased risk of dry skin, aggravating underlying skin defects [26]. Secondly, the positive association of a change in BMI SDS and overweight in preschool years with atopic dermatitis could be explained by immunological changes due to increased body fat, and an association between adipokines and atopic dermatitis has been reported [27].

Anthropometric measures were not associated with allergic rhinoconjunctivitis in accordance with previous studies [28].

In the present study, there was no association between anthropometric measures during childhood and asthma in late childhood, without variation by sex. In 2013, six studies were included in a meta-analysis showing that overweight and obesity in childhood is associated with subsequent asthma. However, the results were inconsistent regarding sex [4]. Recently, in a study including >24,000 children, accelerated weight gain from birth to 3 years was positively associated with asthma by 3 years with risk ratio of 1.22 and at 7 years with risk ratio of 1.13 [9]. Our results do not contradict this, as we may have too few participants to show a significant association of a similar low magnitude.

Physical activity and outcomes

In this cohort, low preschool activity level was positively associated with atopic sensitization at 12.8 years. To our knowledge, this is the first study to show such an association. In a cross-sectional study of 2000 Spanish adolescents using questionnaires, there was no association between physical activity and allergy at 13–17 years [29].

In our study we adjusted for BMI, but BMI underestimates the relative amount of fat tissue in the body composition of children [30]. Thus, the association between low activity and atopic sensitization might be due to a higher body fat percentage in children with a low activity level, independent of weight status, with subsequent changes in adipokines that may influence the development of sensitization [24].

In this cohort, a high level of physical activity at 6–10 years was associated with atopic dermatitis ever at

Table 4 The adjusted odds ratios of asthma in adolescence in 617 Norwegian children by weight/BMI SDS and physical activity after backward stepwise selection of potential confounders (one model for each predictor variable)

Predictor	Outcome variable (final analyses)							
	Asthma ever by first follow-up[a]				Current asthma at second follow-up[b]			
Age	n	OR	95 % CI	LR-p	n	OR	95 % CI	LR-p
Weight SDS								
Birth	580	0.93	(0.72, 1.20)	0.587	439	0.95	(0.71, 1.27)	0.716
BMI SDS								
3 months	520	0.88	(0.64, 1.21)	0.437	411	0.96	(0.67, 1.38)	0.835
6 months	536	1.06	(0.79, 1.41)	0.707	425	0.86	(0.61, 1.20)	0.370
1 year	536	1.00	(0.76, 1.32)	0.998	424	0.78	(0.57, 1.08)	0.127
4 years[c]	454	1.09	(0.80, 1.47)	0.596	361	0.91	(0.63, 1.32)	0.627
First follow-up[d]	558	1.02	(0.79, 1.33)	0.849	426	1.10	(0.81, 1.49)	0.561
Second follow-up[d]	N.A.	N.A.	N.A.	N.A.	421	1.25	(0.90, 1.72)	0.176
Physical activity								
At 3–6 years[e]	454			*0.014*	361			0.475
Normal	275	1.00	Reference		220	1.00	Reference	
Low	57	*3.61*	*(1.56, 8.36)*		48	1.92	(0.66, 5.59)	
High	122	1.34	(0.61, 2.97)		93	1.40	(0.55, 3.55)	
At 6–10 years[f]	558			*0.038*	426			0.177
Normal	351	1.00	Reference		274	1.00	Reference	
Low	92	*2.52*	*(1.24, 5.12)*		69	1.98	(0.80, 4.85)	
High	115	1.02	(0.46, 2.28)		83	1.97	(0.83, 4.67)	

First follow-up: 10.8 years (girls) and 11.8 years (boys); Second follow-up: 12.8 years (both sexes)

Italics numbers indicate statistically significant results

n number of participants, *OR* Odds ratio, *CI* confidence interval, *LR-p* likelihood ratio-test p-value refers to predictor only, *BMI* body mass index (kg/m^2), *SDS* standard deviation score, *N.A.* not applicable

[a] After stepwise backward selection, adjusted for sex, gestational age, mother's preeclampsia and asthma

[b] After stepwise backward selection, adjusted for sex, mother's preeclampsia and mother's asthma

[c] Also adjusted for physical activity at 3–6 years

[d] Also adjusted for physical activity at 6–10 years

[e] Also adjusted for BMI SDS at 4 years

[f] Also adjusted for BMISDS at the first follow-up

first follow-up. This is in accordance with the findings in ISAAC 3, where vigorous physical activity in children 13–14 years was associated with current atopic dermatitis, and was attributed to sweat-induced itch [10]. One possible explanation for an association is that after long-term physical activity, natural killer cell cytotoxicity could be increased, which in turn has been associated with atopic dermatitis [31, 32].

We report an association of low physical activity at both 3–6 and 6–10 years with asthma ever, but not current asthma, in late childhood. In the ISAAC 3 study, several hours of TV viewing was associated with symptoms of current asthma in adolescents [10]. Similarly, studies indicate that physical activity could be protective against the development of asthma [11]. We found no association between physical activity and allergic rhinoconjunctivitis. In ISAAC 3, both associations of vigorous physical activity and a sedentary lifestyle at 13 years with allergic rhinoconjunctivitis were found with odds ratios at 1.25 and 1.17, respectively [10]. With the low number of participants in our study, our results do not contradict these results.

Strengths and limitations

Strengths: The study population is homogeneous regarding socio-economic status and ethnicity. Further, the predictor variables have been sampled by repeated measurements from several ages to examine the window of time in childhood the predictors could possibly affect the development of atopic sensitization and atopic diseases.

However, the study also has some limitations. The present study was not primarily designed to answer the current research questions, but this has been accounted for by including the design variable preeclampsia as a potential confounder, and no confounding was present. BMI may have limited correlation with childhood adiposity [3], and we did not have other adiposity measurements available from the visits at the well-baby clinics. Children who participated in the first follow-up but not in the second follow-up had a higher BMI and more atopic dermatitis. This may have biased our results, as both overweight and atopic dermatitis may be associated with atopic sensitization and other atopic disease. Only the predictors and not the outcomes were measured longitudinally, thus we cannot know if the associations reveal causality, or the direction of the causality. Lastly, due to several statistical analyses, the statistically significant results must be interpreted with care.

Conclusions

The results of this study suggest that BMI and physical activity in early childhood are associated with atopic sensitization, atopic dermatitis and asthma in later childhood. Larger cohorts with repeated measurements of both predictors and outcomes are needed to further elucidate this issue.

Additional files

Additional file 1: Figure S1. Directed Acyclic Graph. Colours of rings: Green = predictor; blue with black dot = outcome; blue = ancestor of outcome; red = potential confounder; black = adjustment set; grey = unavailable/unknown confounders. Red line = biasing path; green line = causal path; black line = closed path. The figure was made by using DAGitty software.

Additional file 2: Table S1. The adjusted odds ratios of asthma in adolescence in 617 Norwegian children by changes in weight/BMI SDS after backward stepwise selection of potential confounders (one model for each predictor variable). **Table S2.** The adjusted odds ratios of atopy in adolescence in 617 Norwegian children according to weight-related anthropometry in adolescence after backward stepwise selection of potential confounders (one model for each predictor variable).

Abbreviations

BMI: body mass index (kg/m^2); IBM SPSS: International Business Machines Corporation Statistical Package for the Social Sciences; IgE: immunoglobulin E; ISAAC: International Study of Asthma and Allergies in Childhood; kU/l: kilo units per litre; MFPR: multiple fractional polynomial regression; SDS: standard deviation score.

Authors' contributions

MRF and KØ participated in the design of the study. KKB finalised the data collection and registration, performed all the statistical analyses and wrote a draft of the manuscript. GEE supervised the statistical analyses. PBJ supervised the planning and the drafting of the manuscript and contributed to the analyses of the data. KØ supervised all parts of the study and writing. All authors read and approved the final manuscript.

Author details

[1] Department of Pediatrics, Stavanger University Hospital, POB 8100, 4068 Stavanger, Norway. [2] Centre for Clinical Research, Haukeland University Hospital, Bergen, Norway. [3] Department of Global Public Health and Primary Care, University of Bergen, Bergen, Norway. [4] Department of Nutritional Sciences, School of Human Ecology, University of Texas at Austin, Austin, TX, USA.
[5] Department of Pediatrics, Haukeland University Hospital, Bergen, Norway.
[6] Department of Clinical Science, University of Bergen, Bergen, Norway.

Acknowledgements

This is a branch of the Stavanger Study at Stavanger University Hospital. We appreciate the important role of Bjørn Øglænd in the planning of the study and collection of data, and the help of paediatric nurses in the outpatient clinic at the department of paediatrics in collecting data. We would also like to thank participating mothers and children.

Competing interests

The authors declare that they have no competing interests.

Funding

"The Stavanger Study" was funded by an internal grant from the National Cancer Institute, NIH and is a part of the MD Anderson Global Programme. The present study was funded by a grant from the Western Norway Health Authority.

References

1. Ng M, Fleming T, Robinson M, Thomson B, Graetz N, Margono C, Mullany EC, Biryukov S, Abbafati C, Abera SF, et al. Global, regional, and national prevalence of overweight and obesity in children and adults during 1980–2013: a systematic analysis for the Global Burden of Disease Study 2013. Lancet. 2014;384(9945):766–81.
2. Schernhammer ES, Vutuc C, Waldhor T, Haidinger G. Time trends of the prevalence of asthma and allergic disease in Austrian children. Pediatr Allergy Immunol. 2008;19(2):125–31.
3. Guibas GV, Manios Y, Xepapadaki P, Moschonis G, Douladiris N, Mavrogianni C, Papadopoulos NG. The obesity-asthma link in different ages and the role of body mass index in its investigation: findings from the Genesis and Healthy Growth Studies. Allergy. 2013;68(10):1298–305.
4. Egan KB, Ettinger AS, Bracken MB. Childhood body mass index and subsequent physician-diagnosed asthma: a systematic review and meta-analysis of prospective cohort studies. BMC Pediatr. 2013;13:121.
5. Boulet LP. Obesity and atopy. Clin Exp Allergy. 2015;45(1):75–86.
6. Glavin K, Roelants M, Strand BH, Juliusson PB, Lie KK, Helseth S, Hovengen R. Important periods of weight development in childhood: a population-based longitudinal study. BMC Public Health. 2014;14(1):160.
7. Eller E, Kjaer HF, Host A, Andersen KE, Bindslev-Jensen C. Development of atopic dermatitis in the DARC birth cohort. Pediatr Allergy Immunol. 2010;21(2 Pt 1):307–14.
8. Anderson EL, Fraser A, Martin RM, Kramer MS, Oken E, Patel R, Tilling K, Study P. Associations of postnatal growth with asthma and atopy: the PROBIT Study. Pediatr Allergy Immunol. 2013;24(2):122–30.
9. Magnus MC, Stigum H, Haberg SE, Nafstad P, London SJ, Nystad W. Peak weight and height velocity to age 36 months and asthma development: the Norwegian Mother and Child Cohort Study. PLoS One. 2015;10(1):e0116362.
10. Mitchell EA, Beasley R, Bjorksten B, Crane J, Garcia-Marcos L, Keil U, Group IPTS. The association between BMI, vigorous physical activity and television viewing and the risk of symptoms of asthma, rhinoconjunctivitis and eczema in children and adolescents: ISAAC Phase Three. Clin Exp Allergy. 2013;43(1):73–84.
11. Eijkemans M, Mommers M, Draaisma JM, Thijs C, Prins MH. Physical activity and asthma: a systematic review and meta-analysis. PLoS One. 2012;7(12):e50775.

12. Ogland B, Vatten LJ, Romundstad PR, Nilsen ST, Forman MR. Pubertal anthropometry in sons and daughters of women with preeclamptic or normotensive pregnancies. Arch Dis Child. 2009;94(11):855–9.
13. Byberg KK, Ogland B, Eide GE, Oymar K. Birth after preeclamptic pregnancies: association with allergic sensitization and allergic rhinoconjunctivitis in late childhood; a historically matched cohort study. BMC Pediatr. 2014;14(1):101.
14. Worldwide variation in prevalence of symptoms of asthma, allergic rhinoconjunctivitis, and atopic eczema: ISAAC. The International Study of Asthma and Allergies in Childhood (ISAAC) Steering Committee. Lancet 1998;351(9111):1225–32.
15. Taylor-Piliae RE, Fair JM, Haskell WL, Varady AN, Iribarren C, Hlatky MA, Go AS, Fortmann SP. Validation of the Stanford Brief Activity Survey: examining psychological factors and physical activity levels in older adults. J Phys Act Health. 2010;7(1):87–94.
16. Alsnes IV, Janszky I, Forman MR, Vatten LJ, Okland I. A population-based study of associations between preeclampsia and later cardiovascular risk factors. Am J Obstet Gynecol. 2014;211(6):657.e1–7.
17. Textor J, Hardt J, Knuppel S. DAGitty: a graphical tool for analyzing causal diagrams. Epidemiology. 2011;22(5):745.
18. Niklasson A, Albertsson-Wikland K. Continuous growth reference from 24th week of gestation to 24 months by gender. BMC Pediatr. 2008;8:8.
19. Juliusson PB, Roelants M, Nordal E, Furevik L, Eide GE, Moster D, Hauspie R, Bjerknes R. Growth references for 0–19 year-old Norwegian children for length/height, weight, body mass index and head circumference. Ann Hum Biol. 2013;40(3):220–7.
20. Brannsether B, Roelants M, Bjerknes R, Juliusson PB. Waist circumference and waist-to-height ratio in Norwegian children 4–18 years of age: reference values and cut-off levels. Acta Paediatr. 2011;100(12):1576–82.
21. Brannsether B, Roelants M, Bjerknes R, Juliusson PB. References and cutoffs for triceps and subscapular skinfolds in Norwegian children 4–16 years of age. Eur J Clin Nutr. 2013;67(9):928–33.
22. Nissen SP, Kjaer HF, Host A, Nielsen J, Halken S. The natural course of sensitization and allergic diseases from childhood to adulthood. Pediatr Allergy Immunol. 2013;24(6):549–55.
23. Dietze J, Bocking C, Heverhagen JT, Voelker MN, Renz H. Obesity lowers the threshold of allergic sensitization and augments airway eosinophilia in a mouse model of asthma. Allergy. 2012;67(12):1519–29.
24. Nagel G, Koenig W, Rapp K, Wabitsch M, Zoellner I, Weiland SK. Associations of adipokines with asthma, rhinoconjunctivitis, and eczema in German schoolchildren. Pediatr Allergy Immunol. 2009;20(1):81–8.
25. Zhang A, Silverberg JI. Association of atopic dermatitis with being overweight and obese: a systematic review and metaanalysis. J Am Acad Dermatol. 2015;72(4):606–16.e4.
26. Nino M, Franzese A, Ruggiero Perrino N, Balato N. The effect of obesity on skin disease and epidermal permeability barrier status in children. Pediatr Dermatol. 2012;29(5):567–70.
27. Machura E, Szczepanska M, Ziora K, Ziora D, Swietochowska E, Barc-Czarnecka M, Kasperska-Zajac A. Evaluation of adipokines: apelin, visfatin, and resistin in children with atopic dermatitis. Mediators Inflamm. 2013;2013:760691.
28. Wang R, Custovic A, Simpson A, Belgrave DC, Lowe LA, Murray CS. Differing associations of BMI and body fat with asthma and lung function in children. Pediatr Pulmonol. 2014;49(11):1049–57.
29. Nova E, Martinez-Gomez D, Gomez-Martinez S, Veses AM, Calle ME, Veiga OL, Marcos A. Influence of health behaviours on the incidence of infection and allergy in adolescents: the AFINOS cross-sectional study. BMC Public Health. 2014;14:19.
30. Brannsether B, Eide GE, Roelants M, Bjerknes R, Juliusson PB. Interrelationships between anthropometric variables and overweight in childhood and adolescence. Am J Hum Biol. 2014;26(4):502–10.
31. Del Giacco SR, Scorcu M, Argiolas F, Firinu D, Del Giacco GS. Exercise training, lymphocyte subsets and their cytokines production: experience of an Italian professional football team and their impact on allergy. BioMed Res Int. 2014;2014:429248.
32. Luci C, Gaudy-Marqueste C, Rouzaire P, Audonnet S, Cognet C, Hennino A, Nicolas JF, Grob JJ, Tomasello E. Peripheral natural killer cells exhibit qualitative and quantitative changes in patients with psoriasis and atopic dermatitis. Br J Dermatol. 2012;166(4):789–96.

22

Development and validation of a standardized double-blind, placebo-controlled food challenge matrix for raw hazelnuts

Marjolein Vandekerckhove[1*], Bart Van Droogenbroeck[1], Marc De Loose[1], Katleen Coudijzer[1], Marc Coppens[3], Philippe Gevaert[4] and Hilde Lapeere[2*]

Abstract

Background: Double-blind, placebo-controlled food challenge (DBPCFC) is considered the gold standard for food allergy diagnosis. However, this test is rarely performed routinely in clinical practice because of various practical issues, e.g. the lack of a standardized matrix preparation. The aim of this study was to develop and validate a convenient DBPCFC matrix, that can easily be implemented in daily clinical practice. The focus of this study was the blinding of hazelnuts, whereby the hazelnuts retained as much as possible their allergenicity and could be mixed homogenously in low-doses to the matrices.

Methods: A basophil-activation test (BAT), microbial tests and an LC-MS/MS test were performed to assess respectively the allergenicity of the used hazelnuts, the microbial stability of the novel developed matrices and the homogeneity of the hazelnuts in the matrices. A sensory test was conducted to validate the blinding of the hazelnuts in the matrices. A pilot DBPCFC study included eight patients as proof of concept.

Results: The BAT-test gave the first insights concerning the retained allergenicity of the hazelnuts. The microbial safety could be assured after 12 months of storage. Sufficient masking was assessed by several sensory tests. Homogeneous hazelnut distribution could be achieved for the different hazelnut concentrations. The DBPCFC's results showed diverse allergic responders (from no reactions to distinct objective symptoms).

Conclusion: A novel stable and validated DBPCFC matrix using raw hazelnuts has been developed that allows easy preparation in a standardized way for convenient use in daily clinical practice.

Trial registration EC Project number: EC/2015/0852; Date of registration: 13 Oct 2015; End date: 01 Feb 2017

Keywords: Double-blind, Placebo-controlled food challenge, Hazelnut allergy, Diagnosis food allergy, Challenge matrix

Background

The double-blind, placebo-controlled food challenge (DBPCFC) is considered the gold standard for food allergy diagnosis. This is however not common practice in the daily clinical setting due to several limitations, such as the lack of standardized preparation of the matrices [1]. One of the limiting factors of the DBPCFC is that the clinical staff must be able to prepare the matrices by themselves, so too labor-intensive preparations (e.g. baking, etc.) are not likely to be used in the routine.

However, from the clinical perspective, this test is useful to e.g. exclude/confirm a possible food allergy when other in vivo/in vitro tests are producing contradictory or inconclusive results, evaluate if patients have outgrown their allergy and to assess the severity of their reactions. For scientific reasons, it can be used to estimate the global

*Correspondence: marjolein.vandekerckhove@ilvo.vlaanderen.be; ilvo@ilvo.vlaanderen.be; hilde.lapeere@ugent.be; Dermatologie@uzgent.be
[1] Technology and Food Science Unit, Research Institute for Agriculture, Fisheries, and Food (ILVO), Burg. Van Gansberghelaan 115, 9820 Merelbeke, Belgium
[2] Faculty of Medicine and Health Science, Department of Dermatology, Ghent University, De Pintelaan 185, 9000 Ghent, Belgium
Full list of author information is available at the end of the article

prevalence of relevant food allergies, to assess the predictive value of other diagnostic methods and to determine specific threshold levels. However, proper validation of these matrices has only been performed in limited studies [2–5]. Further, low allergen dose matrices are needed to determine e.g. the minimum eliciting doses (MED's) of the patients and to include safely severe allergic patients in this test [6]. As reported in 2014 by the Voluntary Incidental Trace Allergen Labelling 2.0 (VITAL) initiative, the MED in 1% of the hazelnut allergic population ($ED_{0.1}$) is estimated to be 0.1 mg hazelnut proteins [6]. However, limited studies have yet been conducted to develop lower dose vehicles whereby the homogeneity was determined.

For hazelnuts, as far as we know, only a low-level matrix was developed using defatted hazelnuts (starting with 3 μg hazelnut proteins) [2]. However, defatting removes oil-body associated allergens which can also provoke severe allergic symptoms [7]. The high-fat content of hazelnuts (± 61% w/w) however makes homogenization and hence masking of the non-defatted nuts difficult.

This project focused on the development and validation of a novel, easy-to-use DBPCFC matrix for raw hazelnuts at low-level, which can be used in a standardized way in daily clinical practice and by multiple centers to allow comparison of test results. This study reports to our knowledge, the first validated matrix containing low doses of raw, non-defatted hazelnuts and no other major allergenic ingredients listed in the Regulation (EU) No. 1169/2011.

Methods

Preparation of the DBPCFC matrices

We developed a powder mix that results in a cold chocolate dessert after the addition of water. The ingredients are listed in Table 1. Blanched raw hazelnuts were ground in a RETSCH ZM200 mill (RETSCH, Düsseldorf, Germany) with a 0.75 mm sieve and afterward rolled with the Exakt 3-wals 80E (Exakt Technologies, Oklahoma, US) at 350 rotations/min. The protein content was determined using Kjeldahl analysis (according to ISO8968-2, conversion factor = 5.18). The rolled hazelnuts were packaged under vacuum conditions and stored in the dark at ambient temperatures (20 °C).

The DBPCFC series were freshly prepared the day itself (± 2–4 h prior start of the challenge) (Table 2). For the verum vehicles first, a dilution series was prepared with suspended hazelnuts in lukewarm water (± 30 °C) (Table 2). Each dilution was shaken vigorously until the hazelnuts were fully suspended prior preparing the subsequent dilution. Each dilution (65 g) was added per portion of powder mix II (= 40.2 g for verum series 5–9; see Table 1) or powder mix I (= 35.0 g for verum series 1–4; see Table 1). To prepare the placebo series, 65 mg lukewarm water was added per portion of powder mix I. All the samples were shaken vigorously and set in at 4 °C for at least 10 min. Of these preparations, the respective

Table 1 Ingredients used for the DBPCFC matrix preparation

Added ingredients	Brand	Powder mix I (g/portion)	Powder mix II (g/portion)
Vanilla sugar[a]	Imperial	10.00	11.00
Brown sugar[a]	Candico	2.50	4.10
Stevia[a]	Pure Via	2.50	2.40
Cacao 100%[a]	Callebaut	8.20	10.70
Cold thickener (Quelli)[b]	Dawn	2.30	1.25
Sunflower Lecithin Sun 400 organic[c]	Lecico	0.30	0.30
Vanilla aroma[c]	Dawn	0.50	0.40
Lemon extract[d]	LorAnn Super-Strength Flavor	0.06	0.09
Cocos extract[d]	LorAnn Super-Strength Flavor	0.10	0.17
Speculaas spices[c]	J. S. Polak	0.28	0.53
Rice flakes Vanille[a]	Olvarit	2.80	2.80
Nutramigen AA[e]	Mead Johnson	5.50	6.50
Total		35.04	40.24

[a] No allergens were mentioned on the product information sheet

[b] Has precautionary labeling on the product information for gluten, eggs, lupine, milk (incl. lactose), soy

[c] Explicitly mentioned that it contains no allergens

[d] No allergens were mentioned on the product information sheet, labeled as gluten-free

[e] Is an amino acid-based formula for babies with a severe cow's milk protein allergy or with multiple food allergies, it's an extensively hydrolyzed formula by breaking down completely the present proteins in amino acids

Table 2 Preparation of the DBPCFC verum dilution series

A. Dilution series of the hazelnuts suspended in water to develop the verum series

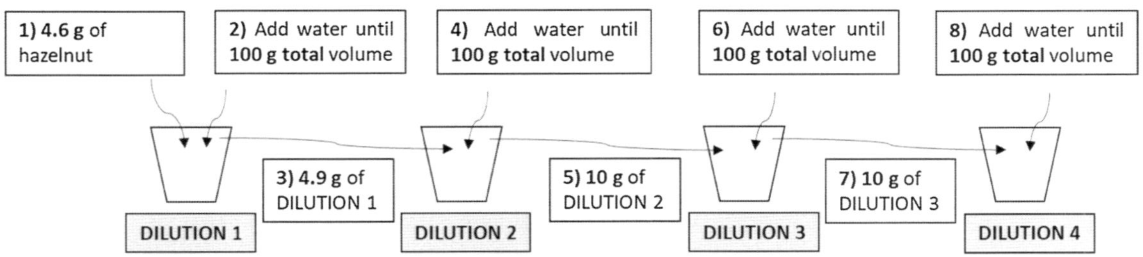

B. Dilution series of the hazelnut DBPCFC verum series

Instructions for preparation/portion				Additional information			
Portion number	Dilution number (65 g)	Powder mix I (g)	Served portion size (g)	Dilution factor of served hazelnuts	Hazelnut (mg)/portion	Hazelnut proteins (mg)/ portion	Ppm (mg/kg) hazelnuts
1	0	35.0	2.50	x	0	0	0
2	4	35.0	2.50	1/10	0.0370	0.005	14.8
3	3	35.0	2.50	1/10	0.3704	0.054	148.0
4	2	35.0	2.50	1/10	3.691	0.535	1476.9
Instructions for preparation/portion				**Additional information**			
Portion number	Dilution number (65 g)	Powder mix II (g)	Served portion size (g)	Dilution factor of served hazelnuts	Hazelnut (g)/portion	Hazelnut proteins (mg)/ portion	Ppm (mg/kg) hazelnuts
5	1	40.2	1.34	1/3	0.04	5.37	27,721.3
6	1	40.2	4.01	1/3	0.11	16.11	27,721.3
7	1	40.2	12.02	1/3	0.33	48.33	27,721.3
8	1	40.2	36.07	1/3	1.00	145.00	27,721.3
9	1	40.2	108.22	1	3.00	435.00	27,721.3

portion sizes were served as listed in Table 2. Similar portion sizes were served in the placebo series as in the verum series.

Assessment of microbial stability

To assess the microbial stability of the materials used, the a_w-values and microbial constitution of both the powder mixes and the rolled hazelnuts were determined. The water activity (a_w) was determined using the Benchtop Water Activity Meter (Pullman, WA, USA). Enumerations of *Escherichia coli* (AFNOR BRD-07/01-07/93 method), *Bacillus cereus* (ISO 7932) and detection of *Salmonella* (ISO 6579) were performed in the ISO 17025 accredited lab for food microbiology at the Belgian National Reference Lab at Research Institute for Agriculture, Fisheries and Food (ILVO, Melle, Belgium).

Assessment of hazelnut allergenicity

To gain the first insights concerning the preserved allergenicity of the blanched rolled hazelnuts, a basophil activation test (= BAT) was performed with three selected hazelnut allergic patients having the following allergic reactions: oral allergy syndrome (= OAS), a late onset of mild urticaria and a severe systemic reaction. Details of the protocol are described in the Additional file 1: BAT protocol.

Assessment of hazelnut homogeneity

LC-MS analysis was performed to confirm the absence of hazelnuts in the powder mixes and to confirm homogenous distribution of the hazelnuts in the different verum concentrations. Two prepared verum series were sampled and analyzed over two separate time periods. Details of the protocol are described in the Additional file 1: LC-MS/MS protocol.

Sensory testing

Sensory tests were performed in two main phases to evaluate the masking of the hazelnuts (panelists were all > 20 years). Panelists with food allergies were not included in this test. In phase Ia and Ib, the tests were performed in the same sensory evaluation booths, by 30 and 31 panelists respectively, who were used to perform sensory tests. A combination of verum samples containing the highest hazelnut concentrations and placebo's (3 and 2 samples per panelist in phase Ia and Ib, respectively) were given sequentially in different orders. After phase Ia, the test was repeated after minor adjustments of the matrices. Between each sample, water and crackers were given. After every tasting, they had to answer if the dessert contained hazelnuts or not, and if yes, by tasting or smelling. In phase II, the same test was performed as in phase Ib, with a consumer's panel (91 panelists). All the tests were analyzed using the Chi^2-test with 95% CI. When there was statistically no difference between the answers of the verum and placebo samples, the hazelnuts were considered sufficient blinded.

DBPCFC pilot study

To validate the usability of the matrices in practice, eight DBPCFC's were performed with patients having a mild hazelnut allergy as proof of concept. For patient details, see Additional file 1: Table S2. The study was approved by the Ethical Committee of the University Hospital (UH) Ghent, and all the patients signed an informed consent prior to the start of the test. Details of the protocol are described in the Additional file 1: DBPCFC protocol.

Results

The rolled hazelnuts (protein content: 14.5% w/w) could be added to the matrices homogenously without leaving visible particulates.

The BAT assays resulted in different half maximal effective concentration values (EC_{50}) for the different patients. For patients A, B and C the following EC50 values were recorded, respectively: 0.34 and 1.6 µg/mL and 0.32 ng/mL hazelnut proteins (see in the Additional file 1: Figure S1). Blood taken from a non-allergic donor gave no activation of the basophils.

The water activity (a_w) of the powder mix and rolled hazelnuts were respectively 0.486 and 0.477. The microbial enumerations were for *E. coli* < 10.0 CFU/g, *Salmonella* sp. 0/25 g and *Bacillus cereus* < 10.0 CFU/g for all the analyzed matrices, even after 1 year of storage at ambient temperatures (20 °C) in the dark.

In addition, no hazelnuts could be detected in the powder mixes after the sensory tests. In Phase Ia (in the sensory lab of ILVO), no significant difference existed between the placebo and verum group ($P = 0.290$). No significant differences were found in smell nor taste between the verum and placebo samples in the group of panelists who detected hazelnuts (resp. $P = 0.286$ and 0.102). In phase Ib (in the same sensory lab), 48% (whereof 40% guessed) of the panel answered correctly for the verum samples and 29% (whereof 44% guessed) thought hazelnuts were present in the placebo matrices. No significant difference was found between the placebo and verum group ($P = 0.096$). Also for smell and taste, no difference was seen (resp. $P = 0.354$ and 0.208). Of the consumer's panel, 30% (whereof 26% guessed) and 35% (whereof 30% guessed) detected hazelnut in the verum and placebo samples respectively, so no significant difference was shown ($P = 0.263$). Also for smell and taste, no difference was seen ($P = 0.581$ and 0.154). For more details regarding the results of the sensorial tests, we refer to Additional file 1: Table S1.

From the LC-MS/MS analysis, a linearity of $R^2 = 0.999$ was obtained after analyzing the different verum series in duplicate, confirming the expected hazelnut presence (see Additional file 1: Figure S2). No hazelnuts were detected in the blanc powder mixes.

The DBPCFC outcomes are summarized in Table 3. During the pilot study, patients 1, 3 and 5 experienced very mild and subjective allergic symptoms at the highest hazelnut dose. Only patients 2 and 4 had distinct objective signs when performing the test. Patient 6 had both for placebo and verum subjective complaints, with similar symptoms of OAS. Patients 8 and 9 experienced no allergic reaction during the test. When results were negative (patients 8 and 9) or questionable (patients 1, 3 and 5), open provocation tests were done which were all positive. However, these reactions were very mild (for patients 3 and 5 e.g. only a mild tingling on the lips or a raw feeling in the throat was experienced after consuming 5 raw hazelnuts).

Table 3 DBPCFC results of the eight patients

Results challenge			
Patient no.	**Dose**	**Signs and symptoms[a]**	**Test outcome**
1	Verum 3–9	Very mild tingling on the lips	+/−; Only mild OAS symptoms; open provocation test needed
	Placebo 1–9	–	–
	Open provocation: ½ hazelnut	Mild tingling on tongue and lips	+/−
2	Verum 4–5	Tingling of the lips, Pruritus Mild urticaria/angioedema of the lips (11 min after verum 4)	+; Test is stopped after dose 5 because of inconvenient allergic complaints
	Placebo 1–9	–	–
3	Verum 9	Very mild tingling on the lips	+/−; Only mild OAS symptoms; Open provocation test needed
	Placebo 1–9	–	–
	Open provocation: 5 hazelnuts	Raw feeling in the throat	+
4	Verum 2–7 Verum 8–9	Pruritus, urticaria lesion in the neck Sneezing, itchy nose	+
	Placebo 1–9	–	–
5	Verum 9	Very mild tingling of the lips	+/−; Only mild OAS symptoms; Open provocation test needed
	Placebo 1–9	–	–
	Open provocation: 5 hazelnuts	Raw feeling in the throat	+
6	Verum 1–9	Very mild tingling of the lips	Verum and placebo challenges gave both mild OAS symptoms. This could be due to the anxiety of the patient during the challenges. Open provocation test is needed
	Verum 9	Gastrointestinal: Nausea	
	Placebo 1–9	Very mild tingling of the lips	
	Placebo 9	Gastrointestinal: Nausea	
	Open provocation: ½ hazelnut	Mild tingling of throat and tongue	+/−
7	Verum 1–9	–	–
	Placebo 1–9	–	–
	Open provocation: ½ hazelnut	Mild tingling of throat and tongue	+/−
8	Verum 1–9		
	Placebo 1–9		
	Open provocation: ½ hazelnut	Urticaria: discrete blister lower lip	+/−

[a] Symptoms and signs were assessed according to the standardized clinical parameters checklist described in the work of Sampson et al. [1]. OAS symptoms/signs were reported extra

+, positive test because of distinct objective signs during the challenge; +/−, results are uncertain because of subjective symptoms during the challenge; −, no reactions were observed during the challenge

Discussion

The main purpose of this work was the development of a DBPCFC matrix for hazelnuts which had to fulfill several criteria like the sufficient masking of the hazelnuts and maintaining as much as possible the allergenicity. Further, easy logistics and preparation, long stability and sufficient palatability of the matrices are required. To include as much as possible different food allergic patients in this test, no other major allergenic food allergens listed in the Regulation (EU) No. 1169/2011 were used as ingredients during the recipe development of these matrices.

In this work, blanched hazelnuts (protein content: 14.5% w/w) were used because the dark testa is difficult to mask, both visually and in taste. For this reason, these were also used in other DBPCFC studies [4]. The nuts were kept at 100 °C for 8 min to remove this testa. Reduced allergenicity of the heat-labile hazelnut Cor a 1 and 2 allergens was only noticed at > 140 °C [8] but not much is known concerning the impact of blanching hazelnuts. Minor or no differences in allergenicity were seen in other blanched tree nuts, however [8]. For the three patients tested, basophil activation was shown, even for the least sensitive patient, presuming a retained allergenic potential of the blanched hazelnuts. However, further research should examine the significant impact of blanching on the hazelnut allergenicity.

To limit the potential impact of further processing on the hazelnut allergenicity, a cold matrix preparation was chosen. The fat content of the verum and placebo matrices were kept at < 25% of the total energy (resp. 13 and 19% of the total energy) so delayed absorption due to a high-fat content will be minimized [4]. The rolled hazelnuts could be mixed in the powder without leaving visible particulates.

The stability of the preparations was assessed by determining the a_w-values and the microbial contamination. The a_w-value can predict the growth of bacteria, yeast, and molds over time. For the hazelnuts and powder mix, these were low enough to inhibit bacterial and mold growth (resp. $a_w \geq 0.91$ and 0.8). In addition, no relevant microbial spoilage was observed by organisms typically associated with confectionery-related food products with low water activity, like hazelnuts, after 1 year of storage at room temperature (20 °C), so an easy logistics of both the powder mixes and rolled hazelnuts can be guaranteed [9–11].

Instead of the most frequently applied triangle test [12], which focuses on differences between matrices whatever the attribution of difference is, the sensory test performed in this study was specifically adapted for its purpose [4], which was comparable with earlier performed sensory tests for DBPCFC matrix validation [3–5], whereby one placebo and verum sample were offered. In this test, the samples were offered sequentially instead of simultaneously, as done in the study of González-Mancebo et al. [5]. When small differences are not linked to the presence of the allergenic ingredient, the samples can be offered sequentially [5]. This represents how a DBPCFC is carried out in clinical practice, whereby the matrices will be given on separate days. We can conclude that considering the followed procedure and the results obtained, the hazelnuts were successfully blinded in our developed matrices. Consequently, the newly developed DBPCFC matrices will minimize the psychological placebo-effects for the patients and the healthcare professionals.

As a proof of concept, DBPCFC's with eight patients were conducted in the clinical setting. The dosage schedule was a combination of semi-logarithmic and logarithmic increases, as performed in an earlier DBPCFC study in 2012 for hazelnuts [2], whereby similar protein portions were administered. This schedule was performed to achieve the top dose with acceptable increments in an acceptable period when starting with low-level protein portions.

The most sensitive patient had already subjective symptoms after the first dose and developed objective signs after the second hazelnut dose (corresponding to 5 and 54 μg of hazelnut proteins, respectively). These findings were comparable with those found earlier whereby 30 μg of hazelnut proteins was the lowest eliciting dose [2]. However, other factors, which were not included in this study, like exercise, alcohol consumption, asthma and anxiety might exacerbate the allergic reactions, so follow-up studies are necessary [13]. Further, the challenges were performed during September–November, and pollen-related food allergies can be worse during and just after pollen season (for birch pollen: ± middle of March until the middle of May) [14]. Different explanations could reason the absence of allergic symptoms for the two negative responders, like possible matrix/processing effects, too low doses of hazelnuts and the removing of the testa. Open provocation tests are therefore of utmost importance at the end of the test. However, psychological effects cannot be excluded then. Since patients with anaphylaxis and children were excluded from this DBPCFC study, further research should be conducted including younger and more severe allergic patients. During the challenges of this work, the patients nor health care professionals could discover the verum series. Most of the patients found the deserts easy to consume.

Conclusion

To conclude, this study reports the production and validation of a novel DBPCFC matrix for raw hazelnuts at low doses, in a format that allows easy logistics and implementation in the common clinical setting.

Abbreviations

DBPCFC: double-blind, placebo-controlled food challenge; MED: minimal eliciting dose; VITAL: voluntary incidental trace allergen labelling; BAT: basophil activation test; LC-MS: liquid-chromatography mass-spectrometry.

Authors' contributions

MV led the project in total. BVD, MDL, KC, and PG made substantial contributions to the conception, design, guidance and follow-up on the research. BVD was also involved in revising the manuscript critically for important intellectual content. MC and HL made substantial attributions for the acquisition, analysis, and interpretation of the data. All authors gave final approval of the version to be published.

Author details

[1] Technology and Food Science Unit, Research Institute for Agriculture, Fisheries, and Food (ILVO), Burg. Van Gansberghelaan 115, 9820 Merelbeke, Belgium. [2] Faculty of Medicine and Health Science, Department of Dermatology, Ghent University, De Pintelaan 185, 9000 Ghent, Belgium. [3] Faculty of Medicine and Health Science, Department of Anesthesiology and Perioperative Medicine, Ghent University, De Pintelaan 185, 9000 Ghent, Belgium. [4] Faculty of Medicine and Health Science, Department of Otorhinolaryngology, Ghent University, De Pintelaan 185, 9000 Ghent, Belgium.

Acknowledgements

The authors wish to express their gratitude to Sarah Blondeel, Raquel Sanz García, Stephanie Duquin and to the lab staff for aiding to execute the experiments. Additionally, we would like to thank ILVO for providing funding to this research.

Competing interests

The authors declare that they have no competing interests.

Funding

We would like to thank ILVO for providing funding to this research.

References

1. Sampson HA, Gerth van Wijk R, Bindslev-Jensen C, Sicherer S, Teuber SS, Burks AW, et al. Standardizing double-blind, placebo-controlled oral food challenges: American Academy of Allergy, Asthma & Immunology–European Academy of Allergy and Clinical Immunology PRACTALL consensus report. J Allergy Clin Immunol. 2012;130:1260–74.
2. Cochrane SA, Salt LJ, Wantling E, Rogers A, Coutts J, Ballmer-Weber BK, et al. Development of a standardized low-dose double-blind placebo-controlled challenge vehicle for the EuroPrevall project. Allergy. 2012;67:107–13.
3. Ronteltap A, van Schaik J, Wensing M, Rynja FJ, Knulst AC, de Vries JH. Sensory testing of recipes masking peanut or hazelnut for double-blind placebo-controlled food challenges. Allergy. 2004;59:457–60.
4. Vlieg-Boerstra BJ, Herpertz I, Pasker L, van der Heide S, Kukler J, Jansink C. Validation of novel recipes for double-blind, placebo-controlled food challenges in children and adults. Allergy. 2011;66:948–54.
5. González-Mancebo E, Díaz Alonso, de Durana MD, García Estringana Y, Meléndez Baltanás A, Rodriguez-Alvarez M, de la Hoz Caballer B, et al. Validation of recipes for double-blind placebo-controlled challenges with milk, egg white, and hazelnut. J Investig Allergol Clin Immunol. 2017;27:40–5.
6. Taylor SL, Baumert JL, Kruizinga AG, Remingtona BC, Crevelc RWR, Brooke-Taylord S, et al. Establishment of reference doses for residues of allergenic foods: report of the VITAL expert panel. Food Chem Toxicol. 2014;63:9–17.
7. Zuidmeer-Jongejan L, Fernández-Rivas M, Winter MG, Akkerdaas JH, Summers C, Lebens A, et al. Oil body-associated hazelnut allergens including oleosins are underrepresented in diagnostic extracts but associated with severe symptoms. Clin Transl Allergy. 2014;4:4.
8. Verhoeckx KCM, Vissers YM, Baumert JL, Faludi R, Feys M, Flanagan S, et al. Food processing and allergenicity. Food Chem Toxicol. 2015;80:223–40.
9. Izurieta WP, Komitopoulou E. Effect of moisture on salmonella spp. heat resistance in cocoa and hazelnut shells. Food Res Int. 2012;45:1087–92.
10. Little CL, Jemmott W, Surman-Lee S, Hucklesby L, de Pinna E. Assessment of the microbiological safety of edible roasted nut kernels on retail sale in England, with a focus on Salmonella. J Food Prot. 2009;72:853–5.
11. Beuchat LR, Komitopoulou E, Beckers I I, Betts RP, Bourdichon F, Fanning S, et al. Low-water activity foods: increased concern as vehicles of foodborne pathogens. J Food Prot. 2013;76:150–72.
12. ISO 4120:2004. International Organization for Standardization, Geneva, Switzerland; 2004. https://www.iso.org/standard/33495.html. Accessed 27 July 2017.
13. Hourihane JO, Grimshaw KE, Lewis SA, Briggs RA, Trewin JB, King RM, et al. Does severity of low-dose, double-blind, placebo-controlled food challenges reflect severity of allergic reactions to peanut in the community? Clin Exp Allergy. 2005;35:1227–33.
14. Hansen KS, Vieths S, Vestergaard H, Skov PS, Bindslev-Jensen C, Poulsen JH, et al. Seasonal variation in food allergy to apple. J Chromatogr B Biomed Sci Appl. 2001;756:19–32.

Health Related Quality of Life among schoolchildren aged 12–13 years in relation to food hypersensitivity phenotypes

Åsa Strinnholm[1,4*], Linnéa Hedman[1,2], Anna Winberg[3], Sven-Arne Jansson[1], Viveca Lindh[4] and Eva Rönmark[1]

Abstract

Background: While Health Related Quality of Life has been investigated among children with IgE-mediated food allergy, less is known about quality of life among children with other types of hypersensitivity to food. The aim of this study was to investigate Health Related Quality of Life (HRQL) in children with and without food hypersensitivity. Further, we compared HRQL between children with different phenotypes of food hypersensitivity.

Methods: In a large population-based cohort of schoolchildren in Northern Sweden, the parents of 2612 (96% of invited) completed a questionnaire. All 125 (5%) children who reported complete elimination of milk, egg, fish or wheat due to food hypersensitivity were invited to a clinical examination and 94 children participated. Of these, 75 children also completed a generic (KIDSCREEN-52) and a disease-specific HRQL questionnaire (FAQLQ-TF). Thereafter, these children were categorised into the different phenotypes: current food allergy, outgrown food allergy, and lactose intolerance. Additionally, 209 children with unrestricted diets answered the generic questionnaire.

Results: The median score of all KIDSCREEN-52 domains were above the population norm of 50 both in children with and without food hypersensitivity. No significant differences in distribution in generic or disease-specific HRQL were found between children with or without food hypersensitivity. There were no significant differences in HRQL between children with different phenotypes of food hypersensitivity. However, children with current food allergy tended to have the lowest HRQL. Further, poor HRQL defined as ≥75th percentile for the disease specific score was significantly more common in the current food allergy phenotype in the domain Emotional impact and the total FAQLQ, compared to the other phenotypes.

Conclusions: In this population-based study, 12–13 year old children reported good HRQL regardless of having food hypersensitivity or not. However, the children with the current phenotype reported lower HRQL than the other phenotypes.

Keywords: Adolescents, Food hypersensitivity, Health Related Quality of Life, Phenotypes of food hypersensitivity, Population-based cohort study

Background

Reported food hypersensitivity (FHS) is common in the Western countries. However, there are large differences in prevalence between studies. In a meta-analysis investigating FHS in 51 studies, the prevalence of self-reported FHS varied from 3 to 35% due to differences in study methods, age of study populations and geographic settings [1]. The high and increasing prevalence of reported FHS [2, 3] may partly be attributed to an increasing awareness about FHS in the population, as well as public interest of different diets [4]. The term FHS includes food reactions of both

*Correspondence: asa.strinnholm@umu.se
[1] Department of Public Health and Clinical Medicine, Occupational and Environmental Medicine, OLIN Unit, Umeå University, 901 87 Umeå, Sweden
Full list of author information is available at the end of the article

immunological and non-immunological origins, and food allergy is a subgroup of FHS [5].

Elimination of foods due to FHS may negatively affect the Health Related Quality of Life (HRQL) [6]. HRQL can be defined as self-perceived health [7] since it is possible to have a chronic disease but still experience a good self-perceived HRQL. Since HRQL is individual and varies with age [6], it is suggested that when applicable, the questionnaires should be completed by the individuals themselves [8]. Usually, children are able to complete their HRQL questionnaire from the age of eight years, given that the questionnaires are age appropriate and that the child have reading skills [9]. Generic HRQL questionnaires are used for comparisons between different diseases, or between subjects with or without a disease [10]. Disease-specific questionnaires investigate HRQL related to a specific disease, e.g. food allergy [11].

The interest in HRQL in children and adolescents with food allergy has increased during the last decades, and a number of disease-specific HRQL questionnaires are now available for children [11, 12], adolescents [13, 14], and parents to children [15–18] with IgE mediated food allergy. However, there is a limited number of HRQL questionnaires available for the wider definition FHS [19, 20]. To our knowledge, no studies have explored HRQL among children with different phenotypes of FHS.

In a population-based cohort of schoolchildren, the paediatric cohort II within the Obstructive Lung Disease in Northern Sweden studies (OLIN), 5% of the children reported complete elimination of cow's milk, hen's egg, fish or wheat due to FHS at age 11–12 years [21]. The aim of the current study was to compare HRQL among children with and without complete elimination of cow's milk, hen's egg, fish or wheat due to FHS, and to study HRQL in relation to different FHS phenotypes. Since milk, egg, fish and wheat are staple foods in Western diet, we hypothesised that avoidance of these foods would have a negative impact on HRQL.

Methods

Study population

In 2006, all children in first and second grade (aged 7–8 years) in three municipalities in Northern Sweden were invited to a longitudinal study about asthma, rhinitis, eczema and FHS [22–24]. The current study was based on a study follow-up in 2010 when the parents of 2612 (96% of invited) children, now in ages 11–12 years, participated in a questionnaire survey [3]. Children in two of the municipalities were also invited to skin prick testing (SPT) with ten common airborne allergens, and 1657 (86% of invited) participated. The SPT were performed by a small group of well-trained research nurses.

Parental questionnaire

The questionnaire included the International Study of Asthma and Allergies in Childhood questions [25] with added questions about symptoms and diagnosis of atopic diseases including FHS [3, 22]. The queries about FHS included; symptoms of FHS in relation to different foods, if elimination of the culprit food was partial or complete, and whether the child had a physician-diagnosis of celiac disease.

Clinical examination

Five percent (n = 125) of the children reported complete elimination of cow's milk, hen's egg, fish and/or wheat due to FHS [21]. During October and November 2010, these children were invited to a clinical examination including a structured interview, specific IgE to the culprit food and a celiac screen test (tissue transglutaminase IgA antibodies) and 94 children (75% of invited) participated [21]. The clinical examinations were performed by the same paediatric allergist (AW). At the time of the clinical examinations, 94 children, 75 (80% of participants) also answered a generic HRQL questionnaire and 74 children answered a disease-specific questionnaire. In addition, a random sample of 320 children without food hypersensitivity was invited to complete the generic HRQL questionnaire during the same period. The questionnaire was sent by mail to the children with unrestricted diet, and 209 (65% of invited) participated. The children were instructed to answer the questionnaire without interference of their parents. The study design and participation are presented in Fig. 1.

Phenotypes of FHS

According to the results of the clinical examination, all children were subsequently categorised into the different FHS phenotypes. Among the 75 children who also answered the HRQL questionnaire the number of children in each phenotypes were: food allergy (n = 23), outgrown food allergy (n = 16) and lactose intolerance (n = 33). Three children could not be categorised to any of the FHS groups: one child was diagnosed as having celiac disease and two children declined participation in blood sampling. The categorisation was performed by the same paediatric allergist (AW) that performed the clinical examinations. The criteria used for the categorisation are presented in a previous study [21].

The generic HRQL questionnaire

HRQL was measured using the Health-related Quality of Life Screening Instrument, KIDSCREEN-52, a generic self-report instrument for children and adolescents aged 8–18 years [10, 26]. The questionnaire

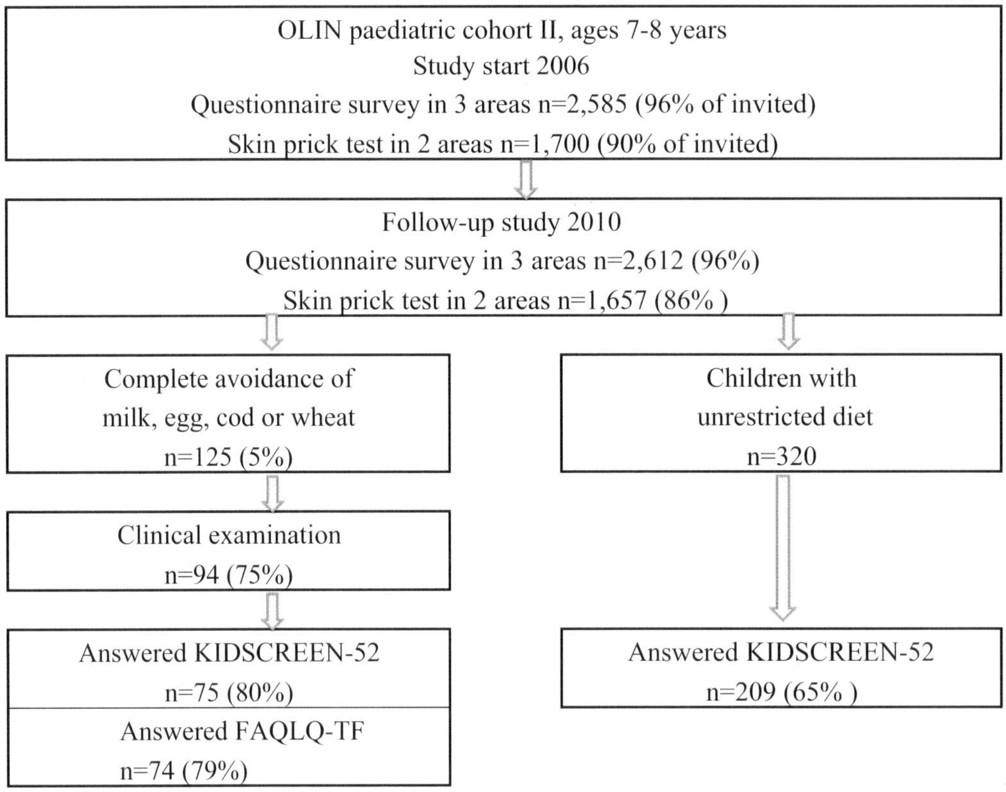

Fig. 1 Study design and participation

has predominantly been used for studies in European countries [27]. The KIDSCREEN-52 measure HRQL in ten domains with underlying items: Physical Well-being (five items), Psychological Well-being (six items), Moods and Emotions (seven items), Self-Perception (five items), Autonomy (five items), Parent Relation and Home Life (six items), Financial Resources (three items), Social Support and Peers (six items), School Environment (six items) and Social Acceptance and Bullying (three items). The responses are given on a five-point scale where 1 is worst HRQL and 5 is the best HRQL. The computerised data was transformed into scales from 0 to 100 for each domain [26]. The instrument, including the Swedish version, has been previously validated [27]. The population norm is a mean of 50 and a standard deviation of ten assuming a normal distributed sample is included. A higher score indicate a better HRQL with 100 indicating the best quality of life and 0 the worst [10, 26].

The disease-specific HRQL questionnaire

Since the children in our study were 12–13 years of age at the time they completed the questionnaires, we used the Food Allergy Quality of Life Questionnaire Teenager Form (FAQLQ-TF). The FAQLQ-TF questionnaire is a self-report instrument for measuring the impact of food allergy on the adolescent's HRQL, at the ages 13–17 years [13]. The FAQLQ-TF questionnaires measure HRQL in three domains with underlying items: Allergen Avoidance & Dietary Restrictions (ten items), Risk of Accidental Exposure (six items) and Emotional Impact (seven items). The responses are given on a seven-point scale. The domain score is the sum of all question scores in the domain divided with number of completed questions in the domain. Total FAQLQ-TF score is the average score of all individual items and each score range from one (minimal impairment) to seven (maximal impairment). A higher score indicate a poorer HRQL. The questionnaire has been translated into Swedish, and used in a previous study [28] but is not yet validated in Sweden. The level of the clinical Minimal Important Difference (MID) is still undecided [29] though, a difference of 0.5–0.7 on a seven point scale has been suggested as clinically relevant [30, 31].

Definitions

Any positive SPT: A positive reaction to at least one of the tested airborne allergens.

Asthma/rhinitis/eczema: Positive response to the question: "Has the child been diagnosed by a physican as having asthma/rhinitis/eczema?"

Food hypersensitivity (FHS): Reported complete elimination of cow's milk, hen's egg, fish and/or wheat due to food allergy or food hypersensitivity.

Heredity asthma/rhinitis/eczema: Reported parental history of asthma/rhinitis/eczema.

Heredity FHS: Reported parental history of food hypersensitivity.

Statistical analyses

The statistical analyses were performed using the Statistical Package of Social Science Software version 22 (SPSS Inc. New York, USA). The Chi square test was used for comparison of categorical data. Since HRQL data was not normally distributed, the Mann–Whitney U test or the Kruskal–Wallis test was used to assess statistical significant differences between groups. A p value <0.05 was considered statistically significant. Poor HRQL was defined as ≥75th percentile for the FAQLQ-TF score and differences between groups were analyzed by Linear by linear association (Mantel–Haenszel).

Results

Basic characteristics of study participants

The prevalence of atopic diseases was significantly higher among children with FHS compared to children without FHS: asthma 25.3 versus 6.2%, rhinitis 28.0 versus 6.2% and eczema 32.0 versus 10.5%, as was family history of FHS, 50.7 versus 21.1% ($p < 0.001$ for all). There were no significant differences between children with and without FHS regarding allergic sensitization to airborne allergens, sex, living conditions, parental smoking or parental socio-economic status (Table 1).

The responders and non-responders to the HRQL questionnaires did not differ regarding sex, atopic diseases, heredity of FHS, allergic sensitization or living conditions. Additional files 1 and 2 shows this in more detail.

Table 1 Comparison of atopic diseases and demographic factors between children with and without food hypersensitivity (FHS)

	FHS n = 75 % (n)	Non-FHS n = 209 % (n)	*p* value
Sex			
Girls	58.7 (44)	48.3 (101)	0.124
Boys	41.3 (31)	51.7 (108)	
Asthma	25.3 (19)	6.2 (13)	<0.001
Rhinitis	28.0 (21)	6.2 (13)	<0.001
Eczema	32.0 (24)	10.5 (22)	<0.001
Heredity FHS	50.7 (38)	21.1 (44)	<0.001
Any positive SPT[a]	46.3 (25)	33.0 (69)	0.069
Living conditions			
Current living			
House	86.1 (62)	79.6 (156)	
Apartment	13.6 (10)	20.4 (40)	0.108
Single parent household	8.0 (6)	10.2 (21)	0.581
Father smoke	13.5 (10)	13.7 (28)	0.967
Mother smoke	10.8 (8)	18.2 (37)	0.139
Parental socioeconomic status			
Professionals	33.2 (24)	24.4 (51)	
Self employed	4.0 (3)	6.2 (13)	
Intermediate non-manual	26.7 (20)	30.6 (64)	
Assistant non-manual	9.3 (7)	11.5 (24)	
Manual workers	14.7 (11)	11.5 (24)	
Manual workers service	8.0 (6)	10.0 (21)	
Unemployed	1.3 (1)	3.3 (7)	0.714

[a] Based on 54 children with food hypersensitivity and 209 children without food hypersensitivity who took part in skin prick testing

Generic HRQL among children with and without FHS

The KIDSCREEN-52 scores vary from 0 to 100, with 100 indicating the best quality of life and 0 the worst. The KIDSCREEN-52 domain specific median scores are presented in Fig. 2. The median value in all domains, among children with and without FHS were around 50 and above. No significant differences in distribution of HRQL were found when comparing children with or without FHS. In the Self-Perceptions domain, the median value tended to be lower among children with FHS compared to children without FHS, although the difference was not statistically significant.

Stratified analysis by sex were performed. Among girls, there was a significant difference between children with and without FHS in the distribution of HRQL in the domain Social Acceptance and Bullying ($p = 0.037$). In the other domains, no differences in distribution of HRQL were found, among neither girls nor boys (Table 2).

Generic HRQL in different FHS phenotypes

HRQL was compared between children with the different FHS phenotypes: current food allergy, outgrown food allergy and lactose intolerance. The KIDSCREEN-52 domain specific scores according to FHS phenotype are presented in Table 3. No significant differences in distribution were found between the phenotypes and the children without FHS. Children with current food allergy tended to have the lowest median values in several domains but the differences were not statistically significant.

Disease specific HRQL in different FHS phenotypes

The FAQLQ-TF responses are given on a seven-point scale where 1 is the best HRQL and 7 is the worst HRQL.

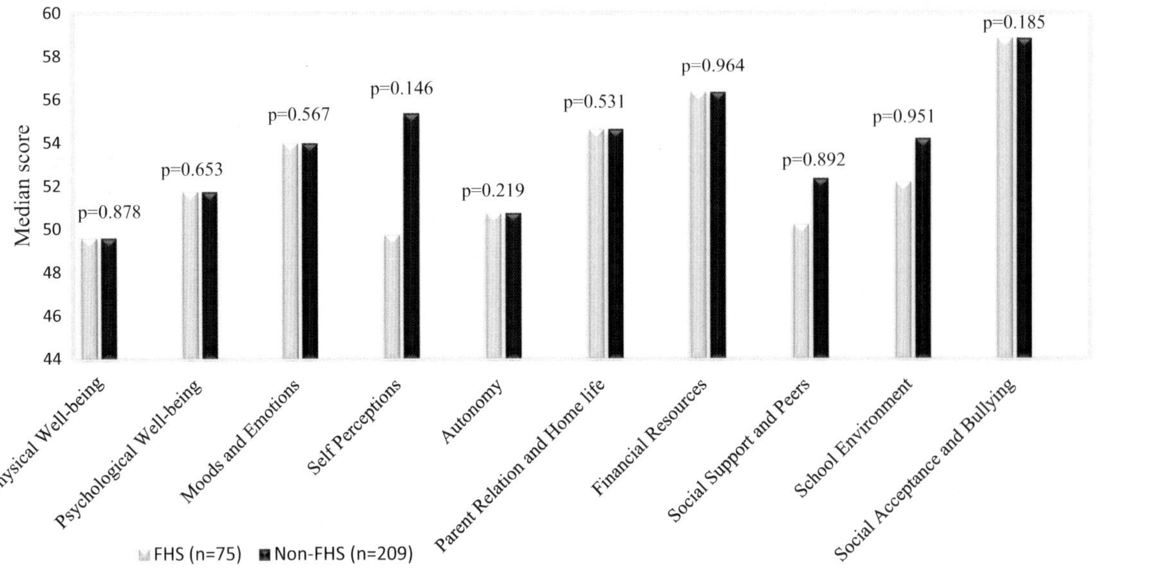

Fig. 2 Median scores in KIDSCREEN-52 domains, among children with and without food hypersensitivity. A higher score indicate better HRQL. Differences between groups was analysed by Mann–Whitney U test

Table 2 Scores in KIDSCREEN-52 domains among girls and boys, with and without food hypersensitivity, respectively

KIDSCREEN-52 dimension	Girls			Boys		
	FHS (n = 44) Median (Q_1–Q_3) Mean	Non-FHS (n = 101) Median (Q_1–Q_3) Mean	p value*	FHS (n = 31) Median (Q_1–Q_3) Mean	Non-FHS (n = 108) Median (Q_1–Q_3) Mean	p value*
Physical well-being	49.6 (42.5–58.4)	49.6 (42.5–55.6)	0.641	49.6 (44.7–52.4)	49.6 (44.7–59.3)	0.521
	50.1	49.5		50.1	51.0	
Psychological well-being	51.8 (47.1–56.8)	51.7 (45.1–57.6)	0.447	51.8 (45.1–57.6)	54.5 (47.1–57.6)	0.172
	53.2	51.6		51.8	53.8	
Moods and emotions	50.2 (45.4–62.1)	54.0 (45.4–62.1)	0.702	54.0 (47.1–70.9)	55.7 (49.1–62.1)	0.982
	52.9	53.5		55.35	56.5	
Self perceptions	49.8 (46.1–56.6)	52.2 (45.3–60.1)	0.879	52.2 (49.8–69.8)	55.4 (52.2–60.1)	0.199
	52.7	52.8		55.8	57.6	
Autonomy	48.7 (45.2–60.5)	50.7 (47.8–56.3)	0.879	53.2 (46.8–60.5)	53.2 (48.7–60.5)	0.646
	51.8	53.6		52.8	54.6	
Parent relation and home life	54.6 (48.0–58.5)	54.6 (47.5–65.9)	0.691	54.6 (47.5–65.9)	54.6 (49.5–65.9)	0.759
	53.8	54.3		54.3	55.4	
Financial resources	56.3 (49.3–62.9)	56.3 (49.3–62.9)	0.945	56.3 (46.6–62.9)	56.3 (49.3–62.9)	0.942
	55.6	55.8		55.3	55.4	
Social support and peers	52.4 (48.3–58.1)	54.9 (47.1–58.1)	0.667	48.3 (45.1–58.1)	50.2 (45.1–58.1)	0.828
	53.8	54.1		51.5	51.8	
School environment	54.2 (50.4–61.9)	54.2 (48.6–61.9)	0.905	52.2(46.9–58.9)	52.2 (48.6–56.4)	0.660
	55.7	56.0		53.1	53.1	
Social acceptance and bullying	58.8 (48.1–58.8)	58.8 (58.8–58.8)	0.037	58.8 (48.1–58.8)	58.8 (48.1–58.8)	0.947
	52.6	55.7		52.6	52.6	

* The statistical significant differences between groups was measured by Mann–Whitney U test

Table 3 Scores in KIDSCREEN-52 domains among children with different food hypersensitivity phenotypes and children without food hypersensitivity

KIDSCREEN-52 dimension	Current food allergy n = 23 Median (Q1–Q3) Mean	Outgrown food allergy n = 16 Median (Q1–Q3) Mean	Lactose intolerance n = 33 Median (Q1–Q3) Mean	Non-FHS n = 209 Median (Q1–Q3) Mean	p value Across 4 groups*
Physical well-being	47.08 (42.53–55.60)	49.63 (40.97–63.06)	49.63 (44.73–55.60)	49.63 (43.08–55.60)	0.896
	48.87	51.46	50.49	50.29	
Psychological well-being	49.34 (45.10–54.49)	54.49 (44.21–68.49)	54.49 (47.12–68.49)	51.78 (47.12–57.60)	0.321
	49.22	53.98	54.79	52.79	
Moods and emotions	51.34 (42.50–62.06)	57.39 (47.64–70.90)	54.02 (47.15–62.06)	54.02 (47.15–62.06)	0.369
	49.94	57.24	55.65	55.07	
Self perceptions	49.76 (46.09–60.11)	52.18 (47.78–69.78)	50.97 (48.28–58.93)	55.38 (49.76–60.11)	0.593
	53.54	55.42	54.26	55.27	
Autonomy	48.69 (40.54–56.27)	53.33 (45.17–60.52)	53.22 (46.85–68.75)	50.77 (48.69–60.52)	0.211
	48.65	53.33	55.09	54.15	
Parent relation and home life	54.65 (47.50–60.36)	56.58 (46.17–65.87)	54.65 (47.50–58.53)	54.65 (47.50–65.87)	0.928
	53.25	55.03	54.33	54.88	
Financial resources	62.86 (46.59–62.87)	52.41 (47.26–62.86)	59.60 (53.39–62.86)	56.35 (49.27–62.86)	0.537
	55.74	53.93	56.75	55.55	
Social support and peers	48.35 (46.66–54.93)	49.30 (44.37–57.33)	54.93 (47.50–67.06)	52.38 (46.66–58.13)	0.463
	50.96	51.39	55.30	52.88	
School environment	52.23 (46.94–58.87)	56.55 (52.22–61.87)	52.22 (48.61–61.87)	54.22 (48.61–58.87)	0.758
	53.46	56.11	55.00	54.82	
Social acceptance and bullying	58.85 (42.19–58.85)	58.85 (48.07–58.85)	58.85 (48.07–58.85)	58.85 (48.07–58.85)	0.556
	50.93	53.22	53.99	54.12	

* The statistical significant differences between groups was measured by the Kruskal–Wallis test

The FAQLQ-TF domain specific scores are presented in Fig. 3. No statistically significant differences in distribution of disease specific HRQL score were found between the different FHS phenotypes. However, the median score in all domains tended to be highest (indicating low HRQL) among children with *current food allergy* compared to *outgrown food allergy and lactose intolerance phenotypes*. Mean and median scores in FAQLQ-TF domains did not differ significantly by sex (Additional file 3).

The proportions of poor HRQL, defined as ≥75th percentile are presented in Fig. 4. Poor HRQL was most common among children with *current food allergy*, and significantly so in the domain Total FAQLQ-score ($p = 0.045$) and Emotional Impact ($p < 0.001$).

Discussion

According to European norms [10, 26], the children aged 12–13 years in this population-based study reported a good generic HRQL and there was no difference in HRQL between children with and without FHS. Further, no statistically significant differences in disease specific HRQL were found between children with the different FHS phenotypes: current food allergy, outgrown food allergy and lactose intolerance. However, the proportion of children having poor quality of life, defined as ≥75th percentile in the disease specific questionnaire, was more common in the current food allergy phenotype compared to the other phenotypes of FHS.

The participants in our study reported a good generic HRQL. Our result is in line with another Swedish population-based study comparing children aged eight years with or without atopic diseases including FHS. Overall, these children reported a good generic HRQL but children with atopic diseases, in particular asthma, had lower HRQL compared with children without atopic diseases [32]. Other factors than the disease itself may have an impact on the HRQL e.g. parental income [33], or being accepted by friends or not [34]. A possible explanation for the good HRQL among children with FHS in our study, and others as well, may be that FHS is common among children in Northern Europe [35]. Thus living with FHS or food allergy might be accepted as a normality and the restricted diet might therefore have a lesser impact on children's daily life [36, 37].

The increased availability of milk and gluten free products in Sweden may affect the HRQL in a positive way e.g. it is easier to prepare meals for children with

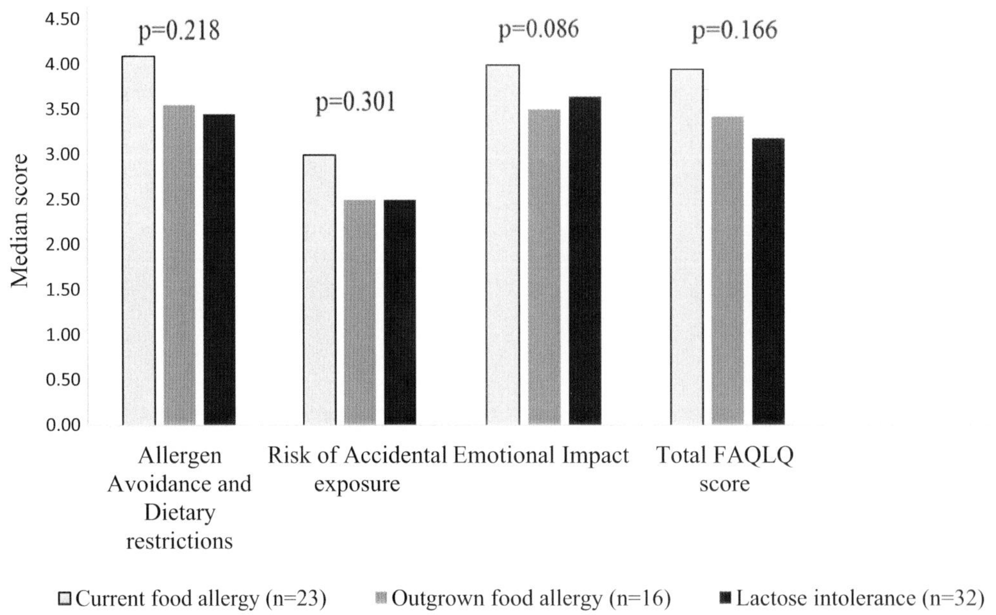

Fig. 3 Median scores in FAQLQ-TF domains, by food hypersensitivity phenotypes. A higher score indicate a poorer HRQL. Differences between groups was analysed by the Kruskal–Wallis test. The score range of FAQLQ-TF is between 1 (best HRQL) and 7 (worst HRQL)

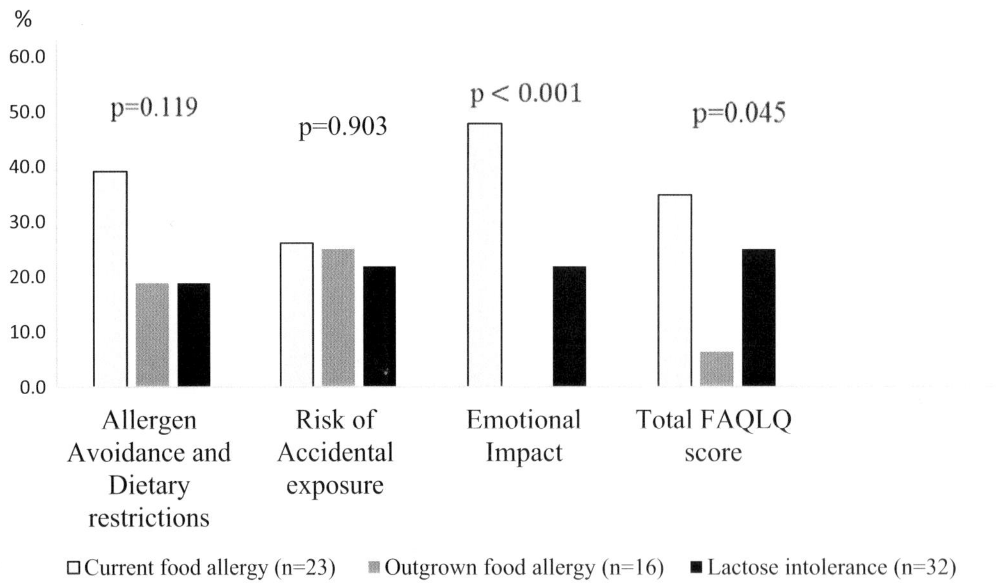

Fig. 4 Prevalence (%) of poor HRQL (≥75 percentile) in FAQLQ-TF domains by food hypersensitivity phenotypes. A higher score indicate a poorer HRQL. Difference between groups was analysed by Linear by linear association (Mantel–Haenszel)

different types of FHS. On the other hand, it probably also increases the awareness of different types of diets. People may regard temporary or non-specific symptoms as symptoms of FHS leading to an un-necessary eliminated diet [4]. Interestingly, the participants in our study showed similar results compared to a Swedish study of randomly selected children aged 11–16 years, with the lowest score in the domain Physical wellbeing [38].

Country of origin may have an impact of HRQL. The Food Allergy Quality of Life Questionnaire-parent form was completed by parents of 1029 food allergic children from different parts of the US. The result was compared with 15 studies from different countries in Europe, using the same questionnaire. The HRQL was more impaired in the US population than the European populations [39]. Thus, it is important that translation and validation of HRQL questionnaires includes lingual as well as cultural translations, due to socioeconomic and cultural differences between countries [40].

To our knowledge, this is the first study investigating HRQL among different phenotypes of FHS in the general population. A number of hospital-based studies have described quality of life in children with IgE-mediated food allergy [13, 33, 41]. In hospital materials, poor HRQL has been related to severe symptoms to foods e.g. anaphylaxis, respiratory or cardiovascular symptoms [33, 41], multiple food allergies [11, 33, 41], comorbidity with atopic diseases [41] or allergy to specific foods e.g. cow's milk and hen's egg compared to allergy to peanuts or tree nuts [33]. In our population-based study, we did not find any statistical significant differences in HRQL between children with and without FHS, which includes a number of different adverse reactions to foods, including food allergy [5]. Food allergy is rarely associated with mortality [42] or daily physical food related symptoms, but the psychological stress of accidently being exposed to the culprit food can be a burden [6, 43]. Many children with FHS do not seek health care due to mild symptoms to foods [44]. Thus, it is likely that those who seek health care due to FHS have more severe symptoms and/or experience a higher impact on their daily life compared to those who do not [45]. This could explain the differing results in HRQL between hospital- based and our population-based study.

In analyses stratified by sex, we found no statistically significant differences in HRQL, except in the domain Social Acceptance and Bullying. In this domain, HRQL was more impaired among girls with FHS compared to girls without FHS, but this difference was not found among boys. It has been shown that adolescent girls generally experience a poorer HRQL compared to boys [46] which is in line with our results. Even though FHS is common among children, it may affect social life and create social exclusion [36] which may lead to bullying. In a previous study, children reported that they had been bullied because of their food allergy, mainly by classmates but also by teachers and school staff [34].

The clinical Minimal Important Difference of the disease specific FAQLQ is not yet decided [29]. We defined poor disease specific HRQL as $\geq$75th percentile and it was most common among children with current food allergy. A possible explanation is that severe symptoms are most common in this phenotype. While respiratory, cardiovascular and severe skin- and gastrointestinal symptoms are relatively common in food allergy [21, 41], lactose intolerance present with milder bowel symptoms [47]. Thus, children with current food allergy are probably more afraid of food reactions compared to children with other phenotypes of FHS associated with milder symptoms.

Interestingly, poor HRQL was also found among children with *outgrown food allergy*. This was however not surprising since these children had a convincing history of food allergy, but they still avoided the culprit food despite tolerance had been achieved [21]. It is well known that tolerance development is common in allergies to foods like egg and milk [48], but children may remain on an elimination diet even if tolerance is achieved [49]. Among our children with FHS, lactose intolerance was the most common phenotype, and these children also reported total elimination to cow's milk [21]. Studies indicate that adolescents with lactose intolerance can drink smaller amounts of cow's milk without symptoms [50]. Hence, after participating in our research program some of the children with FHS could reintroduce the eliminated food, partially or completely [21, 51] which may improve their HRQL. Reasons for staying on a restricted diet are fear of food reactions, difficulties to tolerate taste and textures of the eliminated food and unwillingness to change an approach to food that has become normality [51, 52]. Since reported FHS is common in the population [3, 35] a correct diagnosis and follow-ups is important in order to evaluate persistence of FHS. This evaluation could be performed within the school health care in early school age [53].

Strengths and limitations

The strength of our study is that we compared HRQL between children with and without FHS in the same large population-based cohort and by using both generic and disease-specific HRQL questionnaires. By using generic HRQL questionnaire it was possible to compare HRQL among children with FHS and without FHS [54]. Because the classification of children into different FHS phenotypes was performed after completion of the HRQL questionnaire, the children's responses were not affected by receiving a new diagnosis. Another strength is that the children answered the HRQL questionnaire themselves, since disagreement between child and parent-proxy have been reported [55]. A limitation is that the disease specific questionnaire FAQLQ-TF is primarily developed for IgE-mediated food allergy [13] and does not cover other subgroups of FHS. The Swedish FAQLQ-TF version has not yet been validated but has been used in a previous Swedish study [28]. Regardless, FAQLQ-TF was used in our study because, to our knowledge, there is no available questionnaire in Swedish that is designed to describe adolescents' own perspective of living with FHS. Despite

the current study was based on a large population-based cohort with extremely high participation rate, we were lacking power for some analyses. Regarding the disease-specific HRQL, we found trends with those having current food allergy reporting the lowest HRQL although the differences did not reach statistical significance. Furthermore, the sample size did not allow analyses of HRQL in relation to number of foods avoided.

Conclusions

We hypothesised that total avoidance of milk, egg, fish or wheat due to food hypersensitivity would have a negative impact on HRQL in children, though this could not be verified. Instead, HRQL was similar in 12–13 year-old children with and without FHS in this population-based study. Poor HRQL was most common in the current food allergy phenotype in the domain Emotional impact and the total FAQLQ. Our study emphasizes the importance of identifying children with current food allergy, the FHS phenotype having impaired HRQL.

Abbreviations

FAQLQ-TF: Food Allergy Quality of Life Questionnaire Teenager Form; FHS: food hypersensitivity; HRQL: Health Related Quality of Life; IgE: immunoglobulin E; IQ: interquartile range; KIDSCREEN-52: Health-Related Quality of Life Screening instrument for children and adolescents; MID: clinical minimal important difference; SPT: skin prick testing.

Authors' contributions

ÅS, ER, VL, LH and AW contributed to the study design. ÅS, AW, ER, VL S-AJ and LH contributed to the analysis and interpretation of data. All authors were involved in the discussions and contributed to writing the manuscript. All authors read and approved the final manuscript.

Author details

[1] Department of Public Health and Clinical Medicine, Occupational and Environmental Medicine, OLIN Unit, Umeå University, 901 87 Umeå, Sweden. [2] Division of Nursing, Department of Health Sciences, Luleå University of Technology, 971 87 Luleå, Sweden. [3] Department of Clinical Sciences, Pediatrics, Umeå University, 901 87 Umeå, Sweden. [4] Department of Nursing, Umeå University, 901 87 Umeå, Sweden.

Acknowledgements

Our deepest gratitude to the children and their parents for participating in this study.

Competing interests

The authors declare that they have no competing interests.

Funding

Financial support was provided from the Swedish Heart and Lung Foundation; Swedish Asthma and Allergy Foundation; Visare Norr; a regional agreement among Umeå University, Västerbotten, and Norrbotten Country Council (ALF); State Government Funding for Healthcare Research (FOU); The Swedish Society for Asthma and Allergy Nursing; The Sven Jerring Foundation; The Mayflower Charity Foundation for Children and The Kempe-Carlgrenska Foundation.

References

1. Rona RJ, Keil T, Summers C, Gislason D, Zuidmeer L, Sodergren E, et al. The prevalence of food allergy: a meta-analysis. J Allergy Clin Immunol. 2007;120:638–46.
2. Nwaru BI, Hickstein L, Panesar SS, Muraro A, Werfel T, Cardona V, et al. The epidemiology of food allergy in Europe: a systematic review and meta-analysis. Allergy. 2014;69:62–75.
3. Winberg A, Strinnholm A, Hedman L, West CE, Perzanowski MS, Ronmark E. High incidence and remission of reported food hypersensitivity in Swedish children followed from 8 to 12 years of age—a population based cohort study. Clin Transl Allergy. 2014;4:32.
4. Moore LR. "But we're not hypochondriacs": the changing shape of gluten-free dieting and the contested illness experience. Soc Sci Med. 2014;105:76–83.
5. Johansson SG, Bieber T, Dahl R, Friedmann PS, Lanier BQ, Lockey RF, et al. Revised nomenclature for allergy for global use: report of the Nomenclature Review Committee of the World Allergy Organization, October 2003. J Allergy Clin Immunol. 2004;113:832–6.
6. Saleh-Langenberg J, Goossens NJ, Flokstra-de Blok BM, Kollen BJ, van der Meulen GN, Le TM, et al. Predictors of health-related quality of life of European food-allergic patients. Allergy. 2015;70:616–24.
7. Karimi M, Brazier J. Health, health-related quality of life, and quality of life: What is the difference? Pharmacoeconomics. 2016;34:645–9.
8. Slevin ML, Plant H, Lynch D, Drinkwater J, Gregory WM. Who should measure quality of life, the doctor or the patient? Br J Cancer. 1988;57:109–12.
9. Riley AW. Evidence that school-age children can self-report on their health. Ambul Pediatr. 2004;4:371–6.
10. Ravens-Sieberer U, Gosch A, Rajmil L, Erhart M, Bruil J, Duer W, Auquier P, et al. KIDSCREEN-52 quality-of-life measure for children and adolescents. Expert Rev Pharmacoecon Outcomes Res. 2005;5:353–64.
11. Flokstra-de Blok BM, DunnGalvin A, Vlieg-Boerstra BJ, Oude Elberink JN, Duiverman EJ, Hourihane JO, et al. Development and validation of a self-administered Food Allergy Quality of Life Questionnaire for children. Clin Exp Allergy. 2009;39:127–37.
12. Avery NJ, King RM, Knight S, Hourihane JO. Assessment of quality of life in children with peanut allergy. Pediatr Allergy Immunol. 2003;14:378–82.
13. Flokstra-de Blok BM, DunnGalvin A, Vlieg-Boerstra BJ, Oude Elberink JN, Duiverman EJ, Hourihane JO, et al. Development and validation of the self-administered Food Allergy Quality of Life Questionnaire for adolescents. J Allergy Clin Immunol. 2008;122:139–44.
14. Resnick ES, Pieretti MM, Maloney J, Noone S, Munoz-Furlong A, Sicherer SH. Development of a questionnaire to measure quality of life in adolescents with food allergy: the FAQL-teen. Ann Allergy Asthma Immunol. 2010;105:364–8.

15. Cohen BL, Noone S, Munoz-Furlong A, Sicherer SH. Development of a questionnaire to measure quality of life in families with a child with food allergy. J Allergy Clin Immunol. 2004;114:1159–63.
16. Bollinger ME, Dahlquist LM, Mudd K, Sonntag C, Dillinger L, McKenna K. The impact of food allergy on the daily activities of children and their families. Ann Allergy Asthma Immunol. 2006;96:415–21.
17. Lebovidge JS, Stone KD, Twarog FJ, Raiselis SW, Kalish LA, Bailey EP, et al. Development of a preliminary questionnaire to assess parental response to children's food allergies. Ann Allergy Asthma Immunol. 2006;96:472–7.
18. DunnGalvin A, de BlokFlokstra BM, Burks AW, Dubois AE, Hourihane JO. Food allergy QoL questionnaire for children aged 0–12 years: content, construct, and cross-cultural validity. Clin Exp Allergy. 2008;38:977–86.
19. Mackenzie H, Roberts G, Van Laar D, Dean T. A new quality of life scale for teenagers with food hypersensitivity. Pediatr Allergy Immunol. 2012;23:404–11.
20. Mikkelsen A, Borres MP, Bjorkelund C, Lissner L, Oxelmark L. The food hypersensitivity family impact (FLIP) questionnaire—development and first results. Pediatr Allergy Immunol. 2013;24:574–81.
21. Winberg A, West CE, Strinnholm A, Nordstrom L, Hedman L, Ronmark E. Assessment of allergy to milk, egg, cod, and wheat in swedish schoolchildren: a population based cohort study. PLoS ONE. 2015. doi:10.1371/journal.pone.0131804.
22. Ronmark E, Bjerg A, Perzanowski M, Platts-Mills T, Lundback B. Major increase in allergic sensitization in schoolchildren from 1996 to 2006 in northern Sweden. J Allergy Clin Immunol. 2009;124:357–63.
23. Bjerg A, Sandstrom T, Lundback B, Ronmark E. Time trends in asthma and wheeze in Swedish children 1996–2006: prevalence and risk factors by sex. Allergy. 2010;65:48–55.
24. Strinnholm A, Winberg A, West C, Hedman L, Ronmark E. Food hypersensitivity is common in Swedish schoolchildren, especially oral reactions to fruit and gastrointestinal reactions to milk. Acta Paediatr. 2014;103:1290–6.
25. Asher MI, Keil U, Anderson HR, Beasley R, Crane J, Martinez F, et al. International study of Asthma and Allergies in Childhood (ISAAC): rationale and methods. Eur Respir J. 1995;8:483–91.
26. Ravens-Sieberer U, the European KIDSCREEN Group. The KIDSCREEN Questionnaires—quality of life questionnaires for children and adolescents—handbook. Lengerich: Pabst Science Publisher; 2006.
27. Ravens-Sieberer U, Herdman M, Devine J, Otto C, Bullinger M, Rose M, et al. The European KIDSCREEN approach to measure quality of life and well-being in children: development, current application, and future advances. Qual Life Res. 2014;23:791–803.
28. Protudjer JL, Jansson SA, Middelveld R, Ostblom E, Dahlen SE, Arnlind MH, et al. Impaired health-related quality of life in adolescents with allergy to staple foods. Clin Transl Allergy. 2016;6:37.
29. Salvilla SA, Dubois AE, Flokstra-de Blok BM, Panesar SS, Worth A, Patel S, et al. Disease-specific health-related quality of life instruments for IgE-mediated food allergy. Allergy. 2014;69:834–44.
30. Schunemann HJ, Akl EA, Guyatt GH. Interpreting the results of patient reported outcome measures in clinical trials: the clinician's perspective. Health Qual Life Outcomes. 2006;4:62.
31. Jansson SA, Heibert-Arnlind M, Middelveld RJ, Bengtsson UJ, Sundqvist AC, Kallstrom-Bengtsson I, et al. Health-related quality of life, assessed with a disease-specific questionnaire, in Swedish adults suffering from well-diagnosed food allergy to staple foods. Clin Transl Allergy. 2013;3:21.
32. Covaciu C, Bergstrom A, Lind T, Svartengren M, Kull I. Childhood allergies affect health-related quality of life. J Asthma. 2013;50:522–8.
33. Howe L, Franxman T, Teich E, Greenhawt M. What affects quality of life among caregivers of food-allergic children? Ann Allergy Asthma Immunol. 2014;113:69–74.
34. Lieberman JA, Weiss C, Furlong TJ, Sicherer M, Sicherer SH. Bullying among pediatric patients with food allergy. Ann Allergy Asthma Immunol. 2010;105:282–6.
35. Nwaru BI, Hickstein L, Panesar SS, Roberts G, Muraro A, Sheikh A, et al. Prevalence of common food allergies in Europe: a systematic review and meta-analysis. Allergy. 2014;69:992–1007.
36. MacKenzie H, Roberts G, Van Laar D, Dean T. Teenagers' experiences of living with food hypersensitivity: a qualitative study. Pediatr Allergy Immunol. 2010;21:595–602.
37. Gallagher M, Worth A, Cunningham-Burley S, Sheikh A. Strategies for living with the risk of anaphylaxis in adolescence: qualitative study of young people and their parents. Prim Care Respir J. 2012;21:392–7.
38. Berman AH, Liu B, Ullman S, Jadback I, Engstrom K. Children's quality of life based on the KIDSCREEN-27: child self-report, parent ratings and child–parent agreement in a Swedish random population sample. PLoS ONE. 2016. doi:10.1371/journal.pone.0150545.
39. DunnGalvin A, Koman E, Raver E, Frome H, Adams M, Keena A, et al. An examination of the Food Allergy Quality of Life Questionnaire performance in a countrywide American sample of children: cross-cultural differences in age and impact in the United States and Europe. J Allergy Clin Immunol Pract. 2016. doi:10.1016/j.jaip.2016.09.049.
40. Antolin-Amerigo D, Manso L, Caminati M, de la Hoz CaballerB, Cerecedo I, Muriel A, et al. Quality of life in patients with food allergy. Clin Mol Allergy. 2016;14:4.
41. Protudjer J, Jansson SA, Ostblom E, Arnlind MH, Bengtsson U, Dahlen SE, et al. Health-related quality of life in children with objectively diagnosed staple food allergy assessed with a disease-specific questionnaire. Acta Paediatr. 2015;104:1047–54.
42. Foucard T, Yman IM, Nordvall L. Reduced number of fatal and life-threatening reaction to food. Reporting by the medical profession has resulted in effective measures. Lakartidingen. 2005;102:3465–8.
43. Ostblom E, Egmar AC, Gardulf A, Lilja G, Wickman M. The impact of food hypersensitivity reported in 9-year-old children by their parents on health-related quality of life. Allergy. 2008;63:211–8.
44. Winberg A, West CE, Strinnholm A, Nordstrom L, Hedman L, Ronmark E. Milk allergy is a minor cause of milk avoidance due to perceived hypersensitivity among schoolchildren in Northern Sweden. Acta Paediatr. 2016;105:206–14.
45. Le TM, Flokstra-de Blok BM, van Hoffen E, Lebens AF, Goossens NJ, Dubois AE, et al. Quality of life is more impaired in patients seeking medical care for food allergy. Int Arch Allergy Immunol. 2013;162:335–9.
46. Cavallo F, Zambon A, Borraccino A, Raven-Sieberer U, Torsheim T, Lemma P. Girls growing through adolescence have a higher risk of poor health. Qual Life Res. 2006;15:1577–85.
47. Di Rienzo T, D'Angelo G, D'Aversa F, Campanale MC, Cesario V, Montalto M, et al. Lactose intolerance: from diagnosis to correct management. Eur Rev Med Pharmacol Sci. 2013;17(2):18–25.
48. Skripak JM, Matsui EC, Mudd K, Wood RA. The natural history of IgE-mediated cow's milk allergy. J Allergy Clin Immunol. 2007;120:1172–7.
49. Eigenmann PA, Caubet JC, Zamora SA. Continuing food-avoidance diets after negative food challenges. Pediatr Allergy Immunol. 2006;17:601–5.
50. Usai-Satta P, Scarpa M, Oppia F, Cabras F. Lactose malabsorption and intolerance: What should be the best clinical management? World J Gastrointest Pharmacol Ther. 2012;3:29–33.
51. Strinnholm A, Winberg A, Hedman L, Ronmark E, Lindh V. Reintroduction failure is common among adolescents after double-blind placebo-controlled food challenges. Acta Paediatr. 2016;106:282–7.
52. Strinnholm A, Brulin C, Lindh V. Experiences of double-blind, placebo-controlled food challenges (DBPCFC): a qualitative analysis of mothers' experiences. J Child Health Care. 2010;14:179–88.
53. Kallio P, Salmivesi S, Kainulainen H, Paassilta M, Korppi M. Parent-reported food allergy requiring an avoidance diet in children starting elementary school. Acta Paediatr. 2011;100:1350–3.
54. Flokstra-de Blok BM, van der Velde JL, Vlieg-Boerstra BJ, Oude Elberink JN, DunnGalvin A, Hourihane JO, et al. Health-related quality of life of food allergic patients measured with generic and disease-specific questionnaires. Allergy. 2010;65:1031–8.
55. Upton P, Lawford J, Eiser C. Parent–child agreement across child health-related quality of life instruments: a review of the literature. Qual Life Res. 2008;17:895–913.

A qualitative study exploring parents' experiences with epinephrine use for their child's anaphylactic reaction

Rishma Chooniedass[1*], Beverley Temple[2], Donna Martin[2] and Allan Becker[1]

Abstract

Background: Children with life threatening food allergies live with the constant threat of a fatal reaction, and caregivers must always be prepared to treat with an epinephrine auto-injector (EAI). This interpretive phenomenological study explored parents' perceptions and lived experiences with prescribed EAI use for their child.

Methods: The purposive sample included ten parents of five children under 12 years of age, diagnosed with a food allergy and prescribed with an EAI who recently experienced anaphylaxis. Data sources included digitally-recorded semi-structured interviews and a reflexive journal.

Results: Eight main themes emerged: perception of anaphylaxis, life challenges, isolation, anxiety, hesitation, guilt, influence of health care professionals, and lessons learned. Parents uniformly described multiple life challenges and feelings of isolation, anxiety and hesitation during a reaction that lead to subsequent guilt.

Conclusions: Handling reactions correctly provided parents with confidence to treat subsequent reactions. Witnessing the effects of an EAI and receiving positive feedback from health care providers further strengthened their confidence to quickly and competently intervene in future reactions.

Keywords: Anaphylaxis, Epinephrine, Food allergy, Barriers, Education, Management

Background

Food allergy has increased two to threefold in the last 20 years and is associated with increased anxiety, poor quality of life and increased health care costs including emergency visits and hospital admissions [1, 2]. Approximately 8% of children in North America have a self-reported food allergy [3]. It is estimated that food allergies cost the American economy approximately 25 billion dollars (USD) annually with direct and indirect costs of medical appointments, including loss of family work days [4] and the cost is only increasing as incidence of food allergy rise [1]. This medical condition is of global concern affecting quality of life of both patients and their families.

Presently, there is no cure for food allergies. Avoidance is the primary strategy with epinephrine as the medical treatment recommended for an anaphylactic reaction [5]. Anaphylaxis is a severe allergic reaction that can affect multiple organ systems in the body and can rapidly cause death. Rates of epinephrine use during an anaphylactic reaction are alarmingly low and treatment is often inappropriately managed [6], while treatment in children is often withheld. The reasons for this range from individuals not carrying an epinephrine auto-injector (EAI) when a reaction is occurring, to caregivers not wanting to administer medication if they are unsure of themselves or the situation. Some speculate that injecting epinephrine into their child is a traumatic event which may contribute to the profound lack of treatment [7]. It is crucial to understand the root cause(s) of failing to treat anaphylactic reactions competently in order to better manage the health of children with food allergies.

*Correspondence: rchooniedass@chrim.ca
[1] John Buhler Research Centre, College of Medicine, Faculty of Health Sciences, University of Manitoba, 504H 715 McDermot Ave, Winnipeg, MB R3E 3P4, Canada
Full list of author information is available at the end of the article

Unsworth states, "comprehensive and helpful published advice on patient training (for EAI) is available, but compliance remains poor" [8]. If health care providers are to improve outcomes of anaphylactic reactions, then researchers must identify why caregivers delay or neglect to use EAIs. There is a lack of research exploring experiences and attitudes related to managing food allergies and the use of EAIs [9]. By understanding the thoughts and emotions of parents who have witnessed their child's anaphylactic reaction, health care providers can ensure that caregivers develop the skills, education, and support necessary to make certain that the next reaction is appropriately treated. The purpose of this qualitative study was to describe parents' perceptions and experiences with epinephrine use during a child's anaphylactic reaction.

Methods

This project used steps outlined by Creswell to perform data analysis and interpretation of findings from one-on-one interviews with parents of children living with a life threatening food allergy [10]. Using a purposive sample, a semi-structured, open ended, face-to-face, one-on-one, in person interview was conducted with each participant.

Approvals by the Research Ethics Board (E2015:039) and Health Research Impact Committee (RI2015) were obtained prior to starting the study. Following obtaining consent, demographic data were collected to describe the sample population. Each participant was asked to tell the story of their child's anaphylactic reaction, outlining their experiences, thoughts and feelings during that critical event.

Inclusion criteria

Inclusion criteria were parents and caregivers of children under age 12 with a previous diagnosis of food allergy confirmed by a Pediatric Allergist, who had experienced an anaphylactic reaction that required an emergency room visit within the last 24 months. They must have previously filled a prescription for an EAI. The caregivers were required to speak English.

Exclusion criteria

Exclusion criteria included any caregivers who did not speak English, had an anaphylactic reaction more than 24 months ago, or did not have an EAI. Also, caregivers of children living with another major chronic illness were excluded as this may further negatively affect their perception of health or reasons for use of EAI.

Sampling and recruitment

Participants were recruited by a nurse educator from The Children's Allergy & Asthma Education Centre or via posters displayed at the Children's Allergy Clinic.

Ten participants were recruited. Interviews ranging from 30 to 80 min were conducted in participant homes or workplaces; and recruitment ceased after the tenth interview as no new themes emerged. Data sources included transcripts, field notes, and memos. Audio recordings were collected and transcribed verbatim by an independent transcriptionist. As a form of verification, random copies of transcripts were reviewed by another researcher to ensure that there was congruence in theme development. All data sources were imported into NVivo v11.2 software (2010).

Results

Demographics

Ten parents participated (five females) aged 32–46 years (Table 1). Five children were described in this study who were 3–10 years of age and parents self-reported their child's multiple food allergies (see Table 2). Four of the children were diagnosed within the first year of life, and one was diagnosed at age three. It was not confirmed whether each allergen sensitization caused clinical symptoms as only the most severe anaphylactic reaction within the last 24 months was described.

The length of time participants lived with their child's food allergy ranged from 2 to 9 years. Every child had an EAI and kept it present at all times. All children had experienced an anaphylactic reaction at least two and some up to nine reaction requiring an Emergency Department visit within 24 months. Epinephrine administration from participants ranged from one to six times. As a form of cross verification, data triangulation from hospital charts was obtained to validate participant's recall.

Table 1 Study participant demographics

Variable	Frequency	
	N	Percent
Caregiver		
Mother	5	50
Father	5	50
Employment status		
Employed	8	80
Self-employed	1	10
Unemployed	1	10
Education		
High school	2	20
Post secondary degree	8	80
Household income		
$75,000–$100,000	2	20
$100,000–$125,000	2	20
$125,000–$150,000	2	20
> $150,000	4	40

Table 2 Child demographics

		μ ± SD
Child age		6.3 ± 2.9
Number of allergies		4.6 ± 2.1
Number of anaphylactic episodes		4.9 ± 2.1
EAI uses		3.2 ± 1.9
Variable	**Frequency**	
	N	**Percent**
Age at diagnosis		
≤ 1 year	4	80
1–5 years	1	20
Parent recollection of initial diagnosis		
Allergist	6	60
Emergency doctor	2	20
Nurse practitioner	1	10
Can't recall	1	10

Analysis uncovered a range of thoughts and emotions experienced by parents when their child suffered an anaphylactic reaction that could impact their decision to use an EAI. Figure 1 illustrates the eight main themes that emerged from this study: perception of anaphylaxis, life challenges, isolation, anxiety, hesitation, guilt, influence of health care professionals and lessons learned. This figure represents the external and internal influences on a caregiver's perception. The following section will present the major themes that emerged from the data.

Perception of anaphylaxis

Participants were asked: 'What does the term anaphylaxis mean to you?' They constructed their own meanings based on experiences or what they have been told about anaphylaxis by others.

> *I think we do a great disservice to people with EpiPen videos that show people going into respiratory distress and having red flushed hive-covered faces and dropping to the ground; ... it doesn't always appear that way. (F2)*

This comment serves as a reminder that each reaction is unique, manifesting differently in the same person, even when triggered by the same allergen.

> *things are going to go into hyper overdrive and eventually shut down... You're in a race for time to make sure that things get fixed properly in a timely fashion. (M2)*

The perception that the body's systems "shut down" and using an analogy of a race, exemplifies how rapidly the reaction progresses. It describes how fast anaphylaxis occurs and how quickly caregivers must respond, without relying on specific detailed symptoms.

Life challenges: "logistically expensive nightmare"

Many participants explained how every aspect of their life changed. The obvious and immediate change was avoidance of the suspect allergen. Some participants explained the challenges associated with avoiding allergens. For instance, a caregiver of a child with dairy allergy expressed the additional burden of sourcing foods that do not contain milk and eggs. In addition, it was noted that if the child had multiple food allergies it made avoidance and shopping much more complicated.

Society integrates food into social activities, including family gatherings, meals at restaurants, school, team activities, or celebrations. The task of constantly checking, and re-checking food labels while grocery shopping became an added burden that families had to face on a daily basis. Sourcing alternative foods is possible but requires both more work and necessitates more expense.

> *Dealing with the high cost of these foods is intense, and we are both middle-income earners. Good grief, what do low income people with allergies do? (F2)*

> *At 110 bucks it's like whoa eh, hold on. You know, never mind the ambulance rides... people can't afford that epinephrine. It's expensive. (M1)*

Not only is it a challenge to vigilantly shop for foods that are allergy safe for their children, but the expense is felt in the cost of food, medication, and ambulance fees. Even patients who have stable incomes can feel the burden of paying for an auto injector, further compounded when they are often advised that they should have one for home, school, backpack and other locations. Some participants went as far as discussing that travelling is a major challenge that is best avoided. Preparations for travel included filling multiple prescriptions of EAIs, finding accommodations with a kitchen to prepare meals, and plotting out nearby grocery stores and hospitals.

Isolation, limited social support, misunderstood

Another significant challenge was a change in relationships within the extended family, friends and other support groups. These challenges had the greatest impact on the quality of life experienced by those living with a food allergy and their families.

> *(Anaphylaxis is) basically life or death, it's serious and that you don't take chances. And that people don't understand it unless you've seen your child basically starting to die in front of you don't, they don't get it. And even now, some of our family doesn't quite get it. (F3)*

The frustration becomes evident when one's own family does not understand the implications of anaphylaxis.

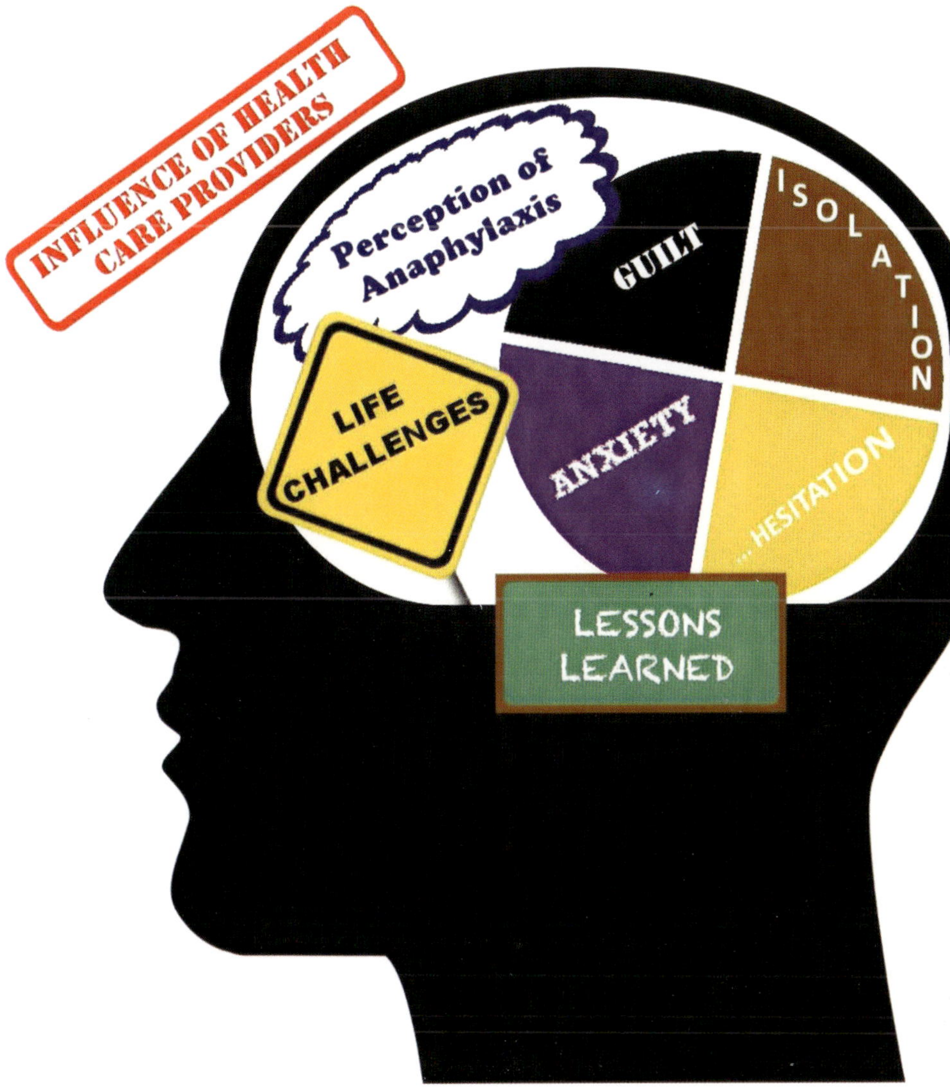

Fig. 1 Emerging themes

Another participant expressed frustration with his family because they continued to put his child at risk of a reaction and he believed that the best action was to avoid visiting their home. The safety of this participant's child is the primary concern, regardless if this meant isolating from family members.

> *It can be lonely. Um, you really find out who your friends are (crying). So you know friends that I had totally been there for just basically vanished the second that she was diagnosed. So because nobody wants their lives to be inconvenienced and food is such a big social aspect. So, things like getting together for play dates or you know all the stuff we used to do before, nobody really wants to do that. (F5)*

Constant anxiety and a visceral fear

Anxiety and fear are parental instincts that intensify when their child has been diagnosed with a food allergy. Participants described a constant feeling of anxiety, both when they are away from their child and even when they are by their side. Some expressed that anxiety may improve with time, but may also stay for years.

> *We're still scared (crying)... Um, we question as parents whether he's going to get to be able to do all the things that we want him to be able to do, because of our own fears. (F4)*

> *It's still a very visceral fear that's always brooding in the back of your mind. What's going on at school?... you're always in a constant state of, alertness to it...*

'Cause I can't be there 24/7... I'll say fear. I'm not going to lie you know. It's this nagging background fear that something's going to happen. (M2)

Parents live with the ever-present possibility of a severe reaction, and the morbidity associated with living in a state of constant uncertainty and anxiety.

(crying) I'm sorry but she was basically dying in the back of the car and I was sitting there in the back with her trying to like wake her up because she was starting to pass out now. (F3)

The traumatic memory relived by this participant is a stark reminder of the seriousness of this situation and reminds her of the mortality of her daughter. This statement evokes the fear and sense of helplessness that parents experience when faced with their child's reaction. Reactions are unexpected, and not being able to control a situation can result in an overwhelming feeling of dread.

It was my fear of hurting my child even though I knew the needle was the right thing. Um, I guess, I think there was even fear of like doing it wrong. (F4)

The fear of what is perceived as inflicting more pain on one's child is a common theme that participants described. Even when parents are witnessing their child suffering a severe reaction, the thought of giving a needle often seems an overly invasive intervention, despite the fact that they recognize it is necessary. This hesitation may cause more harm and is rationalized by the desire not to inflict pain.

Hesitation

Hesitation was a common reaction when uncertainty made participants doubt themselves. Often it was confusion about how the child came in contact with the suspect allergen rather than issues regarding acknowledgment of the reaction. Denial, being reluctant to treat and the urge to wait to see what happens were common responses to an anaphylactic reaction.

Doubt. Self-doubt; do I, am I doing the right thing? Am I over-reacting? Am I under-reacting?... My brain didn't say get me the EpiPen, then I'll take him... I've been trained, I've trained people...as a public health nurse in the schools...but in the moment with the gradual onset that's not this big, exciting, obvious thing...But I was still thinking really? Really? This is warranted?... I was questioning myself while I'm preparing to give it. (F2)

Even in well trained individuals who have experience with anaphylaxis, there is still a hesitation to act, and a sense of down-playing the severity of a situation that can quickly escalate. The inner conflict of self-doubt leading to hesitation is a commonly identified theme among participants. This parent's response to the uncertainty of acting, and how others may view their actions serve to illustrate that caregivers are dealing with more than the critical situation of anaphylaxis. They are dealing with thoughts and fears about how to treat, when to treat, consequences of treating (hurting their child further) and what others will think of their actions. One participant described an EAI as a "horse tranquilizer" because of the size of the device. He described the anxiety associated with using something that large on a small child.

We should have given the EpiPen, but it was the fear of "I'm going to make this worse for my child." Like he's already dealing with the struggling... we just need to get him to the hospital because I don't want to hurt him more. (F4)

Even when they know that a reaction is occurring, there continues to be a reluctance to use epinephrine. Once again, it is evident that hesitation during a stressful moment leads to delay in administration of epinephrine, even when the caregiver is well aware of the correct course of action, partially due to situational stressors or a "kaleidoscope of stressors".

Guilt

A sense of guilt stemmed from many sources. One reason for experiencing guilt was directly due to not treating the reaction. Participants expressed other reasons for feeling guilt, and often identified it was due to the way they had decided to live life and care for their child with a food allergy.

The words we use are probably pretty offensive and probably my kids should go for counselling because he probably feels like some, some kind of leper because we're always talking about contamination and cross-contamination. (F2)

The implications of using terms like contamination (often associated with connotations such as harmful, unclean) make this parent think that her child will feel different from other children.

I should have given it. But then I still didn't give it cause I'm almost there (hospital). And I'm just like oh crap this is serious! I've worked emerge (in the Emergency Department), like I just felt such shame and I felt so stupid. And like me fluffing it off, or you know watch and, watchful waiting, or, you know, you know observation is going to kill him one day and I'm trying to snap out of that. (F4)

Anaphylaxis is one illness in which 'watchful waiting' is a potentially life-threatening decision, and this parent's resultant guilt stems at least in part from following such a course of action.

> *I think I was seriously thinking that like I could lose my son! He could die! Like, this isn't right... I still had the EpiPen. It was still around him. It was on, on his belt. (F4)*

Guilt revolves around the delayed use of the EAI for fear of having to give a needle. This guilt is magnified by how quickly her child improved upon treatment with epinephrine, and further reflects the guilt of what the parent perceives as unnecessary suffering, which could have been avoided if only they had acted sooner. The realization that there is a potential for a child's death is something that cannot be put into words, and, at times, is inconceivable.

Influence of health care professionals

Caregivers are reliant on health care providers for acute and long-term treatment. We trust them because of their profession and rely on them to be proficient and informed on current evidence and best practices. But how do their actions or their reactions affect us?

> *I know from that first time when we got to the hospital and they were like why didn't you give the EpiPen? And they were basically like yelling at us. (F4)*

This participant describes the response from emergency staff and relates feeling berated due to her lack of EAI use. This situation illustrates that parents perceive health care professionals as a source of authority. The manner in which health care providers react to patients and their families can provide a lasting impression, both positive and negative.

> *But then when they (doctors) don't give it either, you know you can say okay because they're in the hospital they can always intubate and start IVs and do all these wonderful things. But hello? Like if you really want to reinforce proper parental management in the community, you got to role model it in the hospital too. (F2)*

When a participant encounters a situation when health care providers do not provide the standard of care for an anaphylactic reaction, it raises doubts in their mind about the competency of the health care provider. The action of a health care professional not administering an EAI undermines the teaching that caregivers have received regarding prompt epinephrine use.

> *So I called her paediatrician and I said, look this is what happening. She started to wheeze and um, he said well just put the phone up to her, up to her mouth so I can kind of hear her breathe... And he says... it likely was a reaction but basically wait until she was having trouble breathing or if she was turning blue before I called 911. (F5)*

Retrospectively this parent realizes the information given was not consistent with the standard of care for an anaphylactic reaction. This results in mistrust of health care professionals and can become a barrier to future care.

> *We had a reaction in Alberta and the hospital is completely different than here (Winnipeg). I mean they were like, well she can still breathe so why are you even here? ...She's got four inch hives on her and she's coughing all the time... with a diagnosis of anaphylaxis you would treat this as anaphylaxis. But they were nah it's fine; go away. (M5)*

This is another example of a patient who encountered inaccurate advice and contrary to what they have been taught. There are health care providers who take initiative to educate caregivers on proper management and treatment of anaphylaxis, and it is disconcerting to encounter other providers who disseminate incorrect information and treatment.

Lessons learned

The best advice might be from someone who has experienced anaphylaxis. Real world advice has both the weight of personal experience and may be more directly relatable to an individual in the same circumstance. This type of education may prove more effective than artificially constructed or simulated examples from health care providers.

> *I have documented most of [her] reactions; I put together a book for her daycare when we had to put her into day care to say this is what all these things look like on the different sites of her body...they told us that they learned more from us than they did URIS (Unified Referral and Intake System in Manitoba that provides health care support for children in community programs). Because they, they hear okay well hives but nobody really knows what hives look like. So you know having, having a resource like that I think would have been really helpful for me to also have somebody tell me what it would be like to; the importance of documenting everything. (F5)*

This family copes with lifestyle changes by becoming proactive and advocating for their child. By providing detailed information on their child's health and possible signs of reaction, they empower themselves and, thus, are better able to deal with the challenges they must face on a daily basis.

Always think anaphylaxis even if there's been a long delay between a potential exposure, even if you haven't seen it. Because if you don't see it, your tendency is to figure out what's wrong and I've been caught in that trap so many times where you're trying to figure out was there an exposure? ...Rather than just recognize the symptoms and respond appropriately. (F2)

The lessons learned from this parent's experience has allowed them to reflect upon and evaluate their initial response and coping skills. Whereas it may be second nature to try to answer the question 'why is my child having a reaction now', experience has taught this participant that the 'why' really is not the important question at the time. Rather, the thought process must be 'my child is having a reaction now and I need to treat it.

I think they're scared that they're going to hurt the child by jamming a needle in them. Or they're scared that they're going to get in trouble for doing something that wasn't necessary, right? So people's fears need to be allayed, that you're not going to get, you won't be held accountable for the cost of an epi, because some people worry about things like this. Or that you've done something medically wrong to the child or something. Just give it. (M4)

Parents relate that one of the key features of coping with the lifestyle changes that come with living with a food allergy is learning to get over the fear of using an epinephrine auto injector. Coping in this case may mean finding ways to mitigate the costs of treatment, and exploring ways to make caregivers more comfortable with the safety of administering an auto injector.

I don't think we realized the force you needed to push with. Which is you know, you get a trainer and it's super loose and um but the big EpiPens you have to push a bit harder. Like the real ones. (M3)

This parent relates real world experience with using an EAI. Specifically, they relate how using an actual devise is not the same as using a trainer, and one way of coping may include becoming more comfortable by practicing with an actual device.

I think they probably do need to hear it from other parents who have been there. Cause it's one thing to hear a nurse say it's no problem or a doctor say just give it, but it's, it's also um, what else are you going to say right? But how about here's someone who's lived it? (M3)

Discussion

Global impact of anaphylaxis

Today, medicine is increasingly concentrating on the importance of quality of life as much as on health outcomes [11]. Participants described that every aspect of their life changed after their child was diagnosed with a food allergy. These findings are congruent with a previous study that identified that parents of children with food allergies found social activities outside the home more stressful [12].

Participants in this study spoke about caring for children with multiple food allergies and stated that life becomes more difficult with each food allergy. This finding echoes other studies that suggest that parents of children with multiple allergies have significantly more anxiety [13]. One participant described that it is not only food that the household needs to avoid, but also nonfood items in the home such as moisturizing creams [14].

Many parents recalled the multiple signs and symptoms of anaphylaxis and they described the helplessness they felt as they witnessed their child's suffering. Despite having an EAI present, most expressed concern with administering a needle to their child, as they perceived that it would contribute to their child's pain. The size of the needle was another component that was emphasized. If one assumes that the needle is the size of the cartridge, then they would certainly assume that the injection would cause significant pain and discomfort. Health care providers should describe the length of the needle found in EAIs, so that caregivers understand it is similar to the needle size used for routine immunizations. It is important for health care providers to inform caregivers that the instantaneous discomfort of a needle will quickly resolve and stop the reaction from progressing (Table 3).

It is known that parental attitudes can influence their children [12]. A study on food allergy showed that maternal anxiety is associated with adolescent distress, possibly due to children learning from parental behavior [15]. Health care providers need to explain to caregivers that it is understandable to feel anxiety, but their child can

Table 3 Barriers to epinephrine use

Emotional barriers	Health care barriers
Fear/anxiety	Limited educators (time and availability)
Guilt	Inconsistent health care information
Hesitation/doubt	Conflicting health care message
Isolation	Lack of consistent support

learn to mimic these unhealthy behaviors. Some participants described no longer visiting the homes of people who put their child at risk of a reaction. Avoiding activities negatively reinforces anxious behaviors [16]. Unintentionally their children, adopt these negative coping skills [17]. These displays of anxious behaviors can affect a child's relationships, school functioning and quality of life. Untreated anxiety in children can predict depression later in life [17]. It is important that health care professionals understand the psychological effects associated with living and caring for a child with food allergies, and if necessary, referrals to mental health practitioners should be supported [18].

Parents relate what they would like to see in the context of an educational tool for anaphylaxis and food allergies. They would appreciate seeing real world examples of reactions and hearing from those who have had the experience of suffering from an anaphylactic reaction or using an EAI and even hearing the subjective experience of those who have been given epinephrine to treat an anaphylactic reaction. It would also be helpful to share experiences of others who have gone through the common feelings of fear, doubt and helplessness when they have been faced with having to treat a loved one suffering a reaction. The consensus is that an educational video that includes real world experience and explores some of the common barriers that families with food allergies are faced with would be a helpful resource. Lanser conducted focus groups to assess the needs of caregivers managing food allergy and found that learning from other families was important [19] and identified the need for videos describing the experiences of others. Haigh and Hardy stated that "the importance of storytelling as the foundation of human experience cannot be overestimated" and can be used as an educational strategy [20]. This method can help other caregivers feel less isolated and prepare them for future challenges they may face. As an outcome of this study, a 3-part parent-led educational video entitled "Food Allergy: Through the eyes of a parent" was developed. This video series highlights parents' stories of life challenges, anaphylactic reactions, and advice for other caregivers. This video is now incorporated into parent food allergy classes at the Children's Allergy and Asthma Education Centre (http://www.caaec.ca) and is available for free on their website (https://www.youtube.com/playlist?list=PLcMGfBsVtJrAgaE5QFsg9gEhtySytDBmS).

Health care professionals

The ways in which hospital staff interacts with caregivers impacts their experience and affects their future actions. Parents have stated that kindness, and clear communication of health care providers can positively impact an Emergency Department visit [21]. One family explained that they were yelled at for not using an EAI and this made them feel guilty and ashamed. It has been shown that negative interactions, such as insensitivity or conflict, have a greater impact on caregivers of children with a food allergy compared to positive social supports [22]. Health care providers must remember that every interaction with a patient and their family is an educational opportunity that should be utilized to teach, review and support.

This study has identified parents' experiences of inconsistent messages from health care professionals. This inconsistency may in part be due to health care professionals treating patients without formal allergy training [23]. It is important to educate patients about the multiple symptoms of anaphylaxis and explain that any combination may occur. Past reactions will not predict future reactions and caregivers always need to be prepared to treat anaphylaxis. If health care providers teach caregivers the importance of a life-saving medication, this message and action should be consistent with the behaviors of health care providers. When caregivers see that this life saving medication is not being used by Paramedics or in the Emergency Department, this creates doubt. Why should caregivers use a needle on their child (causing pain to their loved one) when the health care providers do not use it? Having caregivers' emotions validated by health care professionals provides ongoing support. As part of formal allergy education, there needs to be a mental health component so that caregivers understand that symptoms such as anxiety and fear are common and can be managed. This type of initiative will raise the standards of care in the management of anaphylaxis whether it is in hospitals or the community.

Conclusions

The findings of this study indicate the need for health care professionals to address, educate and prepare parents for the myriad of emotions, thoughts and behavioral responses that are encountered when parents live with children with food allergies. When health care providers teach that these feelings are common, and reinforce the importance of prompt administration of EAIs, caregivers will be reassured that these emotions and doubts are part of the normal process of treating a child. It cannot be overstated that use of an EAI cannot hurt a child and there are no contraindications to their use. Further research into mental health and emotional communication with patient support groups and service delivery of this video or group sessions by parents or advocating parents is needed.

In a system where health care can be delivered by several different professionals, it is imperative that consistent information and treatment is given to all patients. All health care professionals must advocate and demonstrate prompt epinephrine administration. Listening to the experiences of parents who have witnessed their child go through life-threatening reactions can be an invaluable source of experience and this information can be used to help educate, support, and guide other caregivers.

Abbreviation

EAI: epinephrine auto-injector.

Authors' contributions

The original idea for this project came from RC, and was developed further by BT, DM and AB. Data was collected by RC and the analytical framework was developed by RC, BT, DM and AL. Data analysis, and interpretation was done by RC and BT. All authors read and approved the final manuscript.

Author details

[1] John Buhler Research Centre, College of Medicine, Faculty of Health Sciences, University of Manitoba, 504H 715 McDermot Ave, Winnipeg, MB R3E 3P4, Canada. [2] Helen Glass Centre for Nursing, College of Nursing, Faculty of Health Sciences, University of Manitoba, 89 Curry Place, Winnipeg, MB R3T 2N2, Canada.

Acknowledgements

We appreciate the participants who shared their experience. Thanks to Saiful Huq for the development of the image.

Competing interests

The authors declare that they have no competing interests.

Funding

This study was supported by the Manitoba Centre of Nursing Health Research; Kathleen and Winnifred Ruane Graduate Student Research Grant (318056 to RC); and Sigma Theta Tau Xi Lambda Research Award (2016-01 to RC).

References

1. Branum AM, Lukac S. Food allergy among US children: Trends in prevalence and hospitalization. Atlanta: US Department of Health and Human Services, Centers for Disease Control and Prevention; 2008.
2. Cummings AJ, Knibb RC, Erlewyn-Lajeunesse M, King RM, Roberts G, Lucas JS. Management of nut allergy influences quality of life and anxiety in children and their mothers. Pediatr Allergy Immunol. 2010;21(4p1):586–94.
3. Sicherer SH, Sampson H. Food allergy: epidemiology, pathogenesis, diagnosis, and treatment. J Allergy Clin Immunol. 2014;133(2):291–307.
4. Gupta R, Holdford D, Bilaver L, Dyer A, Holl JL, Meltzer D. The economic impact of childhood food allergy in the United States. JAMA Pediat. 2013;167(11):1026–31.
5. Lieberman P, Kemp SF, Oppenheimer J, Lang DM, Bernstein IL, Nicklas RA, Anderson JA, Bernstein DI, Bernstein JA, Fink JN. The diagnosis and management of anaphylaxis: an updated practice parameter. J Allergy Clin Immunol. 2005;115(3):S483–523.
6. Song TT, Worm M, Lieberman P. Anaphylaxis treatment: current barriers to adrenaline auto-injector use. Allergy. 2014;69(8):983–91.
7. Kazak AE, Schneider S, Kassam-Adams N. Pediatric medical traumatic stress. In: Roberts MC, Steele RG, editors. Handbook of pediatric psychology. New York: Guilford Press; 2009. p. 205–15.
8. Unsworth D. Adrenaline syringes are vastly over prescribed. Arch Dis Child. 2001;84(5):410–1.
9. Money AG, Barnett J, Kuljis J, Lucas J. Patient perceptions of epinephrine auto-injectors: exploring barriers to use. Scand J Caring Sci. 2013;27(2):335–44.
10. Creswell JW, Plano Clark VL, Gutmann ML, Hanson WE. Advanced mixed methods research designs. Handbook of mixed methods in social and behavioral research. 2003;209:240.
11. Ravid NL, Annunziato RA, Ambrose MA, Chuang K, Mullarkey C, Sicherer SH, Shemesh E, Cox AL. Mental health and quality-of-life concerns related to the burden of food allergy. Psychiatr Clin N Am. 2015;38(1):77–89.
12. Warren CM, Gupta RS, Sohn M-W, Oh EH, Lal N, Garfield CF, Caruso D, Wang X, Pongracic JA. Differences in empowerment and quality of life among parents of children with food allergy. Ann Allergy Asthma Immunol. 2015;114(2):117–25.
13. LeBovidge JS, Stone KD, Twarog FJ, Raiselis SW, Kalish LA, Bailey EP, Schneider LC. Development of a preliminary questionnaire to assess parental response to children's food allergies. Ann Allergy Asthma Immunol. 2006;96(3):472–7.
14. Laurière M, Pecquet C, Bouchez-Mahiout I, Snégaroff J, Bayrou O, Raison-Peyron N, Vigan M. Hydrolysed wheat proteins present in cosmetics can induce immediate hypersensitivities. Contact Dermat. 2006;54(5):283–9.
15. LeBovidge JS, Strauch H, Kalish LA, Schneider LC. Assessment of psychological distress among children and adolescents with food allergy. J Allergy Clin Immunol. 2009;124(6):1282–8.
16. Rapee R, Wignall A, Spence S, Lyneham H, Cobham V. Helping your anxious child: a step-by-step guide for parents. Oakland: New Harbinger; 2008.
17. Wilson R, Lyons L. Anxious kids, anxious parents: 7 ways to stop the worry cycle and raise courageous and independent children. Deerfield Beach: HCI Publishing; 2013.
18. Roy KM, Roberts MC. Peanut allergy in children relationships to health-related quality of life, anxiety, and parental stress. Clin Pediatr. 2011;50(11):1045–51.
19. Lanser BJ, Covar R, Bird JA. Food allergy needs assessment, training curriculum, and knowledge assessment for child care. Ann Allergy Asthma Immunol. 2016;116(6):533–7.
20. Haigh C, Hardy P. Tell me a story—a conceptual exploration of storytelling in healthcare education. Nurse Educ Today. 2011;31(4):408–11.
21. Nicholas DB, Zwaigenbaum L, Muskat B, Craig WR, Newton AS, Kilmer C, Greenblatt A, Roberts W, Cohen-Silver J. Experiences of emergency department care from the perspective of families in which a child has autism spectrum disorder. Soc Work Health Care. 2016;55(6):409–26.
22. Williams NA, Hankey M. Support and negativity in interpersonal relationships impact caregivers' quality of life in pediatric food allergy. Qual Life Res. 2015;24(6):1369–78.
23. Grabenhenrich LB, Dölle S, Moneret-Vautrin A, Köhli A, Lange L, Spindler T, Rueff F, Nemat K, Maris I, Roumpedaki E, Scherer K. Anaphylaxis in children and adolescents: the European Anaphylaxis Registry. J Allergy Clin Immunol. 2016;137(4):1128–37.

Permissions

All chapters in this book were first published in CTA, by BioMed Central; hereby published with permission under the Creative Commons Attribution License or equivalent. Every chapter published in this book has been scrutinized by our experts. Their significance has been extensively debated. The topics covered herein carry significant findings which will fuel the growth of the discipline. They may even be implemented as practical applications or may be referred to as a beginning point for another development.

The contributors of this book come from diverse backgrounds, making this book a truly international effort. This book will bring forth new frontiers with its revolutionizing research information and detailed analysis of the nascent developments around the world.

We would like to thank all the contributing authors for lending their expertise to make the book truly unique. They have played a crucial role in the development of this book. Without their invaluable contributions this book wouldn't have been possible. They have made vital efforts to compile up to date information on the varied aspects of this subject to make this book a valuable addition to the collection of many professionals and students.

This book was conceptualized with the vision of imparting up-to-date information and advanced data in this field. To ensure the same, a matchless editorial board was set up. Every individual on the board went through rigorous rounds of assessment to prove their worth. After which they invested a large part of their time researching and compiling the most relevant data for our readers.

The editorial board has been involved in producing this book since its inception. They have spent rigorous hours researching and exploring the diverse topics which have resulted in the successful publishing of this book. They have passed on their knowledge of decades through this book. To expedite this challenging task, the publisher supported the team at every step. A small team of assistant editors was also appointed to further simplify the editing procedure and attain best results for the readers.

Apart from the editorial board, the designing team has also invested a significant amount of their time in understanding the subject and creating the most relevant covers. They scrutinized every image to scout for the most suitable representation of the subject and create an appropriate cover for the book.

The publishing team has been an ardent support to the editorial, designing and production team. Their endless efforts to recruit the best for this project, has resulted in the accomplishment of this book. They are a veteran in the field of academics and their pool of knowledge is as vast as their experience in printing. Their expertise and guidance has proved useful at every step. Their uncompromising quality standards have made this book an exceptional effort. Their encouragement from time to time has been an inspiration for everyone.

The publisher and the editorial board hope that this book will prove to be a valuable piece of knowledge for researchers, students, practitioners and scholars across the globe.

List of Contributors

Liane Reeves, Judith Holloway and Carina Venter
Community Nutrition & Dietetic Department, East Oxford Health Centre, Cowley Road, Oxford OX4 1XD, UK
MSc Allergy, University of Southampton, Southampton General Hospital, Tremona Road, Southampton SO16 6YD, UK

Rosan Meyer
Department of Gastroenterology, Great Ormond Street Hospital for Sick Children, London WC1N 3JH, UK

Carina Venter
University of Portsmouth, James Watson West, 2 King Richard 1st Road, Portsmouth PO1 2FR, UK
The David Hide Asthma and Allergy Research Centre, St Mary's Hospital, Newport, Isle of Wight PO30 5TG, UK

Vanessa Garcia-Larsen
Respiratory Epidemiology, Occupational Medicine, and Public Health Group, National Heart and Lung Institute, Imperial College London, Emmanuel Kaye Building, Manresa Road, London SW3 6LR, UK

Stefano R. Del Giacco
Department of Medical Sciences "M Aresu", University of Cagliari, Cagliari, Italy

André Moreira
Faculty of Medicine, University of Porto and Hospital São João, Porto, Portugal

Matteo Bonini
Department of Public Health and Infectious Diseases, Lung Function Unit, Sapienza University of Rome, Rome, Italy
National Heart and Lung Institute, Imperial College London, London, UK

Tari Haahtela
Skin and Allergy Hospital, Helsinki University Central Hospital, Helsinki, Finland

Sergio Bonini
European Medicines Agency, London, UK
Second University of Naples and IFT-CNR, Rome, Italy

Kai-Håkon Carlsen
Department of Medicine and Allergology, University of Oslo, Oslo, Norway

Ioana Agache
Faculty of Medicine, Transylvania University, Brasov, Romania

Nikolaos G. Papadopoulos
Institute of Human Development, University of Manchester, Manchester, UK
Allergy Department, 2nd Paediatric Clinic, University of Athens, Athens, Greece

João Fonseca and Luís Delgado
Laboratory of Immunology, Faculty of Medicine, and CINTESIS (Centre for Health Technology and Services Research), University of Porto and Hospital São João, Porto, Portugal

F. Blanc, H. Bernard, S. Ah-Leung, L. Przybylski-Nicaise and K. Adel-Patient
INRA-CEA, Service de Pharmacologie et d'Immunoanalyse, Laboratoire d'Immuno-Allergie Alimentaire, Bât. 136–CEA de Saclay, 91191 Gif-sur-Yvette, France

P. Stahl Skov
RefLab ApS, Copenhagen, Denmark

A. Purohit and F. de Blay
Hôpitaux Universitaires de Strasbourg, Strasbourg, France

B. Ballmer-Weber and P. Fritsche
University Hospital Zurich, Zurich, Switzerland

M. Fernandez Rivas and I. Reig
Hospital Clinico San Carlos, Madrid, Spain

A. Sinaniotis
University of Athens & "Sotiria" Regional Chest Diseases Hospital of Athens, Athens, Greece

E. Vassilopoulou
University of Nicosia, Nicosia, Cyprus

K. Hoffmann-Sommergruber
Medical University of Vienna, Vienna, Austria

S. Vieths
Paul-Ehrlich-Institut, Langen, Germany

N. Rigby
Institute of Food Research, Norwich, UK

C. Mills
University of Manchester, Manchester, UK

Christophe P. Frossard, José M. Rincon Garriz and Philippe A. Eigenmann
Inflammation and Allergy Research Group and Department of Pediatrics, University Hospitals of Geneva and University of Geneva, 6 rue Willy-Donzé, 1211 Geneva 14, Switzerland

Simone C. Zimmerli
Allergy Unit, University Hospitals of Geneva and University of Geneva, Geneva, Switzerland
EMD Serono, Billerica, MA, USA

José M. Rincon Garriz
Present Address: Fasteris SA, Plan-les-Ouates, Switzerland.

Alexandra F. Santos, Natalia Bécares, Alick Stephens, Victor Turcanu and Gideon Lack
Division of Asthma, Allergy and Lung Biology, Department of Pediatric Allergy, St Thomas' Hospital, King's College London

2nd Floor, Stairwell B, South Wing, Westminster Bridge Road, London SE1 7EH, UK. 2 MRC and Asthma UK Centre in Allergic Mechanisms of Asthma, London, UK

Alexandra F. Santos
Immunoallergology Department, Coimbra University Hospital, Coimbra, Portugal

Gulbenkian Programme for Advanced Medical Education, Lisbon, Portugal

Thuy-My Le, Els van Hoffen, Ischa Kummeling, Carla AFM Bruijnzeel-Koomen, Ans FM Lebens, Titia M Lindner and André C Knulst
Department of Dermatology/Allergology, University Medical Center Utrecht, The Netherlands

Ischa Kummeling, James Potts and Peter G Burney
Department of Respiratory Epidemiology, Occupational Medicine and Public Health, National Heart and Lung Institute, Imperial College London, London, UK

Barbara K Ballmer-Weber
Allergy Unit, Department of Dermatology, University Hospital Zürich, Zürich, Switzerland

Jonas Lidholm
Thermo Fisher Scientific, Uppsala, Sweden

Alan Mackie
Institute of Food Research, Norwich Research Park, Colney, Norwich NR4 7UA, UK

EN Clare Mills
Institute of Inflammation and Repair, Manchester Academic Health Sciences Centre,
Manchester Institute of Biotechnology, The University of Manchester, Manchester, UK

Ronald van Ree
Department of Experimental Immunology and Department of Otorhinolaryngology, Academic Medical Center of the University of Amsterdam, Amsterdam, The Netherlands

Stefan Vieths
Division of Allergology, Paul-Ehrlich-Institut, Federal Institute for Vaccines and Biomedicines, Langen, Germany

Montserrat Fernández-Rivas
Allergy Department, Hospital Clinico San Carlos, IdISSC, Madrid, Spain

Els van Hoffen
Current affiliation: NIZO food research, Ede, The Netherlands

Bodo C. Melnik and Swen Malte John
Department of Dermatology, Environmental Medicine and Health Theory, University of Osnabrück, Sedanstrasse 115, 49090 Osnabrück, Germany

Pedro Carrera-Bastos
Center for Primary Health Care Research, Lund University, Lund, Sweden

Gerd Schmitz
Institute for Clinical Chemistry and Laboratory Medicine, University Hospital Regensburg, University of Regensburg, Josef-Strauss-Allee 11, 93053 Regensburg, Germany

Peter Henneman, Andrea Venema, Femke van Sinderen, Karin van der Lip, Raoul C. Hennekam and Marcel Mannens
Department Clinical Genetics, DNA-diagnostics laboratory, Amsterdam Medical Center, Amsterdam, The Netherlands

Nicole C. M. Petrus and and Aline B. Sprikkelman
Department of Paediatric Respiratory Medicine and Allergy, Emma Children's Hospital, Amsterdam Medical Center, Amsterdam, The Netherlands

Katrine Lindholm Bøgh
National Food Institute, Technical University of Denmark, Søborg, Denmark

Jolanda van Bilsen
TNO, Zeist, The Netherlands

Robert Głogowski
Warsaw University of Life Sciences, Warsaw, Poland

Eva Untersmayr
Department of Pathophysiology and Allergy Research, Medical University of Vienna, Vienna, Austria

Karine Adel-Patient
UMR-INRA-CEA, Service de Pharmacologie et d'Immunoanalyse, Université Paris-Saclay, Gif-sur-Yvette, France

Unni Cecilie Nygaard
Norwegian Institute of Public Health, Oslo, Norway

Ian Kimber
University of Manchester, Manchester, UK

G. Rentzos
Section of Allergology, University Hospital of Sahlgrenska, 413 45 Gothenburg, Sweden

L. Johanson and L. Ekerljung
Krefting Research Centre, Department of Internal Medicine and Clinical Nutrition, University of Gothenburg, Gothenburg, Sweden

E. Telemo
Department for Rheumatology and Inflammation Research, Sahlgrenska Academy, University of Gothenburg, Gothenburg, Sweden

S. Sjölander
R&D, ImmunoDiagnostics, Thermofischer Scientific, Uppsala, Sweden

Isabel J Skypala
Royal Brompton & Harefield NHS Foundation Trust, London, UK

Carina Venter
The David Hide 6. Asthma and Allergy Research Centre, Isle of Wight, UK

Rosan Meyer
Great Ormond Street NHS Foundation Trust, London, UK

Nicolette W deJong
Erasmus MC, Rotterdam, NL, Netherlands

Adam T Fox
Guy's and St Thomas' Hospitals NHS Foundation Trust and Kings College, London, UK

Marion Groetch
Jaffe Food Allergy Institute, Icahn School of Medicine at Mount Sinai, New York, USA

J N Oude Elberink
Department of Allergology, University Medical Centre of Groningen, University of Groningen, Groningen, NL, Netherlands

Aline Sprikkelman
Emma Children's Hospital Academic Medical Centre, Amsterdam, NL, Netherlands

Louiza Diamandi
University of Athens, Athens, GR, Greece

Berber J Vlieg-Boerstra
Emma Children's Hospital, Paediatric Respiratory Medicine and Allergy, Academic Medical Centre, University of Amsterdam, Amsterdam, NL, Netherlands

Sangeeta Dhami
Evidence-Based Health Care Ltd, Edinburgh, UK

Ulugbek Nurmatov
Division of Population Medicine Neuadd Meirionnydd, School of Medicine, Cardiff University, Heath Park, Cardiff, UK

Giovanni Battista Pajno
Allergy Unit, Department of Pediatric, University of Messina, Messina, Italy

Carsten Bindslev-Jensen
Department of Dermatology and Allergy Centre, Odense University Hospital, Odense, Denmark

Wesley Burks
Department of Pediatrics, School of Medicine, University of North Carolina at Chapel Hill, Chapel Hill, NC, USA

George du Toit
Division of Asthma, Allergy and Lung Biology, Department of Paediatric Allergy, MRC and Asthma Centre in Allergic Mechanisms of Asthma, King's College London and St Thomas NHS Foundation Trust, London, UK

Frans Timmermans
Nederlands Anafylaxis Netwerk - European Anaphylaxis Taskforce, Dordrecht, The Netherlands

Aziz Sheikh
Allergy and Respiratory Research Group, The University of Edinburgh, Edinburgh, UK

Isabel J. Skypala
Royal Brompton and Harefield NHS Foundation Trust, Sydney Street, London SW3 6NP, UK

M. Williams
Somerset Partnership NHS Foundation Trust, Somerset, UK

L. Reeves
Oxford Health NHS Foundation Trust, Oxford, UK

R. Meyer
Great Ormond Street NHS Foundation Trust, London, UK

C. Venter
The David Hide Asthma and Allergy Research Centre, Isle of Wight, UK

Rosan Meyer, Robert Dziubak, Heather Godwin, Kate Reeve, Adriana Chebar-Lozinsky and Neil Shah
Department Gastroenterology, Great Ormond Street Hospital for Children NHS foundation Trust, London, UK

Claire De Koker and Ana-Kristina Skrapac
Department Nutrition and Dietetics, Chelsea and Westminster Hospital NHS Foundation Trust, London, UK

Neil Shah
Institute of Child Health, University College London, London, UK

Nicole C. M. Petrus, Raoul C. Hennekam and Aline B. Sprikkelman
Department of Pediatric Respiratory Medicine and Allergy, H7-270, Emma Children's Hospital Academic Medical Center, Meibergdreef 9, 1105 AZ Amsterdam, The Netherlands

Peter Henneman, Andrea Venema, Adri Mul, Femke van Sinderen, Martin Haagmans, Olaf Mook, Raoul C. Hennekam and Marcel Mannens
Department of Clinical Genetics, DNA-Diagnostics Laboratory, Amsterdam Medical Center, Amsterdam, The Netherlands

Joost J Smit, Maarten T Pennings, Karina Willemsen, Manon van Roest and Raymond H Pieters
Immunotoxicology group, Institute for Risk Assessment Sciences, Utrecht University, Utrecht, The Netherlands

Joost J Smit and Maarten T Pennings
Utrecht Centre for Food Allergy, Utrecht, The Netherlands

Maarten T Pennings and Els van Hoffen
Utrecht University Medical Center, Utrecht, The Netherlands

Els van Hoffen
Current affiliation: NIZO food research BV, Ede, The Netherlands

Maarten T Pennings
HU University of Applied Sciences, Utrecht, The Netherlands

Melanie Rae Simpson, Anne Dorthea Bjerkenes Rø, Roar Johnsen, Ola Storrø and Torbjørn Øien
Department of Public Health and General Practice, Norwegian University of Science and Technology, Trondheim, Norway

Anne Dorthea Bjerkenes Rø
Department of Immunology and Transfusion Medicine, St Olavs Hospital, Trondheim University Hospital, Trondheim, Norway

Øystein Grimstad
Department of Dermatology, University Hospital of North Norway, Tromsö, Norway

Melanie Rae Simpson
Det medisinske fakultet, Instiutt for samfunnsmedisin, MTFS, NTNU, Postboks 8905, 7491 Trondheim, Norway

Mark A. Blankestijn, André C. Knulst, Edward F. Knol, Thuy-My Le, Heike Rockmann, Henny G. Otten and Rob J. B. Klemans
Department of Dermatology and Allergology, University Medical Center Utrecht, Utrecht University, Heidelberglaan 100, 3584 CX Utrecht, The Netherlands

Edward F. Knol and Henny G. Otten
Laboratory of Translational Immunology, University Medical Center Utrecht, Utrecht University, Heidelberglaan 100, 3584 CX Utrecht, The Netherlands

Jennifer Lisa Penner Protudjer, Sven-Arne Jansson, Roelinde Middelveld, Eva Östblom, Sven-Erik Dahlén and Staffan Ahlstedt
The Centre for Allergy Research, Karolinska Institutet, Sweden

Jennifer Lisa Penner Protudjer, Roelinde Middelveld, Sven-Erik Dahlén and Staffan Ahlstedt
Institute of Environmental Medicine, Karolinska Institutet, Stockholm, Sweden

Sven-Arne Jansson
Department of Public Health and Clinical Medicine, Umeå University, Umeå, Sweden

Eva Östblom and Ann-Charlotte Sundqvist
Sachs' Children and Youth Hospital, Södersjukhuset, Stockholm, Sweden

Eva Östblom
Department of Clinical Research and Education, Södersjukhuset, Karolinska Institutet, Stockholm, Sweden

Marianne Heibert Arnlind
Swedish Council on Health Technology Assessment, SBU, Stockholm, Sweden
Department of Learning, Informatics, Management and Ethics, and Medical Management Centre, Karolinska Institutet, Stockholm, Sweden

Ulf Bengtsson, Georgios Rentzos and Johanna Åkerström
Allergy Unit, Sahlgrenska University Hospital, Gothenburg, Sweden

Ingrid Kallström-Bengtsson
The Swedish Asthma and Allergy Foundation, Stockholm, Sweden

Birgitta Marklund
Department of Health and Caring Sciences, Linnaeus University, Kalmar, Sweden

Bianca Lötzsch, Sabine Dölle and Margitta Worm
Department of Dermatology and Allergology, Allergy-Center-Charité, Charité - Univer-sitätsmedizin Berlin, Charitéplatz 1, 10117 Berlin, Germany

Stefan Vieths
Paul- Ehrlich-Institut, Langen, Germany

Carina Venter and David M. Fleischer
Section of Allergy and Immunology, University of Colorado Denver School of Medicine, Children's Hospital Colorado , East 16th Avenue, Anschutz Medical Campus, Aurora, CO 80045, USA

Trevor Brown
Children's Allergy Service, Ulster Hospital, Belfast BT16 1RH, Northern Ireland, UK

Rosan Meyer
Department Paediatrics, Imperial College, London, London W2 1NY, UK

Joanne Walsh
Gurney Surgery, Castle Partnership, 101-103 Magdalen Street, Norwich NR3 1LN, UK

Neil Shah
Gastroenterology Department, Great Ormond Street Hospital, London WC1N 3JH, UK

Anna Nowak-Węgrzyn
Jaffe Food Allergy Institute, Icahn School of Medicine at Mount Sinai, New York, NY 10029, USA

Tong-Xin Chen
Department of Allergy and Immunology, Shanghai Children's Medical Center, Shanghai Jiao Tong University School of Medicine, 1678 Dongfang Road, Shanghai 200127, China

Ralf G. Heine
Royal Children's Hospital Melbourne, Murdoch Children's Research Institute, Parkville, VIC 3052, Australia

Michael Levin
Division of Paediatric Allergy and Asthma, Red Cross War Memorial Children's Hospital, University of Cape Town, Room 516, ICH Building, Cape Town, South Africa

Mario C. Vieira
Centro de Gastroenterologica Pediatrica, Department of Paediatrics, Hospital Pequeno Principe, Pontificia Universidade Catolica do Parana, Curitiba, Brazil

Adam T. Fox
Department of Paediatric Allergy, Guys and St Thomas' Hospitals NHS Foundation Trust, London, UK
Division of Asthma, Allergy and Lung Biology, King's College, London, London, UK

Kristine Kjer Byberg and Knut Øymar
Department of Pediatrics, Stavanger University Hospital, POB 8100, 4068 Stavanger, Norway

Geir Egil Eide
Centre for Clinical Research, Haukeland University Hospital, Bergen, Norway
Department of Global Public Health and Primary Care, University of Bergen, Bergen, Norway

Michele R. Forman
Department of Nutritional Sciences, School of Human Ecology, University of Texas at Austin, Austin, TX, USA

Pétur Benedikt Júlíusson
Department of Pediatrics, Haukeland University Hospital, Bergen, Norway

Knut Øymar
Department of Clinical Science, University of Bergen, Bergen, Norway

Marjolein Vandekerckhove, Bart Van Droogenbroeck, Marc De Loose and Katleen Coudijzer
Technology and Food Science Unit, Research Institute for Agriculture, Fisheries, and Food (ILVO), Burg. Van Gansberghelaan 115, 9820 Merelbeke, Belgium

Hilde Lapeere
Faculty of Medicine and Health Science, Department of Dermatology, Ghent University, De Pintelaan 185, 9000 Ghent, Belgium

Marc Coppens
Faculty of Medicine and Health Science, Department of Anesthesiology and Perioperative Medicine, Ghent University, De Pintelaan 185, 9000 Ghent, Belgium

Philippe Gevaert
Faculty of Medicine and Health Science, Department of Otorhinolaryngology, Ghent University, De Pintelaan 185, 9000 Ghent, Belgium

Åsa Strinnholm, Linnéa Hedman, Sven-Arne Jansson and Eva Rönmark
Department of Public Health and Clinical Medicine, Occupational and Environmental Medicine, OLIN Unit, Umeå University, 901 87 Umeå, Sweden

Linnéa Hedman
Division of Nursing, Department of Health Sciences, Luleå University of Technology, 971 87 Luleå, Sweden

Anna Winberg
Department of Clinical Sciences, Pediatrics, Umeå University, 901 87 Umeå, Sweden

Viveca Lindh and Åsa Strinnholm
Department of Nursing, Umeå University, 901 87 Umeå, Sweden

Rishma Chooniedass and Allan Becker
John Buhler Research Centre, College of Medicine, Faculty of Health Sciences, University of Manitoba, 504H 715 McDermot Ave, Winnipeg, MB R3E 3P4, Canada

Beverley Temple and Donna Martin
Helen Glass Centre for Nursing, College of Nursing, Faculty of Health Sciences, University of Manitoba, 89 Curry Place, Winnipeg, MB R3T 2N2, Canada

Index

O

P

R

S

T

U